T0127813

Potbellied Pig
Veterinary Medicine

1st Edition

Potbellied Pig Veterinary Medicine

Kristie Mozzachio, DVM, DACVP, CVA
Mozzachio Mobile Veterinary Services
Hillsborough, NC
United States

ELSEVIER

Elsevier
3251 Riverport Lane
St. Louis, Missouri 63043

POTBELLIED PIG VETERINARY MEDICINE   ISBN: 9780323763592

Copyright © 2023, by Elsevier Inc. All rights reserved

No part of this publication may be reproduced or transmitted in any form or by any means, electronic or mechanical, including photocopying, recording, or any information storage and retrieval system, without permission in writing from the Publisher. Details on how to seek permission, further information about the Publisher's permissions policies and our arrangements with organizations such as the Copyright Clearance Center and the Copyright Licensing Agency, can be found at our website: www.elsevier.com/permissions.

Notices

Practitioners and researchers must always rely on their own experience and knowledge in evaluating and using any information, methods, compounds or experiments described herein. Because of rapid advances in the medical sciences, in particular, independent verification of diagnoses and drug dosages should be made. To the fullest extent of the law, no responsibility is assumed by Elsevier, authors, editors or contributors for any injury and/or damage to persons or property as a matter of products liability, negligence or otherwise, or from any use or operation of any methods, products, instructions, or ideas contained in the material herein.

Senior Content Strategist: Jennifer Catando
Content Development Manager: Somodatta Roy Choudhury
Senior Content Development Specialist: Priyadarshini Pandey
Senior Project Manager: Umarani Natarajan
Publishing Services Manager: Deepthi Unni
Book Designer: Ryan Cook

Printed in India

Last digit is the print number: 9 8 7 6 5 4 3

Working together
to grow libraries in
developing countries

www.elsevier.com • www.bookaid.org

Preface

Miniature, or potbellied, pigs have remained a popular pet over the years and the fad waxes and wanes but never dies out. The pet porcine population does not quite fit into any category—they are too loud and unruly for many small animal practices but too much the revered family member for large animal operations. They are exotic (sort of), yet also a food animal species, much to the chagrin of many owners. Since they can't be pigeonholed, veterinarians across multiple disciplines will be likely to encounter them, yet there is little guidance available.

The intent of this book is to provide a basic reference, a starting point, for those wanting—or at least willing (if "want" is too strong of a word)—to see pet pig patients. While the end result is the culmination of an oh-so-painful "brain dump," I only know what I know, so this book is by no means complete. It's taken the better part of 20 years to come this far with the help of many, many others (veterinarians, owners, minipig enthusiasts around the world, my own pet "guinea" pigs [pun intended]), and I am still only a mediocre clinician. My passion is the collection of information to pass along to those who can take it one step further, and I'm hoping that a written guide will encourage others to give these "black sheep" (yep, another pun) of the pet world a chance!

Acknowledgments

To the many wonderful people who have fielded my every question in the pursuit of all things minipig and who have handled my obsession with grace and good humor (at least to my face), I salute you! Special thanks to the contributors who were willing to tackle this project, despite crazy-hectic-COVID schedules. An especially huge thank you to those who have guided me from the very beginning—Susan Magidson, of Ross Mill Farm, and Dr. Arlen Wilbers, pet pig vet extraordinaire.

Dr. Allen Cannedy

Contributors

Suzanne Burlatschenko, DVM
Industry Representative/Swine Veterinarian
Ontario Swine Research Network
University of Guelph
Southwestern Ontario, Canada

Kristie Mozzachio, DVM, DACVP, CVA
Mozzachio Mobile Veterinary Services, Hillsborough
North Carolina
United States

Lysa Pam Posner, DVM, DACVAA
Professor
MBS
North Carolina State University, Raleigh
North Carolina
United States

Valarie V. Tynes, BS, DVM, Diplomate American College of Veterinary Behavior, Diplomate American College of Animal Welfare
Veterinary Services Specialist
Companion Animal
Ceva Animal Health, Lenexa
Kansas
United States

Contents

Chapter 1

History

Kristie Mozzachio

History

The so-called Vietnamese Pot-bellied Pig was introduced into North America in the mid-1980s by Canadian Keith Connell who first imported a group of European miniature pigs of I and Mong Cai Vietnamese origin into Canada for use in zoos (Connell or CON line); there is no known lineage information for the first group of 18 imported pigs, although the miniature pet pig we recognize today was derived from this group (Blaney 2004). Connell's second import group was dubbed the North American Potbellies (NAP line) and consisted of a broader European base. This group was composed of larger pigs, up to approximately 400 lb (181 kg) and did not contribute to the current population as size made them impractical pets (Blaney, personal communication). American Keith Leavitt later imported from China what came to be called the LEA line, followed by the Royal line imported from England by Harry Espberger; both to add some color into the lineage. The CON, LEA, and Royal are the primary foundation stock of the miniature pet pig currently seen in North America (Magidson 1995).

Originally intended for zoos, the minipig became a surprisingly popular pet among private buyers and prices soared into the thousands of dollars. Organizations such as the North American Potbellied Pig Association (NAPPA) became established, national shows were held, dedicated magazines published, and breeding began for what appeared to be a lucrative endeavor. The original potbellied pigs were typically black and of short stature, with small erect ears, sway back, short nose, wrinkled face, straight tail, and the classic "potbelly" (Blaney 2004; Braun and Casteel 1993; Reeves 1993). Weights ranged up to 250 lb (113 kg), but these pigs were still considered miniature relative to their 500+ lb (227+ kg) farm hog counterparts. Fun fact: "Pinto Pete" was the product of breeding between second generation CON pigs and was an oddly colored black and white pig considered of little value—until the public got a look and started clamoring for him. Had all of the pigs stayed a boring black, maybe we wouldn't be where we are today.

As with all fads, the fervor died down over time and these pet became more affordable for the general population; ownership became more widespread. And again, as with all fads, people eventually tired of these unique pets so many found their way into shelters. Over the ensuing years and continuing to this day, efforts to develop smaller and smaller pet pigs persist and the trendiness of the pet ebbs and flows with each new "breed." Animal shelters and miniature pig rescue organizations remain overwhelmed with each new wave of castaways as a result.

Breeds

So how many miniature pig breeds are there? Well, to answer, one has to define the term *breed*. One definition: "a group of domesticates that, when bred to each other, will regularly produce offspring that are recognizably of that breed, both morphologically and in their aptitudes" (Porter 2002). Given that miniature pigs have few distinguishing features, small size has become the primary goal for any newly touted "breed," and terms such as *teacup, micro-mini, pixie, pocket,* and *thimble* have been used to market these animals. However, of the marketed miniature pet pig breeds (excluding research breeds), only the Vietnamese Pot-bellied Pig is included in one of the most expansive and thorough books on livestock breeds throughout the world (Porter 2002); the many publicized North American minipig "breeds," including the so-called Teacup pig, are notably absent. It is expected that the majority of miniature pet pigs seen today are of mixed origin, with a basis in the Vietnamese breed(s). That said, there are a few that might be considered distinctive local populations, if not a true recognized breed, listed here.

The **Vietnamese Potbellied/Pot-bellied Pig** (Fig. 1.1A) might be considered the "classic" breed and is by far the most well-known, but even this group is a mix rather than a purebred line (Reeves 1993); more of a local type than a true breed, including in their native country (Magidson 1995). Features listed in the breed standards published by NAPPA in the early 1990s include a maximum height of 18 in (45 cm); maximum weight of 95 lb (43 kg) at 1 year of age (author's note: not full-grown for 3 to 5 years); small erect ears; a sway back; and black, black and white, or white coloration (Reeves 1993). This breed is known for its gentle disposition.

The **Juliana** (aka Juliani or Julienne; Fig. 1.1B) pig is also known as the Miniature Painted Pig since coloration is always spotted in a "profuse and random" pattern not in a "piebald pattern" and the base color can be silver, white, red, rust, black, or cream. This breed exhibits a long straight snout, long lean body, small

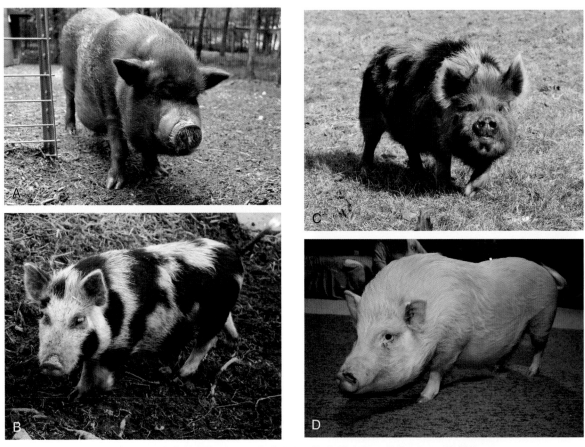

Fig. 1.1 Pet pig breeds: (A) Vietnamese Potbellied Pig (photo credit: Cindy Anne Ford); (B) Juliana; (C) Kunekune; (D) Göttingen;

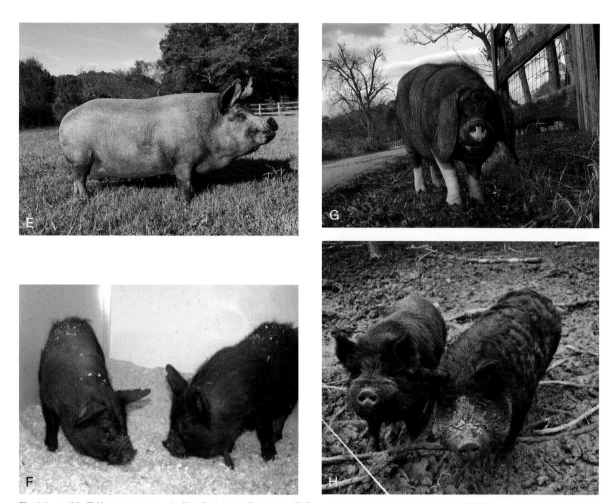

Fig. 1.1, cont'd **(E) Yucatan** (photo credit: Blind Spot Animal Sanctuary); **(F) Panepinto** (photo credit: Linda Panepinto); **(G) Meishan** (photo credit: Blind Spot Animal Sanctuary); **(H) American Guinea Hog.**

erect ears, thick coarse hair coat, 15 to 17 in (38 cm to 43 cm) tall, and without a potbelly or sway back (Juliana Pig Association and Registry 2018). In the authors experience, these pigs tend to be naturally rambunctious and make unruly patients.

The **Kunekune** (Fig. 1.1C) is a New Zealand meat breed first imported into the US in the mid-1990s. It is not a true miniature but, rather, a smaller breed of domestic pig commonly kept as a pet, weighing up to 400 lb (181 kg) and exhibiting distinctive features including large forward-inclined hairy ears, a barrel-shaped torso (the name in the Māori language means "fat and round" or "plump"), a wide forehead, a short upturned snout, thick hair of many colors (black, browns, gingers, creams and with or without spots), and a laid-back personality that makes the breed ideal for petting zoos. Breed characteristics listed by the International Kunekune Hog Registry (Kunekune 2021) now also include the necessity of two wattles at birth (fibrous appendages also called tassels that dangle on either side of the throat and have a tendency to get torn off at times—but provide excellent pulse oximetry readings). Previously described purebred Kunekune pigs were not necessarily wattled.

Several of the miniature pig breeds used in biomedical research, including the Göttingen, Panepinto, and Yucatan (Figs. 1.1D–F) have made their way into pet households but remain relatively uncommon. Some of the smaller commercial breeds such as the Meishan and American Guinea Hog are also sometimes kept as pets (Figs. 1.1G–H).

The American Minipig Association (AMPA) has declared a breed standard for the so-called American Minipig breed that includes features such as 15 to 20 in (~38 to 51 cm) at the top of the shoulders, small erect ears, straight tail with a tassel at the end, healthy coarse hair, and "any variety of colors and markings including but not limited to solid, spots, stripes as an immature color, and agouti as a mature color." They also describe size as "the overall weight of the American Mini Pig should fit its stature as such that the pig is comfortable and able to run and move freely," so there are no weight restrictions that might prevent larger, heavier animals from being considered. Interestingly, a sway back appearance—part of the breed description for the Vietnamese Potbellied Pig—is given as an exclusion. The organization acknowledges a mixture of breeds from around the world that have contributed to the pet now seen in the US and have provided a lovely definition of the "mutt" that is the miniature pet pig seen today.

Food for thought: When wading through the staggering amount of online information generated about the pot-bellied/potbellied/miniature pet pig, it should be remembered that one of the smallest known miniature pig breeds is the Göttingen. This well-established breed, developed in the 1960s with carefully manipulated genetic pedigrees for over the past 60 years (Larzul 2013; Simianer and Köhn 2010), reaches an average adult weight of 45 kg (just under 100 lb). The more recently developed 1990s Panepinto Micropig reaches an adult weight of 25 to 30 kg (55 to 66 lb) (Köhn 2012). Therefore, it stands to reason that "Joe Public breeder" making any claims below this weight is likely full of shit.

Minipig Rescue

Many potential pet pig owners are unaware that minipig overpopulation is a problem, just as it is for other pets such as dogs or cats. Those open to adoption can contact a local rescue, found in nearly every US state and several foreign countries. These organizations

BOX 1.1 PET PIG ADOPTIONS

Just like dogs and cats, overpopulation has led to an abundance of pet pigs available for adoption. In the US, Pig Placement Network (PPN), one of the oldest pet pig rescue organizations, is a good place to start a search for adoptable pet pigs (https://www.pigplacementnetwork.org/). The organization supports a number of rescue groups in vetting the animals, allows posting of adoptable pigs across the country, and has a searchable map for surrendered pigs in need of homes. They also maintain a library of helpful articles and videos for pet pig owners. Pet pigs of all shapes, sizes, and ages (piglets included) are always available for adoption. Potential owners should be made aware of this resource as an alternative to breeder purchase.

can also offer guidance for navigating city, state, and homeowner association ordinances that may not allow miniature pet pigs. Many have already vetted their adoptable animals too, including neutering.

Pig Placement Network in the Northeastern United States is one of the oldest pet pig rescue organizations and, as such, is a reputable source with years of experience (Box 1.1). Smaller rescues or microsanctuaries crop up all the time, but some end up with hoarding situations in need of rescue themselves. Potential owners should research rescue organizations prior to adoption just as they should research breeders prior to purchase. An in-person visit is strongly recommended prior to either purchase or adoption.

BIBLIOGRAPHY

American Minipig Association website. *The American Mini Pig Breed Standard*. https://americanminipigassociation.com/mini-pig-education/what-is-an-american-mini-pig/, 2015. Accessed October 3, 2021.

Blaney J. Personal communication.

Blaney J. History of the US potbellied pig. 6th Annual Pet Pig Symposium. Ames, IA; June 4–6, 2004.

Braun WF, Casteel SW. Potbellied pigs: miniature porcine pets. *Vet Clin North Am Small Anim.* 1993;23(6):1149–1177.

International Kunekune Hog Registry. *Breed Standard*. https://www.internationalkunekunehogregistry.com/breed-standard. Accessed October 3, 2021.

Juliana Pig Association & Registry. *Juliana Pig Breed Standard*. http://www.julianapig.com/BreedStandard.html, 2018. Accessed February 18, 2021.

Köhn F. History and development of miniature, micro- and minipigs. In: McAnulty PA, Dayan AD, Ganderup N, Hastings K, eds. *The Minipig in Biomedical Research*. Boca Raton, FL: CRC Press; 2012:7–15.

Larzul C. *Pig genetics: insight in minipigs. Bilateral Symposium on Miniature Pigs for Biomedical Research in Taiwan and France.* Taïnan, Taiwan; 2013:1–6. hal-00958583.

Magidson R. *History of the Potbellied Pig.* https://rossmillfarm.com/2019/08/history-of-the-potbellied-pig/, 1995. Accessed September 2, 2020.

Porter V. *Mason's World Dictionary of Livestock Breeds, Types and Varieties.* 5th ed. Oxon, UK: CAB International; 2002:211–257.

Reeves DE. History and development of miniature pet pigs in North America. In: Reeves DE, ed. *Guidelines for the Veterinary Practitioner: Care and Management of Miniature Pet Pigs.* Santa Barbara, CA: Brillig Hill, Inc.; 1993:1–6.

Sawyer B. *Where Did Mini Pigs Come From?* Mini Pig Info. 2020. https://www.minipiginfo.com/domestication-history-of-mini-pigs.html. Accessed October 3, 2021.

Simianer H, Köhn F. Genetic management of the Göttingen minipig population. *J Pharmacol Toxicol Methods.* 2010;62:221–226.

Tynes VV. Potbellied pig husbandry and nutrition. *Vet Clin North Am Exot Anim Pract.* 1999;2(1):193–208.

Chapter 2

Behavior

Valarie V. Tynes

Introduction and History

The miniature pigs commonly seen in the pet trade are simply breeds or varieties of the domesticated pig, *Sus scrofa domesticus*. Based on present knowledge, the pig was domesticated from wild boars, after dogs, sheep, and goats, with the earliest known remains of the domesticated pig found in Southwest Asia c. 7000 BC. Under domestication the pig has changed in cranial conformation more than any other domesticated animal except the dog. Domesticated pigs have spread throughout the world and taken on a variety of forms based on the environment and market demands (Epstein and Bichard 1984).

Behaviorally, most domesticated animals share many traits with their ancestral relatives and the pig is no different. The primary differences include an increase in tameness or a decreased fear of humans and a decreased fear of novelty. While an enormous amount of behavioral research exists on domestic pigs, there is much less published data on the behavior of miniature pigs. However, other than their size and conformation, environments they are kept in, and lifestyle, there are no significant behavioral differences in these breeds. There may be minor behavioral differences based on genetics. For example, different breeds of swine are known to have differing levels of aggression or maternal behavior, but the basic behavioral profile remains the same. For the purpose of this chapter, I will extrapolate from what we know of the behavior of the domestic pig and apply it to the miniature pig.

Senses and Communication

The domestic pig evolved from a highly social, forest–dwelling ancestor with largely diurnal activity patterns. Most of their time is spent foraging for food on or under the ground in dimly lit areas while trying to avoid predation. Olfaction and vocalizations developed into their most important sensory modalities with audition playing a slightly less critical role, and vision and visual cues being of least importance to their success.

Understanding how the pig sees the world and how it communicates can give us insight into how to handle it in a way that it perceives as less threatening. This also helps us to better understand the pig's responses to environmental stimuli, and gives us insight into the pig's environmental needs as most behavior problems faced by pet pig owners stem from a failure to meet these needs.

VISION AND VISUAL CUES

The facial musculature of the pig is less differentiated than in other ungulates, so their facial expressions are limited. Without the ability to communicate extensively with visual cues, other sensory modalities become more important. The pig's vision evolved to fit its environmental needs, so it is appropriate for a forest–dwelling, diurnal creature. Ultimately, good vision and complex visual cues are simply not as critical to the pig as its other sensory modalities (Kiley 1972).

Despite the relative insignificance of vision, several studies have demonstrated that pigs' visual acuity is good. Pigs can discriminate between people using visual cues (Tanida et al. 1998) even in dim light (20 lux) (Koba and Tanida 2001). With enough light, pigs will also use visual cues to aid them in navigation in addition to olfactory and spatial cues (Croney et al. 2003). When miniature pigs become obese, they often develop fat deposits in the areas surrounding their eyes and this can result in worsening vision. Pigs thus blinded often become more irritable. It has been hypothesized that this problem can increase aggressive behavior in the pet pig.

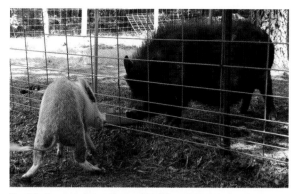

Fig. 2.1 A young pig meets an unfamiliar adult. Note the direct stare, assertive posture, and piloerection of the adult pig. The smaller pig is turning sideways, a likely indication of deference.

Visual cues in pigs are limited to those demonstrating threat and some more subtle cues that appear to signal submission (Fig. 2.1). The typical agonistic threat is an open-mouthed, lateral toss of the head directed toward the threatened individual. It is often accompanied by a short grunt and rarely appears to include a real attempt to bite when directed at humans. Other visual cues that may be seen with aggression can include the hair along the back becoming elevated (although this can be seen in non–aggressive arousal as well) and the tail twitching rapidly.

One of the visual cues in the pig that is believed to signal submission is a turning of the head sideways away from the threat. A subordinate pig may also turn its whole body sideways to signal submission.

OLFACTION

The pig's sense of smell is well developed, and research has demonstrated that a pig can recognize other pigs by the odor of their urine (Meese et al. 1975; Mendl et al. 2002). When pigs investigate conspecifics they concentrate on sniffing the facial region, underside of the belly, and the anogenital region (Meese and Ewbank 1973). Recognition of conspecifics by olfactory cues is important to pigs but not critical. When pigs do not smell familiar to each other there is likely to be some degree of aggression. Similarly, if pigs cannot see each other, they may not be able to recognize each other by smell alone so there may be some degree of aggression. For example, it is not uncommon for a pig to exhibit aggression toward another pig it has lived with for years, simply because the pig was taken to the veterinary clinic for the day. In these cases, the pigs may fight as if they have never met but they usually re–establish their hierarchy quickly with minimal fighting. This further supports the belief that the stimulus for the initiation and continuance of aggression in pigs is multi–sensory in nature (Meese and Baldwin 1975).

Chemical marking is common in wild and feral pigs, especially near their wallows and nests. Pigs apply scent by rubbing their perineal region, head, and sides on the ground in or near the wallow (Graves 1984). When this behavior is repeated by pet pigs in the home, it often leaves a brownish residue on walls and door jambs. This is not a behavior that one should attempt to change in the pig. Rather pet owners should be instructed to protect these areas by moving furniture to block access and/or applying plastic corner guards or protectors (readily available at most home improvement stores) to protruding corners in the home.

TASTE

Research has shown that pigs display a strong preference for glucose, sucrose, fructose, lactose, and saccharin solutions (Kennedy and Baldwin 1972; Houpt and Houpt 1976). These preferences appear to be strongest in the neonate (Houpt and Houpt 1976). However, a great deal of individual variation in preferences has been noted, especially in regard to saccharin. Some pigs appear to strongly prefer saccharin while others seem to find it strongly aversive (Kare et al. 1965).

Pigs do not appear to have a preference for salt solutions as do some other herbivores (Kare et al. 1965). They find very strong salt solutions aversive, but if the solution is not too strong this aversion can be overcome by thirst.

These taste preferences can be useful when it becomes necessary to medicate pigs. Using sweet sticky substances to hide medicine can be extremely effective. Jams and jellies smeared on bread with pills or capsules embedded and then rolled up into a bite-sized ball are usually taken eagerly by most pigs. Following up the medicated "treat ball" immediately with another unmedicated "treat ball" will ensure that if the medicine is bitter, the flavor can be quickly replaced with something else and decrease the chance that pigs develop an aversion to the bread and jam. Most animals can and will develop aversions to foods that they associate with a bitter substance. So if a pig requires regular medication, switching from one sweet flavor to another may be necessary periodically.

AUDITION

The hearing range of the pig is similar to that of most other hoofed mammals who also rely on their hearing to some extent to avoid predation (Heffner and Heffner 1990). The pig's ears are relatively immobile, so localizing sound usually requires that it turns its entire head.

Due to these auditory capabilities, as well as their status as a prey animal, pigs are likely to be easily startled by loud noises (though less likely to develop strong phobias, e.g., thunderstorms, fireworks than a dog). When interacting with pigs, one should speak softly and move slowly so as not to startle them. When startled or frightened, pigs are likely to respond immediately with escape behavior.

VOCALIZATIONS

The pig is an extremely vocal animal with a wide range of calls. The pig's vocalizations are strongly affected by its level of excitement or arousal and several recent studies have found that vocalizations can be very predictive of emotional states and stress (Kiley 1972; Linhart et al. 2015; Villain et al. 2020). In general, amplitude, frequency, and pitch of the vocalizations as well as duration of calls increase as a pig becomes more excited (Kiley 1972; Linhart et al. 2015). See Table 2.1 for a summary of Kiley's findings.

Simply put, grunts, squeals, grunt–squeals, screams, and barks are the most common vocalizations recognized by the majority of researchers (Kiley 1972; Linhart et al. 2015; Garcia et al. 2016; Villain et al. 2020). Grunts are contact calls with an acoustical structure that makes them ideal for short–range communication. Screams are distress calls that are likely to be heard over a longer distance (Linhart et al. 2015). Repeated grunts are common in situations of frustration, especially if the frustrating situation is prolonged

TABLE 2.1 **Vocalizations of the Pig**		
Vocalization	**Description**	**Use**
Common grunt	Low amplitude	Contact call; made while exploring or eating; evoked by any change in the environment
Staccato grunt	Similar but shorter than the common grunt	During similar situations as the common grunt but when excitement is high; before or after squealing sequences; produced when a pig approaches an unfamiliar person
Long grunt	Low to medium amplitude	Typically during tactile stimulation (e.g., belly rubs); when isolated; or before a squealing sequence
Bark	Mouth open; starts at high amplitude then decreases	When startled, frustrated, or generally disturbed; however, playful pigs—most commonly juveniles and young adults—will also bark when they get the "zoomies" (burst of energy in which the pig runs rapidly in short spurts)
High grunt (unique to piglets)	Similar to staccato grunt; higher pitched, usually repeated	More common in younger piglets; evoked by mildly startling stimuli; before suckling and when locating teats
Chirrup (unique to piglets)	Short with rapidly changing pitch	When piglets are picked up; usually before a squeal
Squeal (subadults prior to 6 months)	Constant pitch changes, higher tones	Most common call in piglets; eliciting stimulus is non–specific
Screams	Very loud and tonal; longer with less pitch changes than a squeal	Elicited by any extremely unpleasant situation

Kiley M. The vocalizations of ungulates, their causation and function. *Z Tierpsychol*. 1972;31:171–222.

(e.g., a hungry pig waiting for a meal or treat). They may also be heard from a sow in response to the scream of her piglet, during courtship, or when pigs are isolated. When ambient temperatures drop, there is an increase in high–frequency vocalizations among pigs (Hillmann et al. 2004). Grunts may turn into squeals with increasing emotional distress (Linhart et al. 2015). This is commonly heard when pigs are lifted or restrained. For example, they may grunt upon approach but when lifted, proceed to squealing.

The most common call made by piglets is the squeal (Marchant et al. 2001). Squeals may become screams if the piglet is experiencing a highly aversive event of any kind; screams are extremely characteristic of painful or fearful situations (Kiley 1972). Piglets being castrated without anesthesia produce more high-frequency calls than sham castrated piglets. These calls are especially pronounced during the severing of the spermatic cord further suggesting that high rates of higher frequency calls are a reliable indicator of pain in the pig (Weary et al. 1998).

In general, piglet vocalizations are more easily elicited by startling or frustrating situations; they are likely to squeal when an adult might simply grunt. They also bark more readily. Overall, their vocalizations are more socially facilitated than those of adult pigs (Kiley 1972). In other words, squealing or screaming by one pig can result in squealing and panic by nearby pigs.

Due to the pig's sensitivity to the pitch of vocalizations, one should also avoid speaking in high pitched tones (as we often do when "baby-talking" to dogs and cats). Higher pitches are associated with emotional distress for the pig and pig panic behavior is highly socially facilitated. For this reason, it may be useful to speak at a lower pitch that may translate as more soothing to the pig and less likely to lead to increasing excitement.

Social Behavior of the Pig

Pigs are highly social animals and have a matrilineal social structure when living in natural or semi–natural conditions. In these environments, they live in small groups called sounders that are typically composed of one to two sows and their offspring of the year. Larger sounders may also include females from litters of previous years. The pigs in a sounder appear to be strongly bonded to each other and their behavior is synchronous. The social behavior of wild and feral swine is very similar and is likely representative of normal social behavior in the domesticated pig as well.

NEONATAL AND JUVENILE SOCIAL BEHAVIOR

Neonatal piglets are extremely precocious and can stand, walk, and attempt to nurse within minutes of birth. As soon as they begin walking, piglets begin searching for a teat. Each piglet identifies a particular teat as its own and will aggressively defend the teat from any other piglets. This competitiveness is aided in part by the piglet's sharp "needle teeth," the deciduous corner incisors and tusks that are aimed outward. Most piglets over a day of age will have numerous scratches on their faces from competing with their siblings for a teat. Within about 24 hours after birth, this teat order is well established and fighting between piglets declines significantly (Hemsworth et al. 1976). Once established, the teat order remains relatively stable and is likely to be maintained until weaning (McBride 1963).

Studies of commercial swine have demonstrated the larger the piglet at birth, the more likely it is to attain control of a more productive teat and grow larger than its siblings. Thus, the pigliet maintains a dominant status over its littermates until weaning. Dominance status during the first few weeks of life, however, does not appear to be correlated with dominance after weaning when mixing with other pigs. Body weight appears to play the most significant role in attaining and maintaining dominance after mixing. Larger pigs typically fight more immediately after mixing and gain higher status (Scheel et al. 1977).

ADULT SOCIAL BEHAVIOR

Dominance continues to play an important role in the life of feral, wild, and domesticated swine (Graves 1984). In penned domesticated swine, the dominant animal enjoys more freedom of movement and less restriction of personal space than do more subordinate pigs (Graves 1984).

Whenever unacquainted pigs are introduced, it is likely that initially there will be vigorous fighting in an attempt to establish a hierarchy. Fighting is most

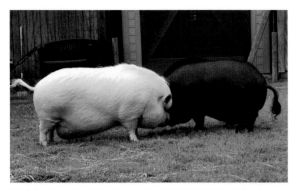

Fig. 2.2 Two unfamiliar pigs meeting for the first time. The pigs are investigating each other's facial area, and the posture assumed is typical of pig-to-pig aggression. The black pig is beginning to demonstrate some piloerection and the slightly stiff, elevated tail that can be indicative of aggressive arousal. The white pig's tail is more obviously elevated, consistent with an aggressive emotional state.

frequent during the first 24 hours and by 48 hours a hierarchy has been established and fighting decreases dramatically. Fighting among pigs usually initially involves both combatants attempting to shove and bite each other about the head and ears (Fig. 2.2). Later, the two pigs may stand with their heads to each other's flank and circle while attempting to bite the other's back legs and flanks (Fig. 2.3). They sometimes circle this way until exhausted. Eventually, one pig will turn to flee and the other pig may chase it, attempting to bite its back legs as it runs away. Losers of fights receive more bites to the rump than winners (McGlone 1985). Bites directed toward the ears are most common with the winning pig directing the most ear bites toward the loser of the fight.

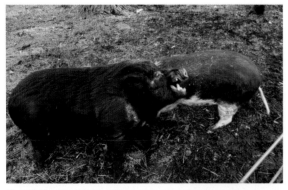

Fig. 2.3 Two pigs fighting. These pigs are at the stage where they are pushing, shoving, and biting at each other.

In some cases, a threatened pig will immediately retreat from the aggressor without fighting. In a few instances two pigs may simply stare at each other for several seconds before one pig retreats, apparently accepting its role as the subordinate. Typically, the dominant pig is responsible for most of the aggression until the hierarchy is stabilized, and most aggressive behaviors are directed toward the pig immediately below the aggressor in the hierarchy (Meese and Ewbank 1973).

Submission in the pig can be difficult to recognize since there does not appear to be a clear sign that turns off an attack by a dominant pig. However, subordinate behaviors may include turning the body 180 degrees to the attacker, running away from threats and attacks, or standing with drooping ears and tail with the back arched (Meese and Ewbank 1973; McGlone 1985).

Aggressiveness has been shown to be a relatively stable temperament trait and is moderately heritable. Measurement of skin lesions or wounding can be used as a measure of aggression among a group of pigs. Lesions around the anterior part of the body (head, neck, and shoulders) are consistent with reciprocated fighting or fighting that involves active participation by two pigs. Lesions around the flank, back, or rump are consistent with a pig being the recipient of aggression by another pig (also referred to as being bullied). The number of anterior skin lesions is genetically correlated with higher levels of reciprocated fighting, and pigs that perform this behavior are also more likely to direct bullying behavior toward other pigs. Therefore, the number of lesions and their locations on pigs can be used as an indicator to help select against aggressive behavior in pigs (Turner et al. 2006, 2008, 2010; D'Eath et al. 2010; Desire et al. 2015a, 2015b). Breeders of miniature pet pigs should be encouraged to breed pigs for good health as well as behavior. See Box 2.1 for tips on acquiring a pet pig.

It should be noted that the mixing of pigs at weaning, as is commonly done in commercial operations, is not natural to the pig. In natural or semi–natural environments, the pig is unlikely to ever be forced into close association with a pig it is not familiar with. Most pigs only ever interact with the members of their own sounder except during breeding season. Confrontations with individuals of other sounders is

BOX 2.1 ACQUIRING A PET PIG

Pet pigs are easily acquired by adoption from a shelter or sanctuary or by purchasing from a breeder.

If acquiring from a shelter or sanctuary:

- Be aware that some pigs are there due to problem behaviors but just as likely, they were given up because they "grew too big" or otherwise failed to meet someone's expectations. Others are given up after people discover that pigs are not allowed by their city or property owners association.
- The pet owner should acquire as much information about the pig's history as possible. In many cases, the pig's behavior improves in a sanctuary setting because it is given a more natural environment and is able to socialize with other pigs.
- The pet owner should be prepared to adopt two pigs if they don't already own one; many sanctuaries will only adopt pigs in pairs because of their strongly held belief that it is in the best interest of the pig and may decrease the incidence of certain behavior problems. There is some evidence to suggest that pigs living in a multi–pig household are less likely to demonstrate human–directed aggression (Tynes et al. 2007).
- If given a proper environment, many of these adult pigs will still bond to a new owner and make excellent pets. A pig should be given time—at least a month—to establish trust and a routine within the new home.

- Sanctuaries may have pigs of all ages available for adoption, including piglets.

If purchasing a pig, a reputable breeder:

- Will not sell a piglet prior to 8 weeks of age
- Will castrate males intended to be pets prior to purchase, possibly spaying females as well
- Will not guarantee the adult size of the pig they are selling
- Will welcome you to visit their breeding facility before and after acquiring your pet
- Will be knowledgeable about pigs and provide the new pet owner with plenty of resources to guide them
- Will express a willingness to take the pig back if the owner finds they can no longer keep it
- Will provide health records for the pig

When visiting a breeder, the buyer should be able to meet at least one parent of the pig they are buying. They should determine the age of the parent because if it is under 3 years of age, its size may not be indicative of the future size of the pig they buy. However, the temperament of the parent(s) and any other relatives of the pig they are planning to buy is very likely to be indicative of their future pet's temperament.

---

usually actively avoided by maintaining distance. Within sounders subordinate pigs avoid confrontations with dominant pigs, and minimal aggression is seen between members of a sounder (Graves 1984). The stability of the hierarchy within sounders is maintained mostly through visual displays with minimal overt aggression.

INTRASPECIFIC AGGRESSION

What does this mean for people who acquire pet pigs? It means that introducing a pig to an unfamiliar pig(s) will likely result in some degree of aggression, regardless of the age of the pigs. The older and larger a pig gets the more likely the aggression will be intense and the pigs will cause some harm to each other. Because aggression between pigs in commercial operations is an important welfare issue, as well as negatively impacting production, many different studies have been performed to examine ways of decreasing intraspecific aggression in swine and some of these can be readily extrapolated to the pet pig.

For example, studies have shown that the presence of places to hide, novel toys, and extra space for introductions can all help decrease the severity of aggression at mixing (McGlone and Curtis 1985; Blackshaw et al. 1997; Spoolder et al. 2000; Hemsworth et al. 2013). Other studies have demonstrated that when there is significant weight asymmetry between pigs at mixing, fights will be shorter with a lower number of bites (Andersen et al. 2000). Studies have also shown that mixed sex groups of pigs fight longer when first introduced as compared to single sex groups (Colson et al. 2006). Keeping this information in mind, the following guidelines should be considered:

- When adding a new pig to a home that already has a pig in it, try to choose a pig that is not extremely close in size to the existing pig. A significant size difference may help the pigs be able to visually "size up" their opponent and fight less to establish a hierarchy.
- When adding a pig, if possible, add a pig of the same sex as the pig already in the home. However, it is possible that since most pet pigs are gonadectomized this guideline may not be important, and anecdotal information suggests that

these sex differences are less likely to be a problem in miniature pet pigs.

- When introducing new pet pigs try to introduce in a large enough area where the pigs can easily escape from one another.
- If the space is a neutral territory with a variety of novel objects in it, this can provide the pigs with a reason to explore the environment rather than just focusing on each other.

A great deal of research has also examined the role that early socialization plays in decreasing aggression between pigs at mixing, and several studies have demonstrated that the opportunity to learn social skills at a young age leads to shorter bouts of aggression when they are mixed at weaning (D'Eath 2005; Kanaan et al. 2008; Kutzer et al. 2009).

Owners of single pet pigs should consider this when thinking about adding a new pet pig. If their current pet has lived its entire life without ever interacting with another pig, its social skills may be particularly poor, making the addition of a new pig to the home more problematic. There may be increased fighting upon introduction and the time to establish a normal hierarchy may be delayed. A pig that lives to adulthood without ever interacting with another pig may not know how to interact normally with a conspecific, resulting in chronic fighting and inability to establish a normal hierarchy. This is another reason why pet owners should be encouraged to acquire two familiar pigs at the same time. Does this mean that owners of single pigs should not add another pig? Absolutely not! The benefits of having a companion

BOX 2.2 TIPS FOR INTRODUCING PET PIGS

- There may be some benefit to allowing pigs to meet on either side of a barrier and interact this way for a day or two. The barrier can allow visual and olfactory contact but not physical contact. Minimal aggressive threats should be seen between the pigs before allowing them to have physical access to each other. If the pigs are exhibiting severe aggressive threats such as charging or ramming the gate repeatedly, they should remain separated visually for another 24–48 hours. For example, keep a closed door between the pigs but allow the pigs to sniff each other under the door.
- If when exposed visually, they continue to threaten each other, separate the pigs with a door and wait another day or two before trying again to allow visual contact.
- Once the pigs can interact at the barrier peacefully, begin observing for signs that one pig may be willing to behave submissively. These signs may be subtle but might include turning away of the head or even walking away when the other pig approaches. Once behaviors like these are witnessed a few times, it is time for the next step.
- When it is time to allow physical contact, the pigs should be introduced in a neutral space if possible (i.e., an area of the yard in which neither pig is housed).
- When performing the initial physical introduction, there should be plenty of space for the pigs to maneuver and for one pig to escape the other if it attempts to do so.
- A certain amount of fighting and minor injuries should be expected. It is likely that intervening too quickly and separating the pigs may in fact decrease the speed with which they can establish their hierarchy and stop fighting.
- Use a sorting panel or board for protection if it becomes necessary to physically separate fighting pigs.

- Verbal praise given to reward certain behaviors (i.e., walking away from confrontation rather than engaging) can help the pigs to associate a pleasant emotional state with the other animal, possibly increasing the speed with which they will accept each other.
- If one of the pigs is consistently trying to escape and avoid fighting, while the other pig is consistently continuing to attack, then temporary separation should be considered. However, the pigs should be returned to a place where they can continue to see, smell, and hear each other, but not harm each other. Pet owners should remain aware, however, that continuing to separate the pigs in this way may slow the process of their hierarchy establishment and contribute to more fighting in the long term.
- After successful introduction, continue to provide separate sleeping areas. Although the pigs will be likely to cohabitate eventually, they may choose to maintain two nesting areas for a period of time.
- Always separate pigs for feeding. This is especially important during the initial introduction.
- Continue to supervise pigs closely for several days after they are allowed to be together full time at home.
- Avoid separating the pigs just because there are minor scuffles. Separation after fighting will only prolong establishment of the hierarchy.
- If the owner wishes to, they can practice redirecting the pigs by calling their names, asking them to come (assuming they have learned that cue), or even just shaking a food bowl. The pigs can then be reinforced for attending to the owner.

far outweigh the risks for the majority of pigs. Owners should simply be prepared for the two pigs to take a bit longer to reach a state of harmony. For more information on introducing unacquainted pet pigs, see Box 2.2.

Interventions that have been used to decrease fighting in pigs after mixing include supplements such as tryptophan, odor masking agents, anti–aggressive drugs such as amperozide and azaperone, and pheromones. While many of these interventions show promise, none have been studied in miniature pigs and more research is needed to determine if practical applications exist. While anxiolytic medications such as trazodone, benzodiazepines, gabapentin, or fluoxetine have received virtually no study in the pet pig; there have been anecdotal reports of their use and efficacy. As a general rule of thumb, pigs can be treated with these medications using doses recommended for dogs.

Pet owners wishing to have pigs as pets should be encouraged to acquire two pigs at the same time, preferably from the same litter or social group (i.e., many sanctuaries have already paired compatible animals), so as to decrease the need to mix unacquainted pigs at a later date. Due to their highly social nature, pigs should never be expected to be the only pig in the home. While they can get along with other animals and certainly bond to people, it is unlikely that the companionship of another species provides them with all of their social needs.

Reproductive Behavior

Problems associated with reproductive or sexual behavior of miniature pet pigs are uncommon and few serious breeders of miniature pet pigs remain. Most pet pigs are gonadectomized early in life. However, there are behaviors associated with sexual maturity that may be seen by owners of pigs who delay gonadectomy and these behaviors can be problematic for the pet owner.

MOUNTING BEHAVIOR

Non–copulatory mounting can occur in either sex of pig regardless of gonadectomy status. While mounting is typically indicative of the presence of testosterone and may suggest that an animal is in fact intact, it can also occur during situations of emotional arousal. Frequent and repeated mounting by intact animals directed toward other intact animals can suggest emotions of conflict or frustration. In these cases, the pigs may have an unstable hierarchy and it is resulting in stress, but pigs do not typically mount each other solely as a display of dominance. If mounting occurs frequently in an apparently neutered male and no other reasons can be identified, the possibility that the pig has a retained testicle should be considered. Other secondary sex characteristics, such as shoulder plate development or scrotal hyperkeratosis (Fig. 4.12), may also be identified and testosterone levels can be measured for confirmation if needed. Females in estrus also frequently exhibit mounting behavior.

CHOMPING OR FOAMING AT THE MOUTH

This is a behavior demonstrated by intact male pigs when sexually aroused or aggressively aroused. The pig chomps or chews repeatedly, working up a large amount of thick, ropey froth (Fig. 4.13). This can be distressing to owners who may fear that their pig is sick or has been poisoned. However, many pigs also perform this behavior when they are anticipating food, albeit to a lesser degree, so the two behaviors should not be confused.

CYCLIC BEHAVIORS IN FEMALE PIGS

When female pigs experience estrus, they often behave more irritably and aggressively. They may also suddenly begin to urinate in the house even when well house trained and become more destructive. These behaviors typically occur in roughly monthly cycles with the pig's behavior returning to normal between the periods of estrus. This regular alteration to a pig's typical behavior provides one more good reason for all female pet pigs to be spayed.

If a pig is acquired when it is already mature, where its previous history may be completely unknown or in doubt, it can sometimes be difficult to determine if the pig has already been spayed. Watching for these regular changes in behavior can be helpful and if they appear spaying is recommended about a week after the signs disappear.

MATERNAL BEHAVIOR

In natural environments, male pigs leave the female groups after breeding and do not assist in caring for the young. About 1 to 2 hours prior to parturition, a female will begin building a nest (Stolba and Wood-Gush 1989). The farrowing nest outdoors can be so well hidden under the pile of vegetation that the sow and piglets may go completely unseen by anyone passing by (Fig. 2.4).

Farrowing may last for a few hours with, usually, no longer than 15 minutes between the birth of each piglet. After the birth of each piglet, the sow may stand and sniff the piglet, but she does not assist the piglet by helping it get out of the birth membranes or by cleaning it. She may eventually consume the placenta, blood, and fluids associated with the birth (Graves 1984).

During the first week piglets rarely leave the nest and the sow returns to nurse them about every 30 minutes. From the second week, piglets follow their dam as she forages, and if startled they will huddle together and run for the nest. If they squeak or squeal, the dam will come running to their aid. During this time, she may display aggression toward any person or animal that approaches too closely. By

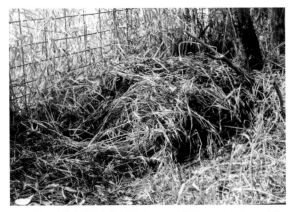

Fig. 2.4 An example of a typical pig nest for farrowing. Toward the left side of the nest, you can just see the sow's head beginning to emerge. (Photo credit: Nancy Shepherd.)

about 3 months of age, the sow nurses the piglets at about 2-hour intervals and by about 88 days of age, she ceases to suckle the litter (Stolba and Wood-Gush 1989).

In the wild, piglets do not disperse from their natal groups until sexual maturity (about 7 to 8 months old) or until the sow is ready to farrow again (Graves 1984).

What is the Best Age to Acquire a Pig?

If purchasing a young pig from a breeder, the prospective pet pig owner should not attempt to acquire the pig prior to about 8 weeks of age. Weaning is a stressful time for young animals due to a sudden change in diet from milk to solids and separation from the sow and littermates. As described, in nature weaning is a gradual process rather than an abrupt one, as it is in most breeding operations. In addition, in the natural environment the female pig may never leave her natal herd. Piglets also continue to learn appropriate social behavior from their siblings and mother even after they are eating solid food. This means that the sudden separation of a new piglet from its herd prior to 8 weeks of age should be avoided if possible. At the time of acquisition, the piglet should already be eating solid food and not require bottle feeding. While research data is limited, it is very likely that bottle–fed piglets are more challenging to raise and do not make the best pets due to their poor social skills.

Early weaned pigs often perform a behavior called belly-nosing, which is an up and down massaging movement using the snout, directing it at other pigs' abdomens. In commercial systems when pigs are weaned abruptly and mixed with unfamiliar pigs, they may even chase other pigs around the pen in an attempt to perform this behavior. In the pet pig this behavior can be very annoying to pet owners especially when their piglet directs this behavior at the owners' arms and legs. In many cases the pig can cause extensive bruising due to this constant nudging of their owners. The persistence of this behavior also demonstrates the degree to which these piglets may be experiencing feelings of deprivation and frustration and provides another important reason for not separating piglets from their herds too early.

Excretory Behavior

Pigs are known for their discriminating elimination behavior. In confinement, they tend to eliminate in one area and prefer to use an area that is as far from their resting space as possible. If they have the space to avoid eliminating near their food and water, they will. However, if confined to a smaller space, pigs will eliminate near their drinking area in an apparent attempt to avoid eliminating near their resting area, suggesting that a clean resting area is a higher priority than a clean drinking area (Baxter 1982/83). Pigs often drink, urinate, and defecate in a close sequence. Therefore, the farther their water is from their resting area, the elimination area will be farther away. In confinement settings this behavior will result in a cleaner pen (Hacker et al. 1994). Generally, pigs prefer to lie in a warmer area and excrete in a cooler area (Hacker et al. 1994). Even in free–ranging pigs, the majority of defecations are situated at least 5 to 15 meters away from the nest sites (Stolba and Wood-Gush 1989).

Pigs adopt a relatively unstable posture when eliminating; they bring their hind limbs and forelimbs close together under their body as opposed to stretching out as many other species do. Males urinate with a more upright stance, but defecation and female urination always assume this cowering–type posture. Tails are usually raised throughout elimination and most pigs wag their tails afterward (Buchenhauer et al. 1982/83). Several studies have suggested that pigs prefer to seek isolation when eliminating. They also have a tendency to back up against a wall or a corner possibly because they feel particularly vulnerable when assuming the posture for eliminating (Baxter 1982/83; Olsen et al. 2001).

HOUSE-TRAINING THE PIG

When pigs are allowed outdoors, they appear to prefer eliminating outdoors. The availability of shade may also increase the chance that they will eliminate outdoors instead of indoors. Owners should be discouraged

from expecting pigs to be "indoors only" and use a litter box all of the time. A pig can be trained to use a litter box, and a litter box, can be very valuable when initially house–training the young pig, but once the pig is an adult it will likely wait until the owner allows it outside to eliminate, as long as the owner has a relatively regular routine. However, even an adult pig may be reluctant to go outside during inclement weather so keeping a litter box available for the pig even after it is completely house–trained is wise. A pig allowed to roam the home unattended at any age may find it convenient to establish a spot for elimination in a room other than where it spends the most time. For this reason and many others, pigs should never be allowed to roam the home unsupervised for a very long period of time. See Box 2.3 for basic house–training instructions for the pet pig and Box 2.4 for providing a litter box for the pig.

Ingestive Behavior

Swine are omnivores and in the wild will spend a significant amount of their waking hours foraging for food. They use their specialized nose to root for edible items below the surface of the soil. Feral swine consume whatever plant material is seasonally available but will also eat earthworms, insects, frogs, snakes, turtles, rodents, and young and eggs of ground–nesting birds. In North America and parts of Europe, acorns and other nuts can comprise around 80% of the vegetable matter in the diet (Graves 1984). Swine will also eat carrion, including carcasses of other pigs, and will readily eat garbage if available.

Pigs naturally have a strongly diurnal pattern of behavior, but daily activity patterns will vary with the season, weather, food availability, and presence of predators. During the summer, they may be more active during early morning and late afternoon but will become more nocturnal as temperatures rise or predation increases. When food is scarce and temperatures are high, pigs rest more, especially during the late afternoon. The amount of food consumed is also affected by temperature, with food consumption decreasing as temperatures increase (Baldwin 1969).

In general, swine prefer to eat several small meals throughout the day. One study of group–housed swine

BOX 2.3 HOUSE TRAINING THE PET PIG

- The first step is understanding that a very young animal (8 to 10 weeks of age) can probably not "hold" its bladder for more than an hour or two at first.
- When first acquired, regardless of age, the pig should never be left unsupervised in the home. The owner should observe constantly so that the pig is not allowed out of sight. When the owner cannot observe, the pig can be confined to an area with a litter box. See *Box 2.4* for more information about providing the pig with a litter box.
- If the pig is ever observed begining to assume the position to eliminate, it should be quickly escorted to the proper area (litter box or outdoors); a sorting panel or even a large piece of cardboard can be used to guide the pig. The owner should then quietly stand by until the pig eliminates and then the pig should be verbally praised or petted for a job well done.
- The pig caught eliminating in the house should *never* be punished, yelled at, or hit. Startling the pig slightly may make it suddenly stop eliminating, allowing the owner to rush the pig outdoors or to a box, but caution is urged when trying to stop the pig from eliminating! If frightened the pig can quickly learn to avoid the owner when needing to eliminate, making the pig more likely to sneak away quietly to eliminate elsewhere. Avoidance of the owner makes house-training extremely difficult since observation of elimination is necessary to provide positive reinforcement.
- The pig should be taken regularly (every 1 to 2 hours) to the preferred place for elimination, either the litter box or outdoors. Piglets are more likely to eliminate after eating and after sleeping so these events should also be followed by trips to the place for elimination.
- Once the pig eliminates, it should be verbally praised.
- As the piglet matures, it can go longer between outings but this should be a gradual process. At 4 months of age, they could be taken out every 3 hours for example. At 6 months, every 4 to 5 hours. However, be aware that all pigs are individuals and there are no time guidelines guaranteed to apply to every pig.
- If in spite of the owner's efforts, if the pig manages to eliminate in the house, the owner should clean the area thoroughly with a cleanser made specifically for pet waste and then try to find a way to prevent the pig's access to this area again.
- If elimination accidents occur in the house, pet owners must ask themselves what they did that allowed the accident to happen so that it can be prevented next time. Pigs do not readily understand that the house is an inappropriate location for elimination. It takes frequent reinforcement for elimination in the right place for the pig to learn to not eliminate in the "wrong" place. Generally, pet owners should not relax their house–training approach until at least 3 months have passed without a single "accident."
- Installation of a pet door with unrestricted access can be an alternative to more time–consuming house–training. Pigs given the option will often choose to eliminate outdoors and need only learn to use a pet door.
- If the pet owner is having difficulty preventing urination in the house, then a urinalysis and physical exam are recommended. Pigs may develop cystitis and begin house soiling. Female pigs in estrus may also house soil.

BOX 2.4 GUIDELINES FOR CREATING A LITTER BOX FOR THE PET PIG

- Any container chosen to serve as a litter box for the pig must be large enough for the pig to step into and turn around completely. The inside surface of the box must be non–slip. If it is not naturally non–slip then bathtub decals or other non–slip surfaces should be added.
- The entrance to the box should be low enough for the pig to step into without much difficulty; one side of a taller box can be cut down if necessary.
- Typical litters like those used for cats should be avoided, especially clay and clumping litters.
- Appropriate litters for a pig litter box may include specialized litters such as pelleted recycled paper litters. Shredded paper, wood shavings, old towels, or potty pads are also frequently used.
- Most of the appropriate litters are not very absorbent, so waste may need to be removed daily and litter changed once or twice weekly depending on the size of the box. The pig
- has an excellent sense of smell, so even when waste is removed enough smell remains to help attract the pig back to the box. A pig will choose to potty elsewhere if the litter box becomes too soiled.
- Locate the litter box against a wall or in a corner when possible.
- Avoid using strong cleansers, such as bleach or pine cleansers, since they may be irritating to the pig's nose and lead to avoidance of the litter box.
- If the pet owner wants to keep the pig indoors much of the time and not have to observe constantly, then the pig's litter box can be confined to a small room or large cage. The space must be large enough that the box can be a few feet away from the pig's resting area, food, and water.
- Pigs forced to stay in a small area without a litter box, longer than they can reasonably hold their bladder and bowels, will learn that it is okay to eliminate where they sleep, making it harder to house–train them.

found that they ate 10 to 12 meals daily and most meals were consumed in under 2 minutes. It is also quite normal for captive swine to alternate between eating and drinking until satisfied (Baldwin 1969). This can pose problems for the owner of a pet pig because it means that the pig can be very messy. Feeding the pig in such a manner that will keep the mess from being a problem (i.e., using a mud tray Fig. 3.4, or shower stall) is easier and more appropriate than trying to stop this normal behavior.

Studies of domestic pigs living in semi–natural environments have found that pigs spend about 52% of the daylight period rooting and grazing and another 23% moving about exploring the environment and foraging (Stolba and Wood-Gush 1989). They tend to investigate edible and non–edible items by sniffing, rooting, biting, and chewing. While some of this behavior may in fact be appetitive (searching for food to relieve hunger, also called extrinsic exploration) some of it is apparently due to curiosity, a strong motivation to gather information about their environment also known as intrinsic exploration. Pigs clearly have a very strong desire to forage and root (Studnitz et al. 2007). While some studies have shown that restricting food will increase foraging behavior, ad libitum feeding does not completely alleviate a pig's motivation to explore (Beattie et al. 2000).

During the fall and winter when food becomes scarce, dominant individuals may defend areas where food is more abundant (Graves 1984). Aggression over food is less common in pet pigs since their food is usually abundant and readily available.

APPLICATION TO THE PET PIG—INGESTIVE BEHAVIOR

Many people feed their pig inappropriately small amounts of food. Sadly, this is often recommended by breeders who tell the new pig owner that these tiny amounts of food are necessary if they do not want their pig to get too big. Many pigs suffer from detrimental developmental effects as well as outright starvation due to this recommendation. Conversely, overfeeding the pig because the owner perceives the obese pig as normal or that their pet is always hungry will lead to obesity that negatively affects the quality of life for many more pigs. The welfare of the undernourished pig and the obese pig are probably equally poor, so educating the pet owner regarding the appropriate

types and amounts of feed to give their pig is an important role for the veterinarian. In addition, they should be instructed HOW to provide feed for their pet so as to increase the pig's opportunity to perform normal highly motivated behaviors such as foraging.

In addition, it has been noted that when food is restricted, pigs will drink more water as if to compensate for the lack of stomach fill (Yang et al. 1981). This often leads to problems with house–training because the pig drinks more water than necessary and then urinates much more frequently than normal.

Many pet pig owners believe that their pet is always hungry due to the constant rooting and exploration. However, it is more likely that the pig is simply exhibiting its normal foraging and exploratory behavior. Chapter 3 on Husbandry and Nutrition provides information on what to feed pigs and also provides some tips for the use of "food puzzles." One cannot overemphasize the importance of HOW to feed the pig. If at all possible, pigs should not be fed food in bowls. Satisfying the pig's need to forage and explore can be partially accomplished by feeding all meals in "food toys" or food puzzles of some type (Fig. 2.5; Fig. 3.10). Anything that requires the pig to "forage" for its food will be mentally stimulating and gives the pig appropriate outlets for this very strong drive. Alternatively, food can be broadcast in the yard as described in Chapter 3. For those concerned about damage to the yard from broadcasting feed, setting

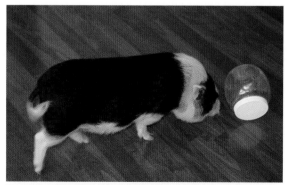

Fig. 2.5 A pig manipulating a homemade foraging toy. Foraging and exploration are normal behaviors in the pig which can be satisfied, in part, by feeding meals in such "food puzzles." Broadcasting feed across the ground (rather than placing in a bowl) is another option. (Photo credit: Valarie V. Tynes.)

aside a "sacrificial" area of the yard could be considered and, if possible, burying the food there. One study demonstrated that when food was buried, sows spent most of their foraging time in the area of buried food and did less damage to the remainder of the enclosure (Bornett et al. 2003).

Exploratory Behavior

Pigs are exploratory animals with a significant amount of their time spent moving about their environment. Studies of activity budgets of wild boars, either captive or free ranging, demonstrate that 16% of their time is spent traveling (Mauget 1981; Blasetti et al. 1988). Part of this time will be engaged in exploring for food. Resting time will increase when food is supplied in abundant quantities (Mauget 1981). Essentially, pigs forage to acquire needed caloric intake when necessary and rest once that caloric intake has been met. This results in a behavior pattern that conserves energy and greatly contributes to the problem of obesity in pet pigs.

Historically, rings have been placed in hogs' noses in order to decrease their rooting and foraging behavior. This has been recognized as a significant welfare problem in part because it appears that rooting is a behavioral need for pigs (Horrell et al. 2001). Pigs that are well fed still root, and pigs with rings in their noses substitute other behaviors for rooting. However, these behaviors are often those that are suggestive of frustration such as increased restlessness, standing inactive, and even increased aggression. See Box 2.5 for information about nose rings in pet pigs.

BOX 2.5 NOSE RINGS

Pet pigs should never have rings placed in their nose. Rooting is likely a behavioral need for the pig and attempting to stop it may lead to frustration and, eventually, other problematic behaviors. When considering acquiring a pet pig, people should keep in mind the words of Hartsock (1984) "…*many management problems of swine stem from our inattention to providing occupation for the pig's nose which trained over evolutionary time for gainful employment gets into every conceivable sort of difficulty when given nothing productive to do.*" One should not try to stop pigs from rooting, they must simply be given appropriate items to root.

Due to concerns about the welfare of ringed pigs, many studies have been performed looking at better ways of decreasing pasture damage in commercial swine. These studies have demonstrated that feeding higher levels of fiber can decrease destruction in paddocks housing sows (Braund et al. 1998) and that when provided with items to root, pigs do less damage to the environment (Edge et al. 2005).

Many studies have also been performed to find ways of enriching the pig's environment so as to decrease frustration, reduce stereotypes and aggression, increase activity, as well as increase overall pig health and welfare. Enrichment in growing pigs has been found to aid in adaption to novel situations, reduce negative behaviors such as belly nosing and tail biting, reduce fearfulness, and improve learning capabilities (Roy 2019).

Analysis of several studies that examined pig behavior in relation to environmental enrichment clearly demonstrates that pigs prefer items that are changeable by manipulating and destroying them (Van de Weerd et al. 2003; Van de Perre et al. 2011; Courboulay 2014). Pigs appear to prefer items that are deformable, destructible, and immobile so that the animals are able to hold and manipulate it (Roy 2019). Like most animals, pigs can quickly habituate to novel objects, so changeability is what appears to keep items novel to the pig. Pigs appear to lose interest in non–destructive items such as tires, chains, bars, and nylon dog bones within a short period of time (Studnitz et al. 2007). Straw and frayed ropes are examples of two items that appear to maintain most pig's interest. In addition, rotation of toys has been shown to aid in maintaining novelty, with different authors suggesting that items be rotated every 2 to 4 days and not presented more frequently than once a week in order to maintain the pig's interest (Gifford et al. 2007; Van de Perre et al. 2011).

Under natural conditions, swine do demonstrate strong site fidelity and the size of their home range will be directly related to food availability. Home ranges varying from 100 to 2500 hectares (247 to 6200 acres) have been documented in free–living swine but they are not defended as a territory (Mauget 1981). Typically, male home ranges will be larger than females (Graves 1984.) These large home ranges should be kept in mind when considering the appropriate housing of the pet pig. This information further supports the importance of providing the pig adequate activities for encouraging exercise.

MANAGING THE PET PIG'S EXPLORATORY BEHAVIOR

The pig's powerful drive to explore their environment by rooting can lead to a great deal of damage when confined to a home. Pigs have been known to root up carpeting and linoleum, shred wallpaper, and chew on drywall. Severely limiting the pig's food, as is often done to "keep the pig small," only increases their drive to forage and explore, potentially leading to more damage in both the yard and the home. In addition, based on research into socialization of commercial swine, it is very possible that some of the other problem behaviors of pigs, such as aggression, could be a result of their being reared in environments that do not allow them to perform their normal species–typical behaviors.

Pet pigs kept outdoors will do a great deal of damage to a yard so they should be given a separate enclosure in which to spend their time rooting if the owner wishes to preserve their landscaping. Limiting yard access in early spring and late fall when the nutrition is underground (e.g., early growing plants, grubs and other insects) can reduce damage. Alternatively, when pet owners have enough space, they can provide two separate "pig yards" and rotate the pig from space to space allowing the grass to recover in each area between visits. Providing the outdoor pig with abundant hay or straw to satisfy their desire to root may decrease their rooting in other areas of the yard, but the pig will still need to be provided with a wallow or other water source for soaking in this enclosure. Otherwise, rooting will also be used to dig a cool place in which to lie. Scattering the pig's daily ration in the area of the enclosure where you wish the pig to root may be helpful at decreasing rooting in other areas. Burying the pig's food there may encourage even more exploration in the one area and result in less destruction to other parts of the yard.

Many pet owners have used "rooting boxes" as a means of directing the pig's exploration toward acceptable items and away from unacceptable items. "Rooting boxes" can be made from plastic wading pools or other plastic boxes appropriate to the pig's size. The "box" should be large enough that the pig can walk

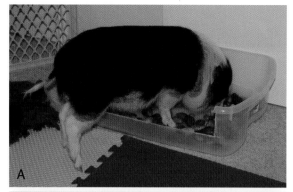

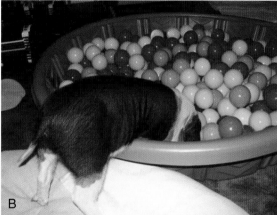

Fig. 2.6 (A) A typical rooting box for a young pig. (B) A larger rooting box containing multiple plastic balls. Rooting is a behavioral need of the pet pig. (Photo credit: Valarie V. Tynes.)

around in it and have an opening cut into the side so that the pig can step into it easily (Fig. 2.6A). Large, smooth river rocks can be placed inside, or plastic balls like those shown in Fig. 2.6B, can be used. If used outside, the box could be filled with topsoil, mulch, or straw. The pig's daily ration and any treats not used for training can be scattered among the material in the box and the pig allowed to forage for it.

Comfort Behavior and Body Care

Pigs are unable to sweat (Ingram 1965), and they consistently maintain a thick layer of body fat. They are, therefore, more sensitive to the effects of heat than to cold and they must change their behavior as needed in order to thermoregulate. When living outdoors, as temperatures start to rise above 59°F (14°C to 15°C), pigs will attempt to cool themselves by staying wet or wallowing in mud (Fig. 3.2). Studies have shown that mud provides evaporative cooling that lasts longer than the cooling provided by plain water alone (Ingram 1965). Studies based on observations of a population of pigs living in a semi–natural environment found that when temperatures rose above 64°F (18°C) pigs spent most of the mid–day hours wallowing in streams and boggy areas (Stolba and Wood-Gush 1989).

The behavior of the pig when they are hot also includes seeking shade and spending more time lying on its sides with its legs outstretched in a fully recumbent position (Andersen et al. 2008). At the same time, the pig will also avoid lying in bedded areas and lying in contact with other pigs (Andersen et al. 2008). In contrast, when temperatures drop the pig will seek a bedded area and spend more time there as well as lying in sternal recumbency. It will also be more likely to choose to lie in contact with other pigs so as to conserve body heat (Andersen et al. 2008).

As temperatures increase to 68°F (20°C) the pig will spend more time rubbing its trunk and hindquarters against objects in its environment suggesting that this may play a role in temperature regulation. This rubbing is likely a form of comfort behavior and probably aids in ectoparasite control as well (Graves 1984). Even in temperatures below 57°F (14°C), the pig will spend a certain amount of time in a wallow if one is available, suggesting that wallowing also plays an important role in skin and hair care.

When necessary and when able, pigs will spend a good part of their day foraging and exploring. The rest of the day they will spend resting and conserving energy. Pigs spend more time resting than any other domestic animal. In semi–natural conditions pigs spend most of their inactive time in day beds. These day beds may simply be a depression in the leaves or soil, but in colder weather piles of vegetation may be used (Graves 1984). Free–living pigs and those living in semi–natural conditions will build communal nests every evening. Most older animals in the group participate in nest building by carrying nest materials to the nest or raking materials in and around the nest. Pigs have been seen to carry materials for up to 20 m to make their nest. These nests can average about 3 m in circumference (Stolba and Wood-Gush 1989).

KEEPING THE PET PIG COMFORTABLE

When temperatures climb to over 70°F (21°C), at a minimum pigs must have adequate shade and a wallow or other sources of moisture will be utilized (Heitman et al. 1962; Blackshaw et al. 1994). Pet pigs will often turn over their water bowl in an attempt to make a cool, wet place to wallow. This can result in their having no drinking water, leading to dehydration and death if it goes unnoticed by owners. Pet pigs living outdoors should be given a place to cool themselves as well as a source of clean, fresh drinking water that cannot be upended (Fig. 3.8). Plastic wading pools can be an excellent means of providing "wallows" for pet pigs.

They should be provided with materials for rooting and nesting. Indoors, pigs will utilize blankets, comforters, or other bedding to make themselves a nest. If not given materials to make a nest, they can become destructive as they attempt to perform these nest–making behaviors in the home. Outdoors, pigs can be provided with straw or old blankets for bedding, and they are highly efficient at making very warm nests for themselves as long as their bedding is protected from rain and other moisture.

Preventing and Managing Other Behavior Problems in the Pet Pig

In addition to those already mentioned, behavior problems that may be seen in the pet pig include aggression to humans and other pets. Minimal research has been done on these subjects about the pet pig so much of the information is anecdotal. Fortunately, pigs learn exactly the same way as any other animal, so the basic rules of behavior science can be applied to them.

HUMAN–DIRECTED AGGRESSION

Only one study to date has been performed looking for possible causes of pet pig aggression directed toward humans (Tynes et al. 2007). This study demonstrated that aggression directed toward humans is relatively common in the miniature pig, but only one significant difference could be found between pigs that demonstrated aggression and those that did not. In the study population, significantly more pigs that lived without a conspecific demonstrated aggression than those that lived with another pig. While it is likely that there are many more factors involved in human–directed aggression, the data from the study suggests that living with a conspecific may help decrease the likelihood of aggression in pigs. Based on our knowledge of pig social behavior, it should not come as a surprise that pet pigs that develop without a conspecific are poorly socialized and, therefore, may not be able to demonstrate entirely normal social behavior toward other pigs or people. The need for adequate socialization is another reason why pigs should never be acquired before 8 weeks of age.

If aggression develops, it usually appears in the form of threats such as charging and snapping (Tynes et al. 2007). However, the threats will escalate to actual bites, with repeated biting in many cases, if responses by people are not appropriate. The threats usually begin when the pig is still young (under 1 to 1½ years) and is often first directed toward visitors to the home, but in other cases will be directed toward members of the home, including the primary caregiver.

No research has been done that demonstrates why so many pigs behave aggressively toward visitors to their home, but one should bear in mind that in natural environments most pigs encounter a limited number of unfamiliar individuals in their lifetime. Therefore, it is possible that introducing pet pigs to every new visitor that comes into the home may be stressful for the pig. They may be attempting to interact in the only way that their normal behavioral profile allows; this normal behavior would typically include avoiding interactions with an unknown individual or aggressing in an attempt to establish a hierarchy between the two. Attempting to respond as a pig would by participating in this interaction is not recommended. In the past, shoving, charging, or vocalizing at the pig has been recommended, but these actions are unsafe and can potentially lead to fear of humans. It is far more rational to either avoid the interactions completely or teach the pig a particular way to respond to visitors to the home. The pig can be taught to sit and stay on its bed and visitors can be instructed to toss treats to the pig. It is possible that positive interactions between pigs and visitors, established while the pig is still young (under 3 to 6 months of age), may allow for

better socialization and decreased aggression toward humans. However, this remains, at this time, an untested hypothesis.

Aggression directed toward humans can stem from a variety of other underlying motivations:

- Fear—If the pet owner does not habituate the pig to gentle handling from a very early age and continues to interact with it in a kind, predictable way, fear aggression may occur. Pigs are prey animals and their initial response to a threat is to attempt to escape. If they are in a situation where they perceive that escape is not possible, they may take a more proactive stance and use aggression to defend themselves (Fig. 2.7). In the author's experience, most cases of fear aggression occurred in pet pigs that have been punished and/or handled very roughly.
- Territorial—While free–ranging pigs do not normally defend territory, they may defend a nest. In some cases, pet pigs have shown aggression directed toward people only when people approach their bed, crate, or confinement area. This is much less common than the other forms of aggression described.
- Pain—A sudden onset of aggression can also be associated with illness or pain in the pet pig just

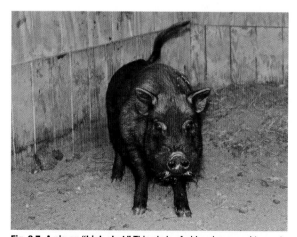

Fig. 2.7 A pig on "high alert." This pig is afraid and prepared to run to avoid a confrontation. His frozen forward–facing posture with its head held high, ears erect, and tail straight is a defensive one; note the dilated pupils. Although an aggressive posture may appear similar, a threatening pig will often flick the tail, chomp at the mouth, and begin to approach, even charge, the object of its attention.

as it can be in other animals. When possible, pigs exhibiting acute onset aggression should always have a thorough physical exam and radiographs, even if sedation is required, so pain can be ruled out.

- Frustration—Some aggression seen in pigs may occur because their environment does not allow them to exhibit their normal range of behaviors.

Pet pigs are less likely to exhibit food aggression than other species, such as dogs. Commercial pigs reared in confinement may demonstrate aggression over food, but this is likely due to overcrowding and the competition that exists in that environment. In the home environment, if a pig is extremely underfed and maintained in a very impoverished environment, frustration associated with food could potentially develop and lead to aggression. See Box 2.6 for tips for preventing and managing aggression.

AGGRESSION TOWARD OTHER SPECIES

It is relatively uncommon for pet pigs to direct aggression toward other species unless they are afraid. When forced to live in a household with other animals, the pig may feel less safe if it cannot simply avoid these other animals. This can be the case in homes that are small or crowded with furnishings, forcing the pig to pass closely by the other pets. Data is limited as to

---

BOX 2.6 TIPS FOR PREVENTING AND MANAGING HUMAN-DIRECTED AGGRESSION IN THE PET PIG

- All pigs should be taught some basic cues such as "come," "sit," or to touch a target. If pigs are allowed on furniture, they can be taught a cue for getting "up" on furniture and "off" on request. Pigs can begin learning these things as soon as they are brought into the home.
- Pigs thrive on routine and training can be accomplished through regularly scheduled, 5-minute training sessions, a minimum of 4 times/week.
- Positive reinforcement training of cues, and the use of these cues, gives the pig and owner a "language" with which to communicate. The pig learns how to get what it wants by politely offering a "sit" for example, and it never gets anything by being pushy, unruly, or aggressive. If it ever fails to respond to a cue, the worst thing that happens to the pig is that it doesn't get the "good thing" that the owner is offering.
- Only positive reinforcement training should be used. Pigs are easily food motivated and also respond well to verbal praise. As such, they are very easy to train by simply reinforcing appropriate and desired behaviors.
- Physical punishment should NEVER be used in an attempt to stop an unwanted behavior. Punishment, including yelling, squirting with a water bottle, hitting, slapping, or shoving will cause the pig to either become afraid of the owner OR attempt to protect its self from the owner's aggressive behavior.
- Once the pig has learned some cues, the pet owner can frequently ask the pig to perform a cue such as "sit" before being given attention, before being let outside or inside, before being fed, or allowed onto the furniture.
- Meetings with strangers in the home should be carefully controlled, especially at first. In the wild, unfamiliar groups of pigs circumvent one another to avoid confrontation, so avoidance should always be an option offered to the pig. If

the pig chooses to approach the visitor, praise can be given. Visitors can also be instructed to *toss* food treats to the pig. This teaches the pig to view strangers as a good thing rather than something to avoid or attempt to run off. If the pig has ever been aggressive in the past, especially around food, then food treats should be avoided.
- If the pig does snap at a person, the pig should be calmly (do not scold the pig) removed from the situation using a sorting panel or board (see Fig. 5.4A) and escorted to the safety of their nest or pen area (effectively a "time-out"). The owner must then ask themselves what could have been done to prevent the situation.
- If the pig begins demonstrating aggressive behavior toward anyone, the situations in which these incidents occur must be identified and the owner's initial focus should be on preventing those situations. For example, if the pig snaps at people who walk by while it is eating, then it needs to be fed somewhere else so that there is no need for people to pass by while the pig is eating. If the pig snaps at visitors to the home, then it may be easier for the pet owner to always put the pig away somewhere *before* visitors arrive. Preventing opportunities for unwanted behavior is a crucial part of an overall behavior modification program.

If the pig is an adult when these problems appear and the pig does not wear a harness and leash or has never been taught any cues, the assistance of a professional may be needed especially if the owner wishes to do more than just prevent opportunities for unwanted behaviors. In that case, the owner should be encouraged to look at the American College of Veterinary Behaviorists website (www.dacvb.org) for a behaviorist that will consult regarding a pet pig. If there are no behaviorists near the pet owner, many will speak with veterinarians by phone and consult and give what advice they can.

what age is ideal for socializing pigs to other species, so if a prospective pig owner has other pets and wishes their pig to get along well with them, the owner should be prepared to aid the process by gradual, positive interactions as soon as possible after bringing the pet pig home.

When problems do occur, usually it is a result of dogs threatening the pig. One should bear in mind that since pigs use fewer visual cues and dogs depend greatly on visual cues to communicate with their respective conspecifics, these two different species do not appear to be very good at "reading" or responding appropriately to the visual cues of the other species. For example, a dog may stare at a pig and maybe even lift its lip, but this will not always result in a pig walking away. They may simply continue with what they were doing. A dog may try to avoid eye contact with a pig and the pig may continue to approach the dog closely, resulting in the dog feeling threatened when that may not have been the pig's intent. Conversely, when a pig wants a dog to leave it alone or a pig wants to defend a resource such as a resting space or food, it will usually snap at a dog and this can be perceived by some dogs as such a severe threat that it will provoke a similar aggressive response in the dog.

Dog aggression toward pigs is worth a special comment. Even though pigs and dogs can get along well, pigs can excite the predatory response in almost any dog if they run and squeal. A pig beginning to run in play may cause a dog to chase, and if the day is hot the pig can quickly succumb to heat exhaustion. If a dog is chasing a pig because predatory behavior has been triggered, a dog may catch the pig and inflict fatal injuries. Sadly, the author is aware of many incidents where owners returned home to find their pig dead from a dog attack. In many of these cases, the dog and pig had lived together for years without problems. When dogs do catch pigs, they often grab them by the neck and shake, resulting in severe tissue damage to the area. These pigs can often be saved if they survive the initial trauma but the scarring can be severe. For this reason, pigs should never be left unattended with dogs.

Psychopharmacology for the Pet Pig

Virtually no data exists on the use of psychotropic drugs for pet pigs. In the author's experience most behavior problems are a result of normal but unwanted behaviors that can be readily managed with owner education, improved environment for the pig, and some behavior modification. On a rare occasion the pig may demonstrate signs of having been so poorly socialized that they truly do not appear to be able to interact normally with other pigs. In these instances, selective serotonin reuptake inhibitors (fluoxetine—1 mg/kg once daily) have been tried and found to be very helpful at allowing the pig to be introduced to other pigs.

A few cases of pigs with very fearful behavior have benefited from selective serotonin reuptake inhibitors. In these pigs, their history was unknown so it was difficult to be certain whether their fearful behavior was due primarily to genetics, a result of poor socialization, or learned behavior. In some cases, pigs may be weaned off medication, but others may need to continue to be medicated. There are simply too few of these cases at this time to be able to say anything with certainty about safety and efficacy.

Training and Behavior Modification

Pet pig owners should be encouraged to avoid all forms of physical punishment with pigs. Slapping the pig, squirting it with water, or even yelling "No" at the pig can lead to fear of the owner and, ultimately, aggression. The bond between the pig and owner needs to be based on trust and predictability not fear or "dominance." It is unlikely that pet pigs demonstrate aggression because they want to be "dominant." They may, however, demonstrate aggression because they are frustrated, conflicted, or anxious. Lack of appropriate environment and confusing interactions with humans likely contribute to the problem as well.

Positive reinforcement training should be instituted immediately after the pig is added to the home. Preventing unwanted behaviors using appropriate management and reinforcing all wanted behaviors will help shape the pig into a trusting and confident companion. Ideally, all pigs should learn some basic cues such as "sit," "stay," and "come." Pigs are highly intelligent and food motivated, so teaching them appropriate behavior is not difficult.

All pet pigs should be trained to wear a harness and walk on a leash while they are still small. Harnesses made for pigs are readily available online and pigs can be habituated to them by using patience and positive reinforcement. All training and behavior management of pigs should focus on the general concepts of preventing unwanted behaviors and reinforcing behaviors that owners wish to see repeated. With attention to providing for the pigs' basic behavioral needs and using appropriate positive reinforcement training to teach the desired behaviors, pigs can be wonderful pets and veterinary patients.

BIBLIOGRAPHY

Andersen HM, Jorgensen E, Dybkjaer L, et al. The ear skin temperature as an indicator of the thermal comfort of pigs. *Appl Anim Behav Sci.* 2008;113:43–56.

Andersen IL, et al. The effects of weight asymmetry and resource distribution on aggression in groups of unacquainted pigs. *Appl Anim Behav Sci.* 2000;68:107–120.

Baldwin BA. The study of behaviour in pigs. *Brit Vet J.* 1969;125:281–288.

Baxter MR. Environmental determinants of excretory and lying areas in domestic pigs. *Appl Anim Ethol.* 1982/83;9:195–200.

Beattie VE, O'Connell NE, Moss BW. Influence of environmental enrichment on the behaviour, performance and meat quality of domestic pigs. *Livest Prod Sci.* 2000;67:71–79.

Blackshaw JK, Blackshaw AW. Shade seeking and lying behaviour in pigs of mixed sex and age, with access to outside pens. *Appl Anim Behav Sci.* 1994;39:249–257.

Blackshaw JK, Thomas FJ, Lee JA. The effect of a fixed or free toy on the growth rate and aggressive behaviour of weaned pigs and the influence of hierarchy on initial investigation of the toys. *Appl Anim Behav Sci.* 1997;53:203–212.

Blasetti A, Boitani L, Riviello MC, et al. Activity budgets and use of enclosed space by wild boars (*Sus scrofa*) in captivity. *Zoo Biol.* 1988;7:69–79.

Bornett HLI, Edge HL, Edwards SA. Alternatives to nose-ringing in outdoor sows 1. The provision of a sacrificial rooting area. *Appl Anim Behav Sci.* 2003;83:267–276.

Braund JP, Edwards SA, Riddoch I, et al. Modification of foraging behavior and pasture damage by dietary manipulation in outdoor sows. *Appl Anim Behav Sci.* 1998;56:173–186.

Buchenhauer D, Luft C, Grauvogl A. Investigations on the eliminative behaviour of piglets. *Appl Anim Ethol.* 1982/83;9:153–164.

Colson V, Orgeur P, Courboulay V, et al. Grouping piglets by sex at weaning reduces aggressive behaviour. *Appl Anim Behav Sci.* 2006;97:152–171.

Courboulay V. Enrichment materials for fattening pigs: summary of IFIP trials. *Cahiers de l'IFIP.* 2014;1:47–56.

Croney CC, Adams, KM, Washington CG, et al. A note on visual, olfactory and spatial cue use in foraging behavior of pigs: indirectly assessing cognitive abilities. *Appl Anim Behav Sci.* 2003; 83:303–308.

da Silva EC, de Jager N, Burgos-Paz W, et al. Characterization of the porcine nutrient and taste receptor gene repertoire in domestic and wild populations across the globe. *BMC Genomics.* 2014; 15:1057.

D'Eath RB. Socializing piglets before weaning improves social hierarchy formation when pigs are mixed post-weaning. *Appl Anim Behav Sci.* 2005;93:199–211.

D'Eath RB, Turner SP, Kurt E, et al. Pigs' aggressive temperament affects pre-slaughter mixing aggression, stress and meat quality. *Animal.* 2010;4:604–616.

Desire S, Turner SP, D'Eath RB, et al. Analysis of the phenotypic link between behavioural traits at mixing and increased long-term social stability. *Appl Anim Behav Sci.* 2015b;166:52–62.

Desire S, Turner SP, D'Eath RB, et al. Genetic associations of short- and long-term aggressiveness identified by skin lesion with growth, feed efficiency, and carcass characteristics in growing pigs. *J Anim Sci.* 2015a;93:3303–3312.

Edge HL, Bulman CA, Edwards SA. Alternatives to nose-ringing in outdoor sows: the provision of root crops. *Appl Anim Behav Sci.* 2005;92:15–26.

Epstein H, Bichard M. Pig. In: Mason I, ed. *The Evolution of Domesticated Animals.* New York: Longman, Inc.; 1984;145–162.

Fraser D. The vocalizations and other behavior of growing pigs in an "open field" test. *Appl Anim Ethol.* 1974;1:3–16.

Garcia M, Gingras B, Bowling DL, et al. Structural classification of wild boar (*Sus scrofa*) vocalizations. *Ethology.* 2016;122: 329–342.

Gifford AK, Cloutier S, Newberry RC. Objects as enrichment: effects of object exposure time and delay interval on object recognition memory of the domestic pig. *Appl Anim Behav Sci.* 2007;107: 206–217.

Graves HB. Behavior and ecology of wild and feral swine (*Sus scrofa*). *J Anim Sci.* 1984;58:482–492.

Hacker RR, Ogilvie JR, Morrison WD, et al. Factors affecting excretory behavior of pigs. *J Anim Sci.* 1994;72:1455–1460.

Heffner RS, Heffner HH. Hearing in domestic pigs (*Sus scrofa*) and goats (*Capra hircus*). *Hear Res.* 1990;48:231–240.

Heitman H, Hahn L, Bond TE, et al. The effect of modified summer environment on swine behavior. *Anim Behav.* 1962;10:15–19.

Hemsworth PH, Rice M, Nash J, et al. Effects of group size and floor space allowance on grouped sows: aggression, stress, skin injuries, and reproductive performance. *J Anim Sci.* 2013;91;4953–4964.

Hemsworth PH, Winfield CG, Mullaney PD. A study of the development of the teat order in piglets. *Appl Anim Ethol.* 1976;2: 225–233.

Hillmann E, Mayerd C, Schön P, et al. Vocalisation of domestic pigs (*Sus scrofa domestica*) as an indicator for their adaptation towards ambient temperatures. *Appl Anim Behav Sci.* 2004;89: 195–206.

Horrell RI, A'Nes PJA, Edwards SA, et al. The use of nose-rings in pigs: consequences for rooting, other functional activities, and welfare. *Anim Welf.* 2001;10:3–22.

Houpt KA, Houpt TR. Comparative aspects of the ontogeny of taste. *Chem Senses.* 1976;2:219–228.

Ingram DL. Evaporative cooling in the pig. *Nature.* 1965;207: 415–416.

Kanaan VT, et al. A note on the effects of co-mingling piglet litters on pre-weaning growth, injuries and responses to behavioral tests. *Appl Anim Behav Sci.* 2008;110:386–391.

Kare MR, Pond WC, Campbell J. Observations on the taste reactions in pigs. *Anim Behav.* 1965;13:265–269.

Kennedy JM, Baldwin BA. Taste preferences in pigs for nutritive and non-nutritive sweet solutions. *Anim Behav.* 1972;20: 706–718.

Kiley M. The vocalizations of ungulates, their causation and function. *Z Tierpsychol.* 1972;31:171–222.

Koba Y, Tanida H. How do miniature pigs discriminate between people? Discrimination between people wearing coveralls of the same color. *Appl Anim Behav Sci.* 2001;73:45–58.

Kutzer T, et al. Effects of early contact between non-littermate piglets and of the complexity of farrowing conditions on social behaviour and weight gain. *Appl Anim Behav Sci.* 2009;121:16–24.

Linhart P, Ratcliffe VF, Reby D, et al. Expression of emotional arousal in two different piglet call types. *PLoS One.* 2015;10(8):e0135414. doi:10.1371/journal.pone.0135414.

Marchant JN, Whittaker X, Broom DM. Vocalizations of the adult female domestic pig during a standard human approach test and their relationships with behavioural and heart rate measures. *Appl Anim Behav Sci.* 2001;72:23–39.

Mauget R. Behavioural and reproductive strategies in wild forms of *Sus scrofa* (European wild boar and feral pigs). In: Sybesma W, ed. *The Welfare of Pigs.* A seminar in the EEC Program of Coordination of research on animal welfare, Brussels. London: Martinus Nijhoff Publishers; 1981:3–13.

McBride G. The teat order and communication in young pigs. *Anim Behav.* 1963;11:53–56.

McGlone JJ. A quantitative ethogram of aggressive and submissive behaviors in recently regrouped pigs. *J Anim Sci.* 1985;61(3):559–565.

McGlone JJ, Curtis SE. Behavior and performance of weanling pigs in pens equipped with hide areas. *J Anim Sci.* 1985;60(1):20–24.

Meese GB, Baldwin BA. The effect of ablation of the olfactory bulbs on aggressive behaviour in pigs. *Appl Anim Ethol.* 1975;1:251–262.

Meese GB, Connor DJ, Baldwin BA. Ability of the pig to distinguish between conspecific urine samples using olfaction. *Physiol Behav.* 1975;15:121–125.

Meese GB, Ewbank R. The establishment and nature of the dominance hierarchy in the domesticated pig. *Anim Behav.* 1973;21:326–334.

Mendl M, Randle K, Pope S. Young pigs can discriminate individual differences in odours from conspecific urine. *Anim Behav.* 2002;64:97–101.

Olsen AW, Dybkjaer L, Simonsen HB. The behavior of growing pigs kept in pens with outdoor runs II: temperature regulatory behavior, comfort behavior and dunging preferences. *Livest Prod Sci.* 2001;69:265–278.

Roy C, et al. Effects of enrichment type, presentation and social status on enrichment use and behaviour of sows with electronic sow feeding. *Animals.* 2019;9:369. doi:10.3390/ani9060369.

Scheel DE, Graves HB, Sherritt GW. Nursing order, social dominance and growth in swine. *J Anim Sci.* 1977;45:219–229.

Spoolder H.A.M., Edwards S.A., Corning S. Aggression among finishing pigs following mixing in kennelled and unkennelled accommodation. *Livest Prod Sci.* 2000;63:121–129.

Stolba A, Wood-Gush DGM. The behavior of pigs in a semi-natural environment. *Anim Prod.* 1989;48:419–425.

Studnitz M, Jensen MB, Pederson LJ. Why do pigs root and in what will they root? A review on the exploratory behavior of pigs in relation to environmental enrichment. *Appl Anim Behav Sci.* 2007;107:183–197.

Tanida H, Nagano Y. The ability of miniature pigs to discriminate between a stranger and their familiar handler. *Appl Anim Behav Sci.* 1998;56:149–159.

Turner SP, Roehe R, D'Eath RB. Selection against aggressiveness in pigs at re-grouping: practical application and implications for long-term behavioural patterns. *Anim Welf.* 2010;19:123–132.

Turner SP, Roehe R, Mekkawy W, et al. Bayesian analysis of genetic associations of skin lesions and behavioural traits to identify genetic components of individual aggressiveness in pigs. *Behav Genet.* 2008;38:67–75.

Turner SP, White IMS, Brotherstone S, et al. Heritability of post-mixing aggressiveness in grower-stage pigs and its relationship with production traits. *Anim Sci.* 2006;82:615–620.

Tynes VV, Hart BL, Bain MJ. Human-directed aggression in miniature pet pigs. *J Am Vet Med Assoc.* 2007;230:385–389.

Van de Perre V, Driessen P, Van Thielen J, et al. Comparison of pig behaviour when given a sequence of enrichment objects or a chain continuously. *Anim Welf.* 2011;20:641–649.

Van de Weerd HA, Docking CM, Day JEL, et al. A systematic approach towards developing environmental enrichment for pigs. *Appl Anim Behav Sci.* 2003;8:101–118.

Villain AS, Hazard A, Danglot M, et al. Piglets vocally express the anticipation of pseudo-social contexts in their grunts. *Sci Rep.* 2020;10:18496. https://doi.org/10.1038/s41598-020-75378-x.

Weary DM, Braithwaite LA, Fraser D. Vocal response to pain in piglets. *Appl Anim Behav Sci.* 1998;56:161–172.

Weary DM, Fraser D. Calling by domestic piglets: reliable signals of need? *Anim Behav.* 1995;50:1047–1055.

Whatson TS. The development of dunging preferences in piglets. *Appl Anim Ethol.* 1978;4:293.

Yang, TS, Howard B, MacFarlane WB. Effects of food on drinking behavior of growing pigs. *Appl Anim Ethol.* 1981;7:259–270.

Chapter 3

Husbandry & Nutrition

Kristie Mozzachio

Husbandry

This section provides some basic guidance to enable a veterinarian to educate owners. While many owners have done extensive research on minipig care, there is much misinformation that might lead them astray. A client handout providing basic husbandry information and some reputable resources for further research is highly recommended. An example can be found at: https://lafeber.com/vet/basic-miniature-pig-care/

ZONING

Owners are often so enamored with their new miniature pig pet that they overlook the fact that pigs are generally considered to be livestock. US city or county ordinances may prohibit the keeping of livestock, and although many now allow miniature pigs as an exception, owners should verify this before adopting a pig, as well as determine whether specific regulations are involved. For example, Seattle, WA, city ordinances (Seattle, WA Municipal Codes 2021) only vaguely refer to "one small potbelly pig" counting towards the limit of three small animals per household, while Raleigh, NC, ordinances specify a maximum of two pigs per household, provided the animals weigh no more than 100 lbs and stand no taller than 22 inches at the shoulder (Raleigh, NC Code of Ordinances 2021). In addition, the restrictive covenants of homeowner associations may supersede those of city or county zoning ordinances. Similar restrictions may exist in other countries as well. In the UK, for instance, there are specific legal requirements for movement and housing of pigs, including pig-walking licenses that involve veterinary inspection of the route for approval (Jackson and Cockcroft 2007). In Austria, miniature pet pigs must be housed with at least one other minipig and "branded for epidemiological reasons and concordantly the local veterinary office has to be informed" (Sipos

et al. 2007). Owners in the US wishing to challenge zoning ordinances can find helpful information and possible resources for legal counsel at: https://www.minipiginfo.com/mini-pig-zoning-ordinances.html Sawyer 2015).

ENVIRONMENT

Miniature pigs do well as either indoor or outdoor pets, although strict indoor confinement (i.e., apartment living) is not recommended and access to the great outdoors should be generous. They are like curious toddlers and need room to explore and engage with their environment; they can be destructive when bored (Fig. 3.1). Pet pigs with adequate outdoor access are mentally and physically healthier, with fewer behavioral problems and better skin, hair, and hoof condition. The ideal environment should promote natural behaviors including rooting, nesting, and exploration (see Chapter 2).

Piglets require warm ambient temperatures and adults tend to prefer mild temperatures as well, with comfortable ranges at approximately 77°F to 86°F (25°C to 30°C) for piglets up to 3 months of age—slightly higher for newborns—and 60° to 75°F (16°C to 24°C) for older animals (Bollen et al. 2000; Froe 1993; Jackson and Cockcroft 2007; Lawhorn 2013); ideal humidity is 50% to 70% (Bollen et al. 2000). However, despite their apparent preference for warmth, pigs lack thermoregulatory sweat glands and are unable to cool themselves via internal mechanisms. They are susceptible to overheating at temperatures exceeding 85°F (30°C) (Lawhorn 2013). Cooling measures are behavioral and include moving into the shade, lying in mud wallows, or rooting into cooler soil to lie down (Fig. 3.2). Wetting the body with a clean water source such as from a pond or pool provides only temporary relief as evaporative cooling is

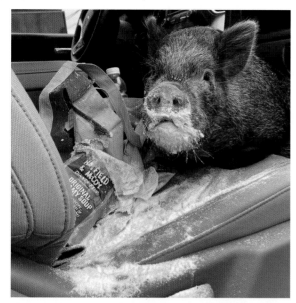

Fig. 3.1 Pet pigs often get into trouble when bored. A proper environment keeps the animal engaged and safely promotes natural behaviors such as rooting, nesting, and exploration. (Photo credit: Kelly Raines.)

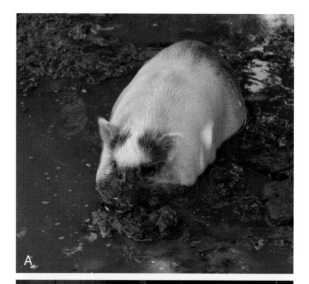

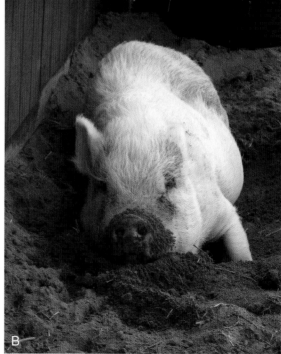

Fig. 3.2 Pigs cannot sweat and are sensitive to overheating at temperatures over 85°F (30°C). Behavioral cooling measures include (A) wallowing in mud—a wet mud coating can cool for several hours while clean water cooling is only temporary— (B) or rooting into cooler soil (A Photo credit: Brittany Sawyer.)

brief, but a wet mud coating can cool the animal for several hours (Signoret et al. 1975). Pigs will often dump a water source in order to create a mud wallow if one is not otherwise provided. Of course, pigs are susceptible to extremes of cold as well.

Pigs are highly social creatures and prefer the company of other pigs, assuming proper introduction, but may get along well with other species including cats or goats, sometimes equids. As a general rule, dogs and pigs should never be left together unsupervised. Donkeys and pigs are not ideal companions as both can be pig-headed and cause intentional injury to one another during spats. Horses, on the other hand, tend to fear pigs and can cause accidental injury due to their large size, and pigs' rooting holes in the pasture can cause injury to the horse as well.

Indoors

Indoor areas should provide adequate traction—carpet, gym or stall mats, or rubber-backed rugs should be provided in areas frequented by the pig. Surfaces such as linoleum, tile, or hardwood are not ideal as slipping can result in fearful behavior or lead to injury. Pigs are particularly prone to injury of the distal humerus during the first 3 or 4 years of life before the physes close, and incomplete ossification at this site may contribute to injury even in the absence of excessive force (Samii and Hornof 2000). Therefore, pet pigs should be discouraged from activity with great impact, such as jumping on and off furniture. Owners can provide pet steps or, better yet, a ramp if they feel the need to have their pet pig on the sofa or bed with them (Fig. 3.3). A ramp is also suggested for entering and exiting a vehicle.

Pigs are readily housebroken and can quickly learn to use a litterbox if the owner desires. Low-sided concrete mixing trays are one option and appropriate substrates include straw, pine shavings, paper pellets, shredded newspaper, or dirt. Pigs can also learn to alert the owner to the need to go outside or use a pet door to access the yard and will typically choose to potty outdoors if given the option (Tynes 2021) (Fig. 3.4).

The pig should be provided a sleeping area with appropriate bedding (see below) that allows them to engage in rooting and nesting behavior. A plastic airline kennel makes an excellent "pig den" and also allows easy confinement if/when transport is necessary (Fig. 3.5). Due to their often-intense nesting behavior—which occurs in both males and females—pet pigs allowed to freely roam the house will pick up anything they deem appropriate and carry the item to their bed including blankets, clothing, throw rugs, even toilet paper pulled from the roll. Pigs with outside access through a pet door may carry leaves and twigs into the house as well.

Outdoors

While there are no standardized guidelines for the exact amount of space required per pig (except by zoning ordinance based on who-knows-what), a size of 8 × 15 feet (2.4 × 4.6 m) per pig is considered the minimum, although ≥50 square feet (15 square meters) per pig is recommended (Froe 1993; Lawhorn 2013) and several factors should be considered: The area should be large enough to allow separate eating, sleeping, and toileting areas; there should be adequate space to root or graze; adequate shade is necessary since pigs are prone to sunburn and overheating; ideally, there should space to roam and explore. Some pigs are grazers while others will till the land if given

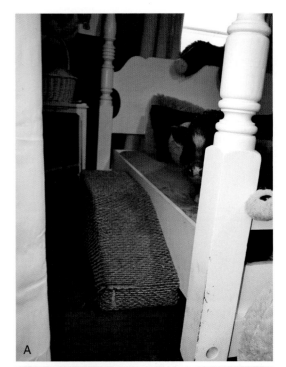

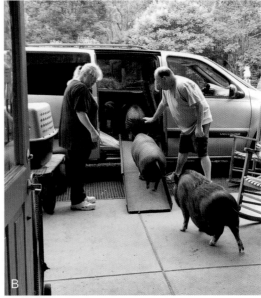

Fig. 3.3 (A) pet ramp or steps are recommended to prevent pigs from jumping to access a bed, sofa or vehicle. (B) Injury to the distal humerus is common prior to physis closure and potentially complicated by incomplete ossification, making the animals prone to injury at this site, even without excessive force.

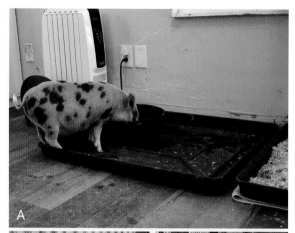

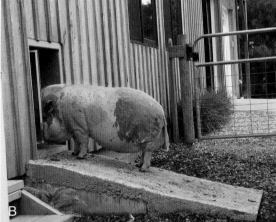

Fig. 3.4 Pet pigs are readily housebroken. (A) Large, low-sided trays can be filled with pine shavings and used as a litter box indoors, but most pigs given pet door access (B) prefer to potty outside if given the option.

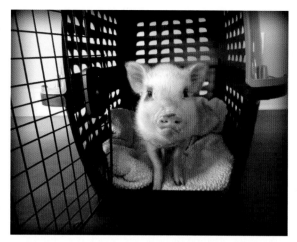

Fig. 3.5 One indoor housing option is to create a "pig den" using a solid plastic airline kennel—preferable to wire cages as pigs are prone to accidental hoof injuries in these. Providing rubber-backed mats or other traction, plus a few food treats, will encourage the pig to readily use the space, and such a kennel allows easy confinement if/when transport is necessary. (Photo credit: https://lifewithaminipig.com/meet-oscar/.)

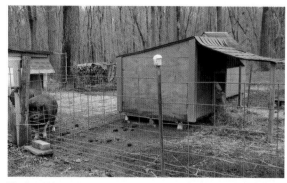

Fig. 3.6 This small straw-bedded wooden pig house features a raised floor, removable plastic weather strips at the entrance to reduce drafts in winter, and an overhang that allows the pig to exit to eat or potty during inclement weather. Hog panels are used to divide pig pens and feature separations that are closer together towards the bottom to discourage inquisitive snouts; the bottom portion of the panel can be buried to prevent pigs from rooting underneath. It should be noted that hog panels are useful for confining/separating pigs but are too short to discourage predators.

the opportunity. Owners must consider that a pig can easily destroy a yard. This will likely determine whether a pet is allowed free-range access or must be confined within a pig-friendly area that may be devoid of greenery, at best, and something resembling a cratered moonscape, at worst. The pig pen must be suitably fenced, as much to prevent predator access as to keep the pig confined. Hog panels are a relatively inexpensive option designed to keep pigs confined and feature separations that are closer together towards the bottom to discourage inquisitive snouts. However, these panels are only about 2.8 feet (0.85 m) tall which is inadequate to

discourage predators. Hog panels are best used to create a separate pen area(s) (Fig. 3.6) within an otherwise adequately fenced yard (i.e., chain link +/− electric wire at the top and bottom). Another use for hog panels is to create two or more separate grazing areas in which access is rotated to diminish destruction as each natural area can be allowed to recover between pig visits. Fencing may need to be partially buried in the ground to prevent pigs from rooting underneath.

HOUSING

Outdoor housing should provide adequate protection from the elements and should include a raised floor, low or ramped access, adequate ventilation but free from drafts, and dry bedding as appropriate for the weather (i.e., deep straw or hay in which the pig can completely bury itself in colder temperatures, pine shavings in warmer weather). The house should also be readily accessible for cleaning or if the pig is sick or injured and non-ambulatory. In addition to the main roof structure, a protective awning (Fig. 3.6) will encourage the pig to come out to eat or potty during inclement weather. With a deeply bedded, draft-free, dry house, preferably insulated in colder climates, pigs should be able to tolerate freezing temperatures without issue, especially if there are two or more pigs. If a supplemental heat source is needed, commercially available electric piglet heating pads may be preferable to heat lamps for safety reasons, although the pet should be monitored to be sure the cord isn't chewed or frayed and the pig at risk of electrocution. Another safe option is to fill heavy duty plastic containers (i.e., empty laundry detergent bottles) with hot water, wrap in towels, and place into the house; heat will slowly dissipate and can make the pig more comfortable for short bouts of frigid weather. Whatever the heat source, the area should allow room for the pig to move away if too warm.

BEDDING

A suitable bedding material should be provided for nesting as this is a basic behavior that should be encouraged and is observed in both sexes (Tynes 2021). If blankets are used, fleece may be the best option as it is most resistant to tearing; however, be forewarned that nothing is completely pig proof. Blankets should be checked frequently for tears and replaced when small pieces are at risk of accidental ingestion. Straw or hay are also suitable and pine shavings are common as well, although pigs often prefer to fully immerse themselves within bedding substrate if possible, or

at least bury the head (Fig. 3.7). Hay/straw should be changed frequently (i.e., monthly) as break down creates unhealthy levels of dust in the shelter; however, damp or wet bedding should be changed immediately. Do not, under any circumstances, use a down comforter. Trust me on this.

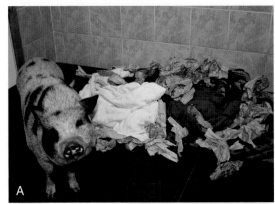

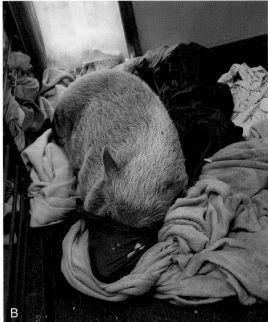

Fig. 3.7 Both male and female minipigs will nest, and suitable bedding should be provided to allow them to engage in this natural behavior. Fleece blankets are most resistant to tearing and adding plain brown paper on a regular basis can be a blanket-sparing option (A) as the pigs will preferentially rip and nest with the paper. Many pigs prefer to fully immerse themselves within bedding substrate, or at least cover the snout (B).

WATER

Drinking

Fresh water should be available at all times. Pigs often play in their water and frequently dump bowls for the fun of it or to cool off on a hot day. Finding a low-sided, non-tip water bowl that can withstand a pig snout is no easy feat, but options include a large weighted bowl with outward-sloping sides, a bowl anchored to a fence or other permanent structure, a bowl partially buried in the ground, or a livestock water trough with a low pan (Fig. 3.8). A bowl placed within the center of a tire is another creative option. Pigs that empty their water source on a hot day are at risk of salt toxicity if the situation is not quickly remedied. Owners should be forewarned that many pigs do not consume a lot of fluid outside of mealtimes. Water can be added to meals to encourage intake if there is concern, but this should never be in lieu of access to fresh water.

Cooling

In addition to shade or fans, water can be provided for cooling in hot weather. Pigs cannot sweat and rely on evaporative cooling to maintain body temperature (Signoret et al. 1975; Tynes 2021). A plastic child's wading pool (with bathtub decals added for traction and one side cut down for ease of access) is one option; there are also pools made specifically for pigs that feature heavy duty, non-slip vinyl and low, padded sides (Fig. 3.9). Providing a mud wallow (or better yet, allowing the pig to create one) is an excellent means of providing prolonged evaporative cooling as well as protection from the sun and insects. Note: Pigs that rinse off in clean water may be more susceptible to sunburn, so it is recommended that pools be placed in shaded areas.

ENRICHMENT

Pigs do not "play" in the way a dog or cat might but are intelligent animals that can get into trouble if not adequately engaged. Items that best maintain the interest of a pig are those that are "ingestible, odorous, chewable, deformable, and/or destructible" (Van de Weerd et al. 2003) as well as clean and, most importantly, novel (Grandin 1989). Enrichment generally involves food or exploration, although pleasurable

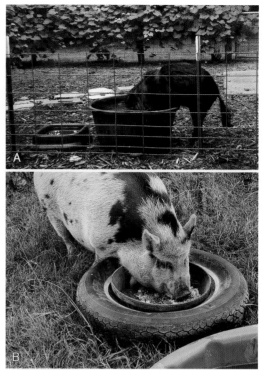

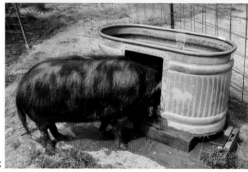

Fig. 3.8 Pigs are at risk of salt toxicity if deprived of water, usually due to tipping of bowls on a hot day. Options for waterers include (A) a weighted bowl with sloped sides to discourage tipping, (B) placement of a bowl within a tire to help anchor, (C) or use of a stock tank with a low pan (expensive and not available in all areas). Larger containers are less likely to be dumped out but may be too tall for the pig to easily access (A). (https://www.stockandfield.com/.)

interactions with humans (i.e., belly rubs, head or back scratch) are also a form of enrichment. Pig entertainment options include:

- Broadcast food pellets over a clean area to allow foraging behavior in order to consume meals.

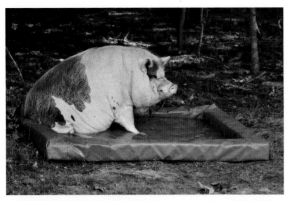

Fig. 3.9 Pools made specifically for pigs feature heavy duty, non-slip vinyl and low, padded sides and can be purchased at: http://gfxlizard.com/FinalPaHeartland/. While clean pool water allows for brief evaporative cooling, a wet coating of mud can cool for several hours; however, this may be objectionable to owners of indoor pets. Pigs that rinse in clean water are also especially susceptible to sunburn, so pools should be placed in a shaded area and sunscreen applied as needed. (Photo credit: Leanne Jones.)

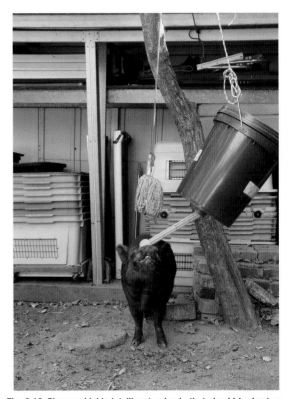

Fig. 3.10 Pigs are highly intelligent animals that should be kept engaged and preferred "toys" are those that can be manipulated, chewed, and of course, dispense food treats. This homemade treat dispenser is one option that meets piggy approval. A variety of other options can be found at: https://www.minipiginfo.com/mini-pig-enrichment.html. (Photo credit: Marcie Christensen.)

- For indoor pets, pellets can be sprinkled into/onto a "rooting box" or mat (Fig. 2.6). Commercially available mats can be purchased online, or owners can use a kiddie pool or other deep-sided container filled with large plastic balls, large river rocks, crumpled paper, and/or hay. Obviously, items small enough to pose a choking hazard should not be used nor should sand be used as unintentional ingestion is likely to occur.
- Offer snacks in a food-dispensing toy (Fig. 3.10) that requires manipulation, such as a Kong toy smeared with peanut butter or treats placed within a closed cardboard cereal box.
- Regularly provide novel or "renewed" (same item but fresh addition) nesting materials such as plain brown paper (Fig. 3.7A) or fresh straw as pigs enjoy tearing and/or maneuvering these items.
- Allow access to a novel area that has not been explored in the recent past such as a new area of the yard or a different room in the house.
- Hang knotted ropes or hay-dispensing objects where the pig can manipulate them, and rotate items used on occasion.
- Mount a nylon brush for rubbing/scratching.

- Leash train and take for walks (Fig. 3.11).
- See https://www.minipiginfo.com/mini-pig-enrichment.html (Sawyer 2020) for more enrichment ideas.

Nutrition

Miniature pigs are "easy keepers" to say the least. They are omnivores that will eat and thrive on anything but also gain excess weight easily. Owners frequently develop elaborate meal plans that involve fruit chopping, salad preparation, and cooking to the pig's preference. None of this is necessary but must be considered in formulating a diet plan if compliance is to be expected.

Although swine nutrition has been extensively studied and detailed guidelines published (National Research

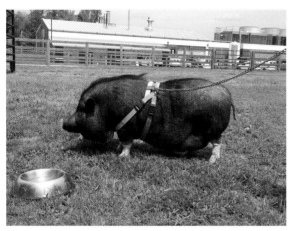

Fig. 3.11 Pig-specific harnesses feature a clip at both the neck and girth for ease of getting it on and off. Although training a prey animal to tolerate restraint takes patience, a pet pig will readily comply once it becomes evident that harness and lead indicate novel exploration activity.

Council 2012), these refer to commercial breeds fed ad libitum for rapid growth. While basic nutritional requirements are the same, data from studies in miniature pigs used in research can be more appropriately applied to the pet population. One major takeaway from these studies is that miniature pigs do not voluntarily limit feed intake based on energy requirements and that ad libitum feeding leads to obesity. It has been reported that 60% ad libitum intake is sufficient to prevent obesity, supply nutrients, and maintain health (Bollen et al. 2005); in other words, pigs will eat almost twice what they need if given the option. And this is why the pig is my spirit animal.

FEEDING GUIDELINES

What to Feed

A balanced commercial feed is recommended as it is easy to adjust the amount to achieve good body condition while meeting the dietary requirements of the animal. Pelleted forms are most common and are easier to digest than ground forms (Nahrwold 1993). In addition, non-pelleted feeds containing coarsely ground corn or seeds that pass intact in the feces may lead to coprophagy, which is otherwise uncommon. A number of miniature pig feeds are available online or through local farm supply stores and include Mazuri®, Manna Pro®, Nutrena®, and Champion in the US; all-purpose livestock feed or some equine feeds are also suitable, although all-purpose feeds tend to have unspecified, lower quality "by-product" ingredients. Protein content should ideally be about 12% to 14% for pigs over 5 months of age (16% to 20% for younger piglets), and while fat content of miniature pig formulations is typically 2% to 4%, anecdotal evidence from owners suggests that higher fat content helps improve naturally dry, flaky pig skin. Higher fat content is more commonly found in some equine feeds (i.e., senior) given to pet pigs, but a supplement added to any base diet can be used. Feed can be top-dressed with a food oil such as coconut, almond or flaxseed, or any product labeled for the canine and given at the same dosage (i.e., Welactin®) may suffice. Fiber content in adult feed should be at least 14% to provide satiety (Holtz 2010) and cereal grains like corn, wheat, or oats, as well as soybean meal or hulls, are usually the primary ingredients. Although pigs can subsist on feed formulated for farm hogs, it is not recommended for a number of reasons: these feeds are formulated for rapid gain and ad libitum feeding and, if the amount is restricted, nutrient concentrations may be insufficient (Helke et al. 2015); some contain antibiotics or additives to increase weight gain; there has also been at least one report of Vitamin D toxicity in potbellied pigs fed a commercial swine ration (Wimsatt et al. 1998), suggesting that macro and micro mineral composition of some hog feeds may be inappropriate for the pet population.

Miniature pig feeds are typically categorized as starter (aka creep feed or youth), grower (aka active adult), or maintenance rations, with decreasing protein and increasing fiber content as the pig matures. Starter rations might best be reserved for breeders as piglets adopted post-weaning (7 to 8+ weeks of age) can be immediately started on a grower or active adult ration. Maintenance rations can be started quite early, even immediately post-weaning, as most pets are neutered at a young age and many live sedentary lifestyles (Tynes 1999).

Roughage is also recommended and can be obtained through grazing or feeding greens; some pigs will also eat hay. This helps maintain a healthy GI tract and provides "fill," so the pig is satiated. For animals lacking natural grazing access, leafy greens or green vegetables are a good choice, but it has also been reported that resistant starches (i.e., uncooked oats, plantains or green/unripe bananas, beans, legumes) allow for better, prolonged satiety (Souza da Silva 2013) and, therefore, might make good snacks in small quantities (Box 3.1). Although pigs have been shown to demonstrate a preference for sugary foods (Signoret et al. 1975), these types of snacks add calories with short-lived contentment, just as they do in humans, and should be kept to a minimum. It is important to note that pet pigs can gain excessive weight on pasture so pelleted rations should be modified as needed. Forage items like fruits and, especially, acorns or other nuts easily lead to excessive weight gain and should be removed from the environment if causing an issue.

Dog and cat foods are inappropriate for pet pigs and can cause serious health issues such as salt toxicity (Holbrook and Barton 1994). Table scraps or junk food like potato chips can have a similar effect and should be avoided. And also remember that miniature pet pigs are still considered swine and subject to livestock feeding regulations, although these may be difficult to enforce in pet households. This means that it is illegal to feed items with meat or other mammalian by-products, which includes dog and cat food; even stricter rules may apply in some regions, forbidding table scraps of any kind.

Fresh water should be available at all times, although pigs tend to be prandial drinkers that (messily) consume most of their daily intake during meals (Ball 2012). Pigs also demonstrate a cool to tepid temperature preference, consuming less if water is too warm or cold (Tynes 1999). While water can be added to pelleted feed and may be necessary to slow rapid ingestion or prevent choking in some animals, this should not be in lieu of access to fresh water.

How Much to Feed

Pigs easily gain weight, and obesity has historically been a common health problem of this pet, so food must be carefully rationed. General maintenance ration guidelines (Box 3.2): Young piglet: ½ cup per 15 to 25 lb body weight per day; adult: 1 cup per 50 to 80 lb body weight/day (Boldrick 1993). Don't feed ad lib. A miniature pig should readily eat all feed provided. If food is left behind, the pig is being overfed or has a medical issue.

Label feeding instructions on most commercial miniature pig feeds are incorrect and will lead to obesity. Mazuri® Mini Pig Mature Maintenance 2021, for example, recommends as much as 9 cups (1300 g) per day for pigs over 150 lb with an additional ½ cup for each 10 lb of body weight over 150 lb. This is a massive amount of food! Most feeding guidelines suggest anywhere from 1% to 3% body weight per day (Holtz 2010; Manna Pro® 2021 product label; Nahrwold 1993; Nutrena® 2021 product label) which can still be somewhat high and lead to excessive gain. Although livestock are often fed on a percent body weight basis, this assumes the ability to measure (or at least accurately estimate) body weight, and pet pig owners may be confused by the concept and calculations. I prefer to specify a measurable amount that is familiar to the owner, and 2 cups (400 g) total per day for a healthy average-sized adult pig (80 to 160 lb; 36 to 73 kgs) in good body condition is a general rule of thumb.

While feeding to an appropriate body condition is necessary with all pets, this concept may require further explanation as many pet pig owners wrongly believe that pigs are naturally fat and will purposely feed

BOX 3.1 HEALTHY SNACK OPTIONS FOR POTBELLIED PIGS

While a commercially available miniature pig feed is recommended as a base diet, the following are healthy snacks that can provide better satiety, especially if given multiple times throughout the day which more closely approximates natural feeding behavior. Caloric content must still be considered in determination of amount (i.e., lettuces can be given in abundance while starchy foods should be fed in smaller quantities).

- Grazing
- Leafy greens
- Green vegetables such as cucumbers or green beans
- Frozen peas
- Beans
- Green/unripe bananas or plantains (yellow bananas are high in sugar)
- Uncooked oats

BOX 3.2 HOW MUCH TO FEED A MINIPIG

General guidelines for maintenance feeding of commercial miniature pig feeds:

- Young piglet: ½ cup per 15–25 lb (7–11 kg) body weight per day
- Adult: 1 cup per 50–80 lb (23–36 kg) body weight/day

to achieve an obese body condition. Body condition/weight check may be needed at least twice a year, more often if weight gain or loss is intended, to keep the pig on track for weight goals. Adjustments to the diet may be needed seasonally (i.e., increased amount with cold weather) or with other mitigating factors such as illness, advancing age, or lactation. Additionally, as dominance may influence access to feed, separate feeding areas may be necessary for multi-pig households if appropriate body condition cannot be maintained in a group setting. Pigs fed together will frequently switch bowls as well as move back and forth between food and water bowls. This is normal and acceptable as long as all pigs maintain an appropriate weight.

Pregnancy and Lactation. While pregnant females can be fed normal maintenance rations, energy requirements increase during lactation. One general recommendation is to increase from 1 cup twice daily (BID) maintenance to 1.5 cups BID a few days after farrowing and continuing to slowly increase; dividing total feed into 3 to 4+ meals provides better fill and greater contentment, especially as larger quantities may make the sow feel bloated and uncomfortable. Litter size helps determine the total feed increase needed and is roughly ½ additional cup per piglet per day within the first 2 weeks and continuing for 6 weeks post-farrowing (Magidson, personal communication). A highly digestible starter ration can be provided to the piglets at around 10 days of age and should be placed such that piglets can access but not the sow (creep feeding). Piglets may find a softened mush easier to ingest initially and should be eating well by 4 to 5 weeks of age; food should be provided fresh and only in a quantity that the piglets will consume per feeding (Nahrwold 1993). Fresh water should also be provided for piglets, and the sow will drink a tremendous amount of water as well (1 gallon/sow/day is a good rule of thumb for average intake and increases to as much as 6 gallons/day with lactation [Brumm 2006]). When weaning is desired at 6 to 8 weeks post-farrowing, the sow should be removed from the piglets and reduced to maintenance rations (Burlatschenko and Magidson, personal communication).

As a general rule, piglets should gain approximately 1 lb/week for the first year of life (Magidson, personal communication) and attain about half their adult weight by 1 year of age (Wilbers 2013).

How Often to Feed

Pigs are natural foragers and, in the wild, spend a good part of the day procuring food (Tynes 2021). Even domestic pigs on pasture spend as much as 6 to 7 hours daily seeking and eating food (Signoret et al. 1975). However, this is impractical in most pet households and twice daily feeding is most common. One enrichment suggestion that allows the pig to engage in natural foraging behavior is to give at least a portion of each meal scattered over the ground or in a food-dispensing toy. My personal pigs get about half of their feed mixed with water in a bowl and the other half broadcast across the yard. Each meal takes at least 30 minutes and the hope of finding a missed pellet often provokes foraging behavior outside of mealtimes. Commercially available rooting mats for indoor use can be purchased online, or owners can fill a plastic kiddie pool with large river rocks or plastic balls and sprinkle food among them (Fig. 2.6).

BODY CONDITION SCORE

Body condition scoring for pigs is based on the 5-point scale used in commercial swine (Ramirez and Karriker 2019) (Box 3.3). A score of 1 is emaciated, 5 obese, and 3 or slightly under ideal. However, these standards lean towards rounder, fuller builds in meat-producing animals, while the less muscular build of a miniature pig should aim for a not-quite-so-rounded, more angular condition (Wilbers 2005). As conformation varies, feeding to a certain body condition frequently proves to be a difficult concept for owners to grasp. In addition, the public perception of the pig lends to overfeeding to achieve obesity. Even the most well-researched owners may believe a body condition score of 4 or 5 to be the goal for a healthy pig. This is

BOX 3.3 POTBELLIED PIG BODY CONDITION SCORING

> Minipig body condition score is based on the 5-point scale used in commercial swine, with 3 or slightly under considered ideal. Both written and pictorial descriptions of minipig body condition scores can be found at the following link: https://www.minipiginfo.com/mini-pig-body-scoring.html

a well-seated misconception and care must be taken to explain the features of the minipig at a healthy weight.

Ideal Body Condition

At an ideal weight (Fig. 3.12A), the pig's eyes should be visible. Some conformations have deep-set eyes that may not be as readily visible, but the eyes should never be fully obscured. In most breeds, the ears should be erect. Small jowls cover the jawline should lead cleanly into a distinct neck. Ribs should be palpable but not visible; hips should be well rounded but palpable with firm pressure, and the iliac crest barely visible from the topline. In other words, there should be a visible waist looking down at the top of the pig, not a rectangular shape or, even worse, an oval. The base of the tail should not be folded into the flesh. The belly should not drag the ground.

Underweight

A skinny pig (Fig. 3.12B) is similar to any other species and may appear gaunt in the face with sunken eyes and a prominent jawline, ribs and/or spine may be

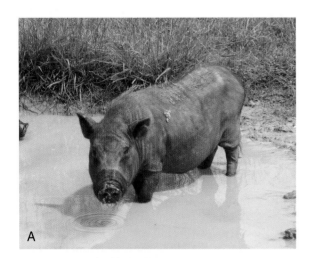

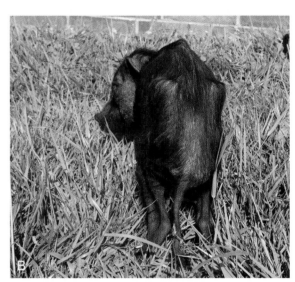

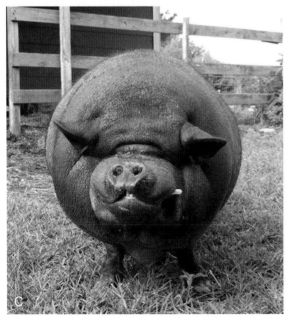

Fig. 3.12 Body condition score (BCS) in pigs is based on a 5-point scale. (A) At an ideal condition of 3 or slightly under, the eyes are visible (even if deep-set), ears are upright, jowls are without excessive folds, and the hip points are just visible. (B) With an emaciated BCS of 1, the spine and hips are readily visible (or palpable if hidden by hair), the jawline is prominent, and the animal may exhibit a hunched posture, drooping ears, and dull eyes. (C) At an obese BCS of 5, subcutaneous fat deposition may completely obscure the eyes and push the ears into a horizontal position rendering the pig "fat blind/deaf".

visible or easily palpable if covered by hair, hip bones are prominent. In severe cases, the animal may exhibit a hunched posture, with the hind limbs tucked under the body. They may be dull eyed and slow moving with generalized piloerection and dull, coarse hair.

Feeding an Emaciated Pig. As with any other species, food must be carefully introduced to a starving pig to prevent "refeeding syndrome"—a condition recognized in humans and other species that can cause gastrointestinal issues such as diarrhea, vomiting, or loss of appetite as well as severe metabolic disturbances that can lead to death (Cook et al. 2021; Khoo et al. 2019). Based on guidelines reported for human patients (Reber et al. 2019), small, frequent meals of quality feed given at about ⅓ maintenance ration together with water and electrolytes +/− vitamin and trace mineral supplementation is a good start that might best allow the animal to metabolically adjust. More severe cases may require hospitalization.

Overweight

Pigs are capable of gaining weight to the point that subcutaneous fat accumulation pushes the normally upright ears lateral and forward, effectively blocking transmission of sound into the ear canal and rendering the pig hearing impaired (Fig. 3.12C). Facial fat folds can literally obscure the eyes such that the globe cannot be physically accessed; as pigs compensate well with other senses, owners may be unaware that their pet has become mechanically blind. The face may be rotund with deep crevices on the forehead and/or pendulous jowls bearing multiple folds; the belly is also pendulous and may drag the ground in extreme obesity. The tailhead is buried in dimpled folds of skin.

Dieting the Obese Pig. As with any species, it is far easier to prevent weight gain than it is to diet an obese animal. The metabolism of the pig seems to slow significantly in obesity, and weight loss may require marked reduction in feed in addition to controlled exercise. At Ross Mill Farm & Piggy Camp just outside of Philadelphia, PA, USA, there is a program in which obese animals board for the recommended year to be placed on a strict diet prior to return home. Feed is often reduced to as little as ¼ cup twice a day, a quarter of maintenance ration; an exercise regimen

complements the diet. In this manner, a markedly obese animal that can barely maintain sternal recumbency and walks only a few steps before resting can eventually achieve an acceptable body condition. This weight loss program has been highly successful for many years and there seem to be no medical issues with such severe feed restriction. Alternatively, a less intense restrictive diet can be formulated, with weight loss occurring over a longer period.

BIBLIOGRAPHY

Ball RS Husbandry and management. In: McAnulty PA, Dayan AD, Ganderup N, Hastings K, eds. *The Minipig in Biomedical Research.* Boca Raton, FL: CRC Press; 2012:24–26.

Boldrick L. Nutrition. In: *Veterinary Care of Pot-Bellied Pet Pigs.* Orange, CA: All Publishing Company; 1993:33–39.

Bollen JA, Hansen AK, Rasmussen HJ. Husbandry. In: *The Laboratory Swine.* Boca Raton, FL: CRC Press LLC; 2000:17–29.

Bollen PJA, Madsen LW, Meyer O, Ritskes-Hoitinga J. Growth differences of male and female Göttingen minipigs during ad libitum feeding: a pilot study. *Lab Anim.* 2005;39(1):80–93.

Brumm M. Patterns of drinking water use in pork production facilities. *Nebraska Swine Rep.* 2006:10–13. https://digitalcommons.unl.edu/coopext_swine/221. Accessed February 18, 2021.

Burlatschenko S. *Personal Communication.*

Cook S, Whitby E, Elias N, et al. Retrospective evaluation of refeeding syndrome in cats: 11 cases (2013–2019). *J Feline Med Surg.* 2021:1–9.

Froe DL II. Environment and housing of miniature pet pigs. In: Reeves DE, ed. *Care and Management of Miniature Pet Pigs.* Santa Barbara, CA: Brillig Hill, Inc.; 1993:13–19.

Grandin T. *Effect of Rearing Environment and Environmental Enrichment on Behavior and Neural Development in Young Pigs.* 1989. http://hdl.handle.net/2142/21967. Accessed February 18, 2021.

Helke KL, Ezell PC, Duran-Struuck R, Swindle MM. Biology and diseases of swine. In: Fox JG, Anderson LC, Otto GM, et al., eds. *Lab Animal Medicine.* 3rd ed. San Diego, CA: Elsevier, Inc.; 2015:700.

Holbrook TC, Barton MH. Neurologic dysfunction associated with hypernatremia and dietary indiscretion in Vietnamese pot bellied pigs. *Cornell Vet.* 1994;84(1):67–76.

Holtz W. Pigs and minipigs. In: Hubrecht R, Kirkwood J, eds. *The UFAW Handbook on the Care and Management of Laboratory and Other Research Animals.* 8th ed. Ames, IA: Universities Federation for Animal Welfare; 2010:484.

Jackson PGG, Cockcroft PD. *The pet pig. Handbook of Pig Medicine.* Philadelphia, PA: Elsevier Limited; 2007:212–219.

Khoo AWS, Taylor SM, Owens TJ. Successful management and recovery following severe prolonged starvation in a dog. *J Vet Emerg Crit Care (San Antonio).* 2019;29(5):542–548.

Lawhorn B. *Management of Potbellied Pigs & Feeding and Nutrition of Potbellied Pigs.* Merck Veterinary Manual; Revised June 2013. https://www.merckvetmanual.com/exotic-and-laboratory-animals/potbellied-pigs/management-of-potbellied-pigs. Accessed February 18, 2021.

Magidson S. *Feeding Guidelines.* Ross Mill Farm; Published May 20, 2020. https://rossmillfarm.com/2020/05/feeding-guidelines/. Accessed February 18, 2021.

Magidson S. *Personal Communication.*

MannaPro®. *Potbellied Pig Feed Product Facts.* https://www.mannapro.com/cattle-swine-other/feed/potbellied-pig-feed. Accessed February 18, 2021.

Mazuri® *Mini Pig Mature Maintenance Product Sheet.* 2021. https://pims.purinamills.com/BusinessLink/media/Mazuri/ProductSheet/5Z4C.pdf?ext=.pdf. Accessed October 3, 2021.

Nahrwold DF. Nutrition in miniature pet pigs. In: Reeves DE, ed. *Guidelines for the Veterinary Practitioner: Care and Management of Miniature Pet Pigs.* Santa Barbara, CA: Brillig Hill, Inc.; 1993: 21–26.

National Research Council. *Nutrient Requirements of Swine.* 11th rev. ed. Washington, DC: National Academies Press; 2012.

Nutrena® Country Feeds Mini Pig Feed. 2021. https://www.nutrenaworld.com/product/country-feeds-mini-pig-feed. Accessed February 18, 2021.

Raleigh, NC Code of Ordinances, Sec. 12-3004.—Definitions, domesticated animal. Municode. 2021. https://library.municode.com/nc/raleigh/codes/code_of_ordinances?nodeId=DIVIICOGEOR_PT12LIRE_CH3AN_ARTAGEPR_S12-3004DE. Accessed October 2, 2021.

Ramirez A, Karriker L. Herd evaluation. In: Zimmeran JJ, Karriker LA, Ramirez A, et al., eds. *Diseases of Swine.* 11th ed. Hoboken, NJ: John Wiley & Sons, Inc.; 2019:8–9.

Reber E, Friedli N, Vasiloglou MF, et al. Management of refeeding ayndrome in medical inpatients. *J Clin Med.* 2019;8(12):2202.

Samii VF, Hornof WJ. Incomplete ossification of the humeral condyle in Vietnamese pot-bellied pigs. *Vet Radiol Ultrasound.* 2000;41(2):147–153.

Sawyer B. *Are You Zoned for a Pig?* Mini Pig Info. 2015 https://www.minipiginfo.com/mini-pig-zoning-ordinances.html. Accessed February 18, 2021.

Sawyer B. *Minipig Enrichment: Activities for Your Pig.* Mini Pig Info. 2020 https://www.minipiginfo.com/mini-pig-enrichment.html. Accessed February 18, 2021.

Seattle, WA Municipal Codes, 23.42.052—Keeping of Animals. Municode. 2021. https://library.municode.com/wa/seattle/codes/municipal_code?nodeId=TIT23LAUSCO_SUBTITLE_IIILAUSRE_CH23.42GEUSPR_23.42.052KEAN. Accessed October 2, 2021.

Signoret JP, Baldwin BA, Fraser D, Hafez ESE. The behaviour of swine. In: Hafez ESE, ed. *Behaviour of Domestic Animals.* London: Baillière Tindall; 1975:295–329.

Sipos W, Schmoll F, Stumpf I. Minipigs and potbellied pigs as pets in the veterinary practice—a retrospective study. *J Vet Med A Physiol Pathol Clin Med.* 2007;54(9):504–511.

Souza da Silva C. *Fermentation in the Gut to Prolong Satiety: Exploring Mechanisms by Which Dietary Fibres Affect Satiety in Pigs* [PhD thesis]. Wageningen, NL: Wageningen University; 2013.

Tynes VV. Miniature pet pig behavioral medicine. *Vet Clin North Am Exot Anim Pract.* 2021;24(1):63–86.

Tynes VV. Potbellied pig husbandry and nutrition. *Vet Clin North Am Exot Anim Pract.* 1999;2(1):193–208.

Van de Weerd HA, Docking CM, Day JEL, et al. A systematic approach towards developing environmental enrichment for pigs. *Appl Anim Behav Sci.* 2003;84(2):101–118.

Wilbers AM. Handling pet pigs as patients. In: *NAVC Conference Proceedings.* 2013. https://www.vetfolio.com/learn/article/handling-pet-pigs-as-patients. Accessed February 18, 2021.

Wilbers AM. Obesity, structure and body score. 7th Annual Potbellied Pig Symposium; 2005; Knoxville, TN.

Wimsatt J, Marks SL, Campbell TW, et al. Dietary vitamin D toxicity in a household of pot-bellied pigs (Sus scrofa). *J Vet Intern Med.* 1998;12(1):42–44.

Chapter 4

Reproduction

Dr. Suzanne Burlatschenko

Overview of the Female Reproductive System

The miniature pet pig attains sexual maturity earlier than domestic swine, with the female attaining puberty between 3 and 6 months of age. Estrus (aka heat) cycles occur every 21 days in minipigs, as in domestic swine, and pigs will reproduce at all times of the year. Reddening and swelling of the vulva can be observed at the beginning of estrus (Fig. 4.1), followed by behavioral changes such as restlessness; a sticky mucoid discharge may be observed. Note: Bloody discharge is abnormal, but owners often fail to report a problem as they interpret the "piggy period" as normal. A pig in heat may become more vocal and may attempt to mount or nip, and these estrus behaviors can be misinterpreted as aggression but are cyclic in nature. During ovulation the pig will "lock up" (stand stiffly) if hand pressure is placed on the back. Some females may urinate more frequently and in different areas outside of the litterbox—a behavior designed to attract a boar and commonly mistaken for urinary tract infection. Estrus signs typically last 2 to 3 days. Most owners will elect to have their female pig spayed as estrus behaviors may become quite annoying and particularly unacceptable, with temporary loss of housebreaking in indoor pets.

The reproductive tract type of the female pig is a bicornuate uterus, and all parts but the uterine body are very long (Fig. 4.2). Ovaries appear "cystic," but this is normal follicular development; a large thin-walled bursa covers each ovary, and the fallopian tubes are long and coiled in the caudal abdomen. Uterine horns are extremely long and may resemble intestine but palpate more firmly

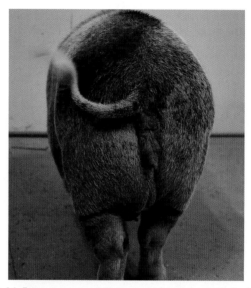

Fig. 4.1 Estrus occurs every 21 days in miniature pigs and lasts about 2 to 3 days, with reddening and swelling of the vulva commonly observed (pictured), with or without a sticky mucoid discharge. Estrus behaviors, including mounting, nipping, and most importantly, urine marking, often prompt owners to pursue spay.

and exhibit faint longitudinal striations. The broad ligament is fan-shaped and highly vascular, becoming increasingly thickened with fibrous connective tissue as the pig ages (Fig. 4.3). The cervix is thick, elongated, and interdigitating. Miniature pigs have 6 to 8 pairs of teats.

Defects of the female genital system are not uncommon in commercial swine, although they are uncommonly reported in the pet population. They include duplication of the vagina, cervix, and uterine horns; aplasia of the uterus, cervix, vagina, and vulva; and intersexuality. True intersexes (known as hermaphrodites) have both ovarian and testicular tissue.

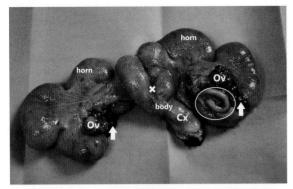

Fig. 4.2 The female minipig reproductive tract consists of cystic-appearing ovaries *(Ov)* covered by a thin red bursa *(arrows)*, long oviducts *(circled)*, long uterine horns, long cervix (Cx; only proximal tip pictured), and short uterine body. "X" marks the uterine bifurcation.

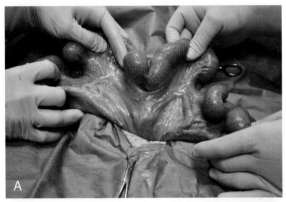

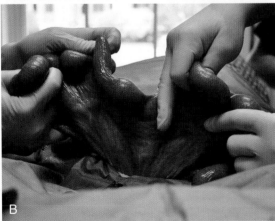

Fig. 4.3 A female ages, the broad ligament becomes increasingly fibrous, masking the large blood vessels throughout (A). Backlighting allows better visualization during spay surgery, illuminating any thin connective tissue regions that lack large blood vessels (B).

Pseudohermaphrodites will usually present with the external genitalia of the female but have the internal genital organs of the opposite sex (Kirkwood et al. 2012).

Female miniature pigs are uniquely prone to complications of the reproductive tract, if the tract is left intact and the animal is never bred. Unspayed female pigs develop cystic endometrial hyperplasia (CEH), leiomyomas or leiomyosarcomas, and, less frequently, pyometra; abnormalities are very common in aging, nulliparous animals, with pathologic changes starting as young as 5 years of age (Ilha et al. 2010; Mozzachio et al. 2004) (Fig. 4.4). Pigs with uterine tumors may present with abdominal distention (Fig. 4.5), discomfort, or vaginal bleeding, although many animals exhibit no clinical signs. Anorexia may or may not be present but is more likely in advanced disease (Mozzachio et al. 2004). Diagnosis is facilitated by ultrasound or other imaging, and treatment is removal of the reproductive tract. Early ovariohysterectomy is, therefore, indicated in the miniature pig. Ovariectomy is not recommended as there are multiple reports of neoplasia in the uterus of aged females many years post-spay (Fig. 4.6). Uterine adenocarcinoma is most common in these animals, and although metastasis is rare, treatment involves a second surgery to remove the remainder of the reproductive tract. Incidence is unknown.

GESTATION AND FARROWING

Gestation length ranges from 113 to 115 days. Placentation is of the epitheliochorial type, which is similar to that of humans (Swindle 2016). Piglets that are born earlier than 110 days mostly succumb to respiratory distress syndrome from decreased compliance and residual lung capacity (Caminita et al. 2015).

The mammary glands will become engorged before giving birth (known as farrowing); about 48 hours prior to parturition there may be a serous secretion, changing to a milky secretion within 24 hours of farrowing. Prior to farrowing, the female will become restless and begin nesting. Feed intake will drop. Some pigs may shiver as contractions are occurring. Piglets are born singly at approximately 15- to 30-minute intervals, with the farrowing occurring over a total of 3 to 4 hours on average (Helke et al. 2015). Placental expulsion signals the end of the farrowing process.

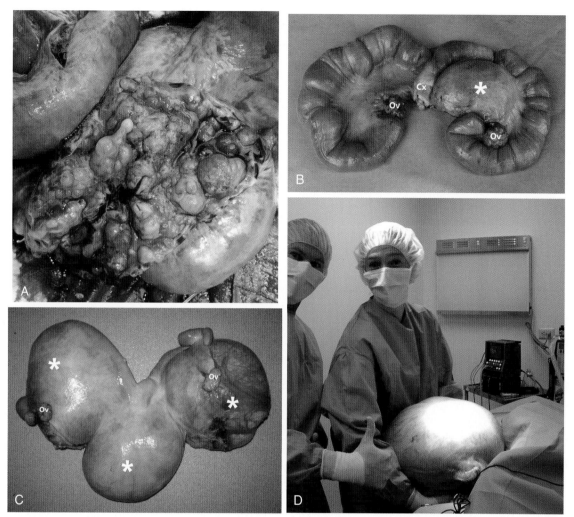

Fig. 4.4 Uterine pathology is extremely common in nulliparous pigs, and many animals exhibit abnormalities by about 6 to 7 years of age. (A) Cystic endometrial hyperplasia is the most common abnormality comprised of numerous cysts along the mucosal surface. (B) Focal uterine leiomyoma in the broad ligament of a 6-year-old pig (*). (C) 3 discrete leiomyomas (*) in a 16-year-old pig. (D) A 50 lb (23 kg) uterine leiomyoma in a 10-year-old pig. *Ov*, ovary; *Cx*, cervix.

Miniature pigs have an average of 6 to 8 piglets in a litter (range 1 to 15). Piglets are born precocious and will find their way to the mammary glands shortly after birth (Fig. 4.7).

A nesting box and pen should be prepared ahead of time for the sow and piglets. The dimensions of the pen will depend on the size of the pig and should include a box for the piglets with a low barrier that keeps piglets inside but allows the sow to enter and exit easily. A heat lamp should be hung in the box to provide warmth, as piglets do not thermoregulate for several days. They have no brown fat from which to metabolize for heat production and rely on shivering for thermogenesis (Herpin et al. 2002).

The newborn piglet requires an environmental temperature of about 90°F (32°C) to maintain body

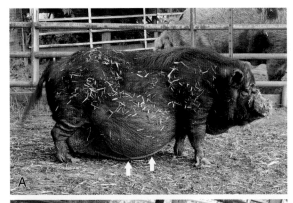

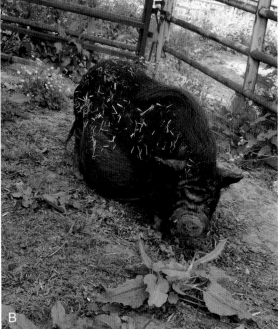

Fig. 4.5 Abdominal distension (A) may be observed in females with uterine neoplasia but can be difficult to interpret as a potbellied appearance is typical. However, engorgement of the subcutaneous abdominal vein *(arrows)* is common with abdominal pathology, though not specific for uterine tumor(s). Viewed from a different angle (B), the mass-like distension of the abdomen is more apparent.

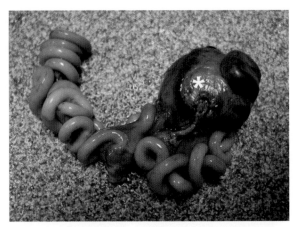

Fig. 4.6 Ovariohysterectomy is recommended over ovariectomy as there are multiple reports of neoplasia in the uterus of aged females many years post-spay. This uterine adenocarcinoma (*) was identified in the atrophied uterus of a 14-year-old pig that had been ovariectomized at 6 months of age; the pig initially presented for an episode of intense vaginal bleeding.

temperature. A box deeply bedded with coarse shavings or straw, along with a heat lamp, will suffice. Note: Care should be taken if using straw as sleeping piglets may become buried, prone to crushing if the sow is unaware of their presence (Magidson, personal communication). Care should also be taken so that the sow does not have access to the heat lamp. The lamp should be hung high enough so that the sow is not overheated or burnt if she nurses underneath it. Placement of the box away from drafts is important, especially if one is used in a barn environment. A sample farrowing box is seen in Fig. 4.8. Note the rails on the sides of the box—they help to prevent the sow from crushing the piglets when they are very young.

Piglets weigh approximately 1 lb (0.5 kg) at birth and should gain approximately 1 lb/week for the first year of life (Magidson, personal communication). They are typically born with a domed head, which is a normal appearance.

Miniature piglets do not require supplemental iron after birth, unlike domestic swine (Amalraj et al. 2018) as they usually have access to the outdoors and will acquire iron naturally through foraging in dirt and eating plants. Other domestic swine procedures, such as needle teeth clipping or tail docking, are not typically performed. Given the very different conditions under which miniature pet pigs are raised, problems such as inter-piglet fighting or tail biting are not typically observed, rendering these procedures unnecessary.

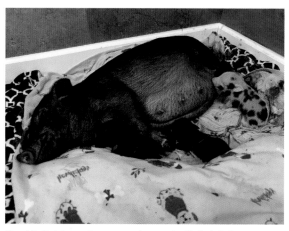

Fig. 4.7 Piglets are born precocious and will find their way to the mammary glands shortly after birth. Note the deeply bedded farrowing box with sides just high enough to keep piglets confined but allow the sow to enter and exit. (Photo credit: Blind Spot Animal Sanctuary.)

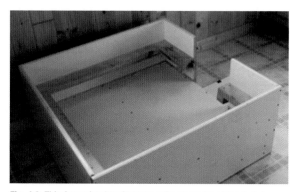

Fig. 4.8 This farrowing box features rails along the sides to help prevent the sow from crushing young piglets. The box should be deeply bedded with blankets, straw or shavings and placed in a draft-free area; a heat lamp may be needed for warmth as piglets are unable to thermoregulate for several days. (Photo credit: Dr. Suzanne Burlatschenko.)

Most miniature pigs are weaned around 6 to 8 weeks of age. Supplemental feed may be supplied to the piglets in the form of creep feed (aka starter or youth), which is a dense, highly digestible feed designed to introduce the piglets to solid food. This can be introduced when the piglets are about 10 days old and should be supplied in an area that the sow cannot access. Fresh water should be in plentiful supply for the lactating sow, and the piglets

should also have easy access to water, especially when they begin eating prepared feed. For specific feeding guidelines for lactating sows and piglets, see Chapter 3.

Dystocia

Most miniature pigs will farrow without assistance, but occasionally a piglet may become lodged (Fig. 4.9). Indicators are a restless sow, contractions with no progress, an extended interval from the birth of the last pig, and placental tissue not being passed. Due to the overall small size of the pig, it is very difficult to manually assist births as is done in large domestic swine. If there is concern regarding a lodged piglet, an ultrasound will confirm the presence of a piglet and its relative location. Ultrasound is preferred to avoid stressful transport if portable radiography is unavailable. However, if C-section is considered likely, the sow may require transport if the surgery will not be performed in the field.

Occasionally, a sow may tire during the birthing process and contractions may cease. If an extended period of time has passed between piglets with no progress, oxytocin (5 to 10 U) may be administered intramuscularly (IM) to aid delivery—assuming verification that the vaginal canal is patent (i.e., no piglets have become lodged). As this is a powerful hormone, giving more will not elicit a larger effect. Oxytocin should never be administered if no pigs have been born as the cervix may not be fully dilated and there is a serious risk of uterine rupture.

If there is a pause in farrowing, gently coaxing the sow to get up and move around may assist with movement of piglets through the uterus. The pig may urinate and/or defecate, which will provide some relief.

If the sow has been experiencing contractions for 3 to 4 hours with no progress, a C-section may be indicated. In this author's experience, a C-section is rarely necessary in miniature pet pigs. It is most commonly indicated in females bred at a very young age, before reaching adult size. C-section can be performed via different approaches including abdominal midline, but the right flank (parallel and just dorsal to the mammary gland and cranial to the inguinal canal) has the advantage of allowing the piglets to

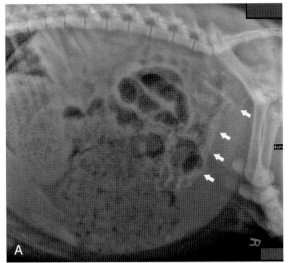

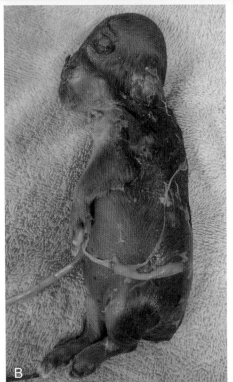

Fig. 4.9 Dystocia occurs occasionally in miniature pigs, especially in females bred at a very young age. This female was unintentionally bred by her littermate at 6 months of age, and after passing a single deformed fetus, the second fetus became lodged at the pelvis (A; arrows). Following surgical removal, the second fetus was also noted to be malformed (B).

nurse with less risk of dehiscence (Braun 1993; Lawhorn 2013).

Maternal Hysteria

Agitation and maternal aggression are not uncommon in swine giving birth. The miniature pig sow should be approached cautiously when she is entering the farrowing process. Pigs may charge at the owner or attempt to bite before, during, and after farrowing; the use of a board between the person and the pig is useful to avoid injury on both sides. It is best to give the sow quiet and privacy as overstimulation can upset the animal and produce or exacerbate these negative behaviors.

Maternal hysteria occurs mainly in animals farrowing for the first time. Aggression/hysteria may include snapping at piglets or even savaging the piglets. If unsure of the pig's attitude, piglets may be temporarily placed in a box with bedding and a heat lamp or other source of warmth (hot water bottle) until the sow appears to be resting comfortably.

Maternal aggression is also distressful to owners. It is usually managed by administration of azaperone (Stresnil) at the rate of 1 mg/lb (2.2 mg/kg) given IM. Most sows will settle within a short period of time and continue farrowing. If farrowing is complete, as evidenced by passage of placental tissue, then the piglets can be put back on the pig once she has shown signs of sedation. The sow will then usually allow the piglets to nurse. If azaperone is unavailable, acepromazine may be used at 0.05 to 0.1 mg/kg IM. Acepromazine is less effective than azaperone, however, the latter is unavailable in the United States.

Congenital Anomalies

Anomalies at birth are periodically seen in swine and may include inguinal hernias, umbilical hernias, cryptorchidism, atresia ani, cleft palate, polydactyly, or syndactyly (Fig. 4.10). Cardiac defects, the most common of which is the ventricular septal defect, are occasionally observed and can result in heart murmur, poor growth, exercise intolerance, and early death; however, depending on severity, the piglet may "outgrow" the problem. These conditions have a heritable component. That being said, umbilical hernias are also seen with navel abscessation and subsequent failure

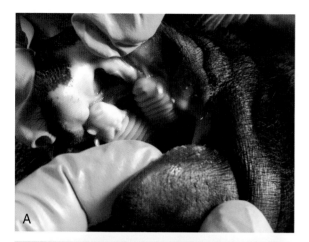

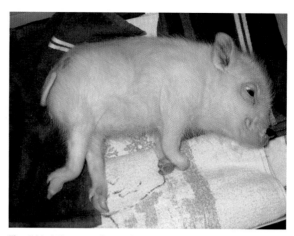

Fig. 4.11 Arthrogryposis may be caused by exposure to toxic plants, such as tobacco stalks or jimsonweed. (Photo credit: Gary Peterson.)

OVARIOHYSTERECTOMY

Spaying the miniature pig is a relatively straightforward surgery in the younger female, with a notable difference being that the horns coil in the caudal abdomen near the uterine body necessitating a caudal midline approach (i.e., as for cystotomy). Spay may be performed as early as 6 to 8 weeks of age. Older females may present greater difficulty as many have a large amount of fat, and those in estrus are best postponed as vasculature is even more prominent than usual. Ovariectomy is not recommended as older pigs may present with uterine pathology that requires a second spay procedure (Fig. 4.6). Surgical details and anesthetic protocols are discussed in separate chapters (see Chapters 8 & 9).

PREGNANCY TERMINATION

Given the overwhelming number of owner-surrendered pet pigs and continued emergence of hoarding cases with animals numbering into the hundreds, pregnancy termination may be requested to prevent more births. To induce estrus or terminate pregnancy, dinoprost tromethamine (Lutalyse®), a synthetic prostaglandin F2α, can be given as two injections (8 and 5 mg in a 25-kg pig) 12 hours apart (Lawhorn 2013). The corpora lutea (CL) required to maintain pregnancy are susceptible after Day 16 of gestation through term, as the CL is essential for the entire gestation period in

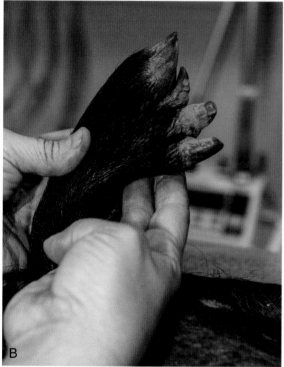

Fig. 4.10 Cleft palate (A) and polydactyly (B) are congenital defects; inguinal and umbilical hernias, atresia ani, and cryptorchidism have also been identified. (Photo credit [B]: Jennifer L. Davis.)

of the closure of the abdominal wall. Other conditions such as arthrogryposis (Fig. 4.11) may be caused by exposure to toxic plants, such as tobacco stalks or jimsonweed (Ramirez 2012).

swine (Schlafer and Foster 2016). Estrus should occur 3 to 7 days post-injection. After pregnancy termination and recovery, it is recommended that the animal be spayed in order to prevent future pregnancies.

Overview of the Male Reproductive System

The male miniature pig can reach puberty as early as 2 months of age, and male and female littermates (and sow) should be separated prior to this time to prevent unwanted pregnancy. Physical features of the intact male that become increasingly obvious with age are long wiry facial hair, thick tail tassel, dense fibrous shoulder plates, and thickening (hyperkeratosis) of the scrotum (Fig. 4.12). Male behavior traits are influenced by sexual maturity and include excessive salivation, lip-smacking, and "huffing" vocalizations, as well as "kneading" the ground with the forelimbs. Other traits such as territorial marking with urine, sexual behaviors such as mounting (Fig. 4.13) and repeated ejaculation, and aggression towards humans—not to mention the strong, offensive odor emitted by intact

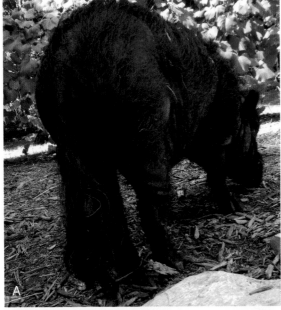

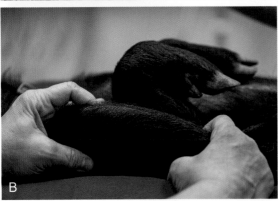

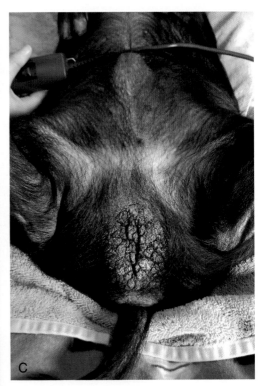

Fig. 4.12 Physical features of the intact male that become more obvious with age are thick tail tassel (A), dense fibrous shoulder plates (B), and thickening (hyperkeratosis) of the scrotum (C). (Photo credit [B]: Jennifer L. Davis.)

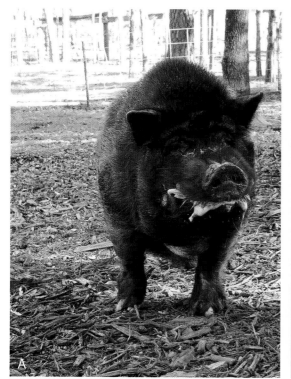

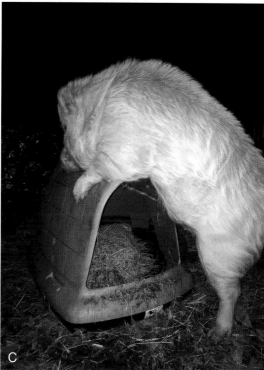

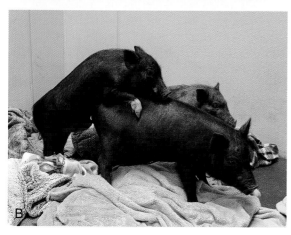

Fig. 4.13 Behavioral traits of intact males include excessive salivation (unrelated to anticipation of food) (A) as well as mounting any object, animate or inanimate (B and C). (Photo credit [C]: Pigtopia.)

boars—are more problematic. Therefore, it is preferred that the male undergoes castration prior to puberty and the onset of undesirable behaviors (Østevik et al. 2012).

The male reproductive system is similar to that of other livestock with a few exceptions. The penis forms a sigmoid flexure, which is important anatomically

when working with conditions such as a urethral stone. The tip of the penis is corkscrew shaped (Fig. 4.14) and frequently unsheathed in sexually active boars; however, following castration, unsheathing of the penis is not observed except with medical issues such as intense pushing with urinary tract obstruction. There is a preputial diverticulum in the

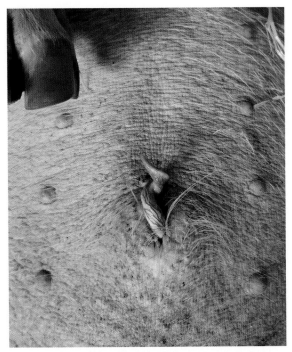

Fig. 4.14 The tip of the penis is corkscrew shaped and frequently unsheathed in sexually active boars; following castration, unsheathing of the penis is abnormal and should be investigated.

sheath near the orifice, normally filled with a malodorous fluid.

The testicles in the miniature pig are located relatively close to the body, unlike domestic boars. Both testicles should be palpated to ensure that there is indeed a testicle present. As mentioned beforehand, the cryptorchid condition is not uncommon in swine. If a cryptorchid boar is presented for neutering, be sure to ascertain which testicle is undescended so that the surgical procedure is conducted on the correct side. Never remove the descended testicle without also removing the undescended testicle (see also Chapter 9).

Closure of the external inguinal rings is not necessary during normal castration surgery; in fact, more post-procedure complications were noted in one study and were felt to result from manipulation of the ring tissue. This then resulted in post-operative swelling, which was not seen in pigs who did not undergo inguinal ring closure (Salcedo-Jiménez et al. 2020). However, the ring should be palpated, and if too large

(i.e., a finger can be inserted), closure may be warranted to prevent herniation post-castration.

Occasionally a scrotal hernia may be present. This condition is easily detected and the surgical repair is performed during castration. Closure of the external inguinal rings would be indicated in this condition.

Intact boars kept for breeding purposes should be kept in separate housing than humans. Boars emit a strong odor and can be unpredictably aggressive, although this behavior is much less common in miniature pigs as compared to commercial swine. Two boars may live together for companionship, but boars should not be routinely grouped with other boars as fighting will ensue. Additionally, boars develop distinctive tusks, which can cause serious injury to humans or other animals.

CASTRATION

Castration is recommended for non-breeding males as testicular tumors, frequently cancerous, are common in aged boars (Fig. 4.15), in addition to undesirable behaviors and odor as described earlier.

Castration techniques for the male pig are similar to those used for canine castration and neuter is typically performed at 8 to 12 weeks of age (Lawhorn 2013). Prescrotal or scrotal approaches can be used with either open or closed technique for removal of each testicle. Consideration should be given to how the pig is housed as to which approach is taken. A scrotal approach may be preferred for pigs living in a barn environment with bedding (such as straw or shavings) that could possibly contaminate the incision. However, there is more drainage associated with a scrotal technique. A prescrotal approach is acceptable for those pigs who will be dwelling in a home and is the most common approach used in pets.

Surgical details and anesthetic protocols are discussed in separate chapters (see Chapters 8 & 9). Analgesia during surgery is recommended, and there are references in the literature regarding post-operative analgesia (Salcedo-Jiménez et al. 2020).

Cryptorchid Surgery

In domestic swine, a homozygous recessive gene has been postulated to be associated with cryptorchidism. One study involving the progeny of cryptorchid boars

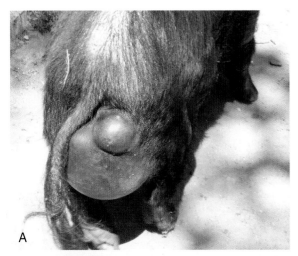

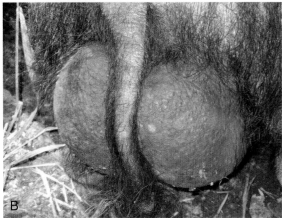

Fig. 4.15 Castration is recommended for non-breeding males as testicular tumors are common in aged boars and may be unilateral (A) or bilateral (B). While some tumors are benign, many are cancerous with lung metastasis ultimately leading to death. (Photo credit [A]: Refuge GroinGroin.)

found that between 10.9% and 31.4% of male progeny had a retained testicle (Anderson and Mulon 2019).

The undescended testicle should be removed surgically, as its presence will promote undesired boar behavior including aggression, and unwanted pregnancy can occur if the animal is housed with an intact female. Retained testicles may also become cancerous.

Prior to surgical removal of the retained testicle, it is essential to determine on which side the testicle is retained. If there is one testicle descended, careful palpation will determine if it sits on the right or the left; anecdotally, the left testicle is more likely to be retained (Skelton et al. 2021; Wilbers, personal communication) and typically sits just inside the inguinal canal. Rarely, a pig can be monorchid with only one identifiable testis. If the descended testicle has been removed, it will be more difficult to locate the undescended testicle. Ultrasound examination can be used to locate the undescended testicle (Østevik et al. 2012). A laparoscope, if available, will assist in the location and removal of the testicle (Rosanova et al. 2015).

Two other approaches to cryptorchid surgery have also been described. A paramedian approach on the ipsilateral side is a classic surgery. However, an inguinal approach has also been described for removal of retained testicles in domestic swine (Scollo et al. 2016). Regardless of surgical choice, the retained testicle is exteriorized and removed.

CHRONIC PENILE PROLAPSE

Penile prolapse (Fig. 4.16) has been reported in a number of species, including the Vietnamese potbellied pig, with one litter reported as a congenital condition in that all of the male piglets in the litter exhibited penile prolapse. The condition is postulated to occur due to ineffective preputial muscles or paralysis of the retractor penis muscle (Reig et al. 2019).

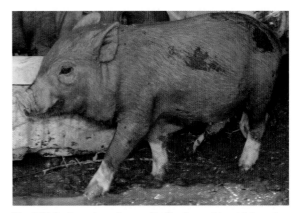

Fig. 4.16 Penile prolapse is occasionally observed in miniature pigs. Initial treatment may involve use of hygroscopic agents and lubrication to replace the penis within the sheath, followed by a purse-string suture around the preputial orifice to hold in place. If unsuccessful, surgical intervention may be necessary, although continued medical management (along with castration) may allow a young pig to outgrow the condition. (Photo credit: https://www.minipiginfo.com/)

Massage and lubrication may be tried, along with hygroscopic agents to place the penis back in the sheath if it is not traumatized or otherwise damaged. The penis should also be evaluated for foreign material (i.e., hair ring) that may be contributing. Under anesthesia, a purse-string suture is placed around the preputial orifice to hold the penis in the sheath. Reig reports that this technique may not be viable if there is paralysis of the retractor penis muscle, in which case surgical intervention may be required. This author had a case of persistent penile prolapse in a 2-month-old neutered miniature pig that was not resolved successfully with purse-string suturing. The owner elected to manage the prolapsed penis with hygroscopic agents and elevation using a home-made "codpiece" to avoid further trauma; the condition resolved successfully over the course of approximately 2 months.

Surgical options have been described in other species and include enlargement or narrowing of the preputial orifice, preputial advancement, phallopexy, and preputial muscle myorrhaphy. A description of surgical correction using phallopexy with or without urethropexy is provided by Reig. Both approaches were determined to be successful at follow up.

PERSISTENT FRENULUM

The frenulum is a piece of tissue that holds the penis to the inside of the prepuce. It usually atrophies in domestic male swine between 4 and 6 months of age, and the penis thus separates (St. Jean and Anderson 2004). Occasionally the frenulum persists, resulting in the inability of the intact boar to fully extend the penis. The affected boar may be anesthetized, and the frenulum simply cut with a pair of scissors. There is usually minimal bleeding afterwards.

BIBLIOGRAPHY

Amalraj A, Matthijs A, Schoos A, et al. Health and management of hobby pigs: a review. *Vlaams Diergeneeskundig Tijdschrift.* 2018; 87(6):347–358.

Anderson DE, Mulon PY. Anesthesia and surgical procedures in swine. In: Zimmeran JJ, Karriker LA, Ramirez A, et al., eds. *Diseases of Swine.* 11th ed. Hoboken, NJ: John Wiley & Sons, Inc.; 2019: 179–196.

Braun Jr W. Reproduction in miniature pet pigs. In: Reeves DE, ed. *Guidelines for the Veterinary Practitioner: Care and Management of Miniature Pet Pigs.* Santa Barbara, CA: Brillig Hill, Inc.; 1993: 27–39.

Caminita F, van der Merwe M, Hance B, et al. A preterm pig model of lung immaturity and spontaneous infant respiratory distress syndrome. *Am J Physiol Lung Cell Mol Physiol.* 2015;308(2): L118–L129.

Helke KL, Ezell PC, Duran-Struuck R, et al. Biology and diseases of swine. In: Fox JG, Anderson LC, Otto GM, et al., eds. *Lab Animal Medicine.* 3rd ed. San Diego, CA: Elsevier, Inc.; 2015:700–704.

Herpin P, Damon M, Le Dividich J. Development of thermoregulation and neonatal survival in pigs. *Livest Prod Sci.* 2002;78:25–45.

Ilha MRS, Newman SJ, Van Amstel S, et al. Uterine lesions in 32 miniature pet pigs. *Vet Pathol.* 2010;47(6):1071–1075.

Kirkwood RN, Althouse GC, Yeager MJ, et al. Diseases of the reproductive system. In: Zimmerman JJ, Karriker LA, Ramirez A, et al., eds. *Diseases of Swine.* 10th ed. Ames, IA: Wiley-Blackwell; 2012: 329–347.

Lawhorn DB. *Reproduction of Potbellied Pigs.* Merck Veterinary Manual; Revised June 2013. https://www.merckvetmanual.com/exotic-and-laboratory-animals/potbellied-pigs/reproduction-of-potbellied-pigs. Accessed February 2021.

Magidson S. Personal communication.

Mozzachio K, Linder K, Dixon D. Uterine smooth muscle tumors in potbellied pigs (Sus scrofa) resemble human fibroids: a potential animal model. *Toxicol Pathol.* 2004;32(4):402–407.

Østevik L, Elmas C, Rubio-Martinez LM. Castration of the Vietnamese pot-bellied boar: 8 cases. *Can Vet J.* 2012;53(9):943–948.

Ramirez A. Differential diagnosis of diseases. In: Zimmerman JJ, Karriker LA, Ramirez A, et al., eds. *Diseases of Swine.* 10th ed. Ames, IA: Wiley-Blackwell; 2012:18–31.

Reig L, Hill JA, Mitchell A, et al. Surgical treatment of chronic penile prolapse in Vietnamese pot-bellied pigs: 5 cases (2016–2017). *Vet Surg.* 2019;48(5):890–896.

Rosanova N, Singh A, Cribb N. Laparoscopic-assisted cryptorchidectomy in 2 Vietnamese pot-bellied pigs (Sus scrofa). *Can Vet J.* 2015;56(2):153–156.

Salcedo-Jiménez R, Brounts SH, Mulon PY, et al. Multicenter retrospective study of complications and risk factors associated with castration in 106 pet pigs. *Can Vet J.* 2020;61(2):173–177.

Schlafer DH, Foster RA. Female genital system. In: *Jubb, Kennedy & Palmer's Pathology of Domestic Animals.* Vol 3. St. Louis, Missouri: Elsevier, Inc.; 2016:358–464. 6th ed. doi:10.1016/B978-0-7020-5319-1.00015-3.

Scollo A, Martelli P, Borri E, et al. Pig surgery: cryptorchidectomy using an inguinal approach. *Vet Rec.* 2016;178(24):609–613.

Skelton JA, Baird AN, Hawkins JF, et al. Cryptorchidectomy with a paramedian or inguinal approach in domestic pigs: 47 cases (2000–2018). *J Am Vet Med Assoc.* 2021;258(10):1130–1134.

St. Jean G, Anderson DE. Surgery of the swine reproductive tract. In: Fubini SL, Ducharme N, eds. *Farm Animal Surgery.* St. Louis, MO: Saunders; 2004:565–576.

Swindle MM. The reproductive system. In: Swindle MM, Smith AC, eds. *Swine in the Laboratory: Surgery, Anesthesia, Imaging and Experimental Techniques.* 3rd ed. Boca Raton, FL: CRC Press, Taylor and Francis Group; 2016:191–211.

Taverne Marcel, Noakes David E. Parturition and the Care of Paturient Animals and the Newborn. Veterinary Reproduction and Obstetrics. Elsevier; 2019:115–147.

Chapter 5

Handling and Restraint

Kristie Mozzachio

Overview

Restraint is arguably the most difficult—and unique—aspect of dealing with miniature pig patients. In general, less restraint is best and will result in less obnoxious squealing and less stress for all involved. Remember that pigs are a prey animal—restraint occurs only with predation, and the pig will respond accordingly. They are also stubborn and, given their tremendous strength, do best when coaxed rather than forced. A restricted amount of space, secure footing, and a quiet, calm environment is the optimum starting point, and owners should be forewarned of potential squealing. It should also be noted that pigs avoid moving into dimly lit areas, can be frightened by excessive movement, and balk at visual changes in flooring like a distinct threshold into a room or a floor grate, much like a horse (Grandin 1986). They can be difficult to propel forward unless an uninterrupted surface is provided (i.e., long carpet runner or a string of similarly colored mats).

Of course, the ideal method of restraint is individual to the patient. Young, fit, healthy pigs can tolerate most techniques, but an old arthritic animal may require gentler methods. Injectable sedation on an obese patient may not be ideal due to fat deposition of drugs, so oral sedatives, inhalant anesthesia, and/or a sling device may be best. Restraint options include the following.

BELLY RUB

While obviously not a means of true restraint, a well-socialized pig might be amenable to a relaxing belly rub in a comfortable, non-threatening environment (Fig. 5.1). With the pig in lateral recumbency, a physical exam can easily be performed, and injections given, especially if subcutaneous (Box 5.1).

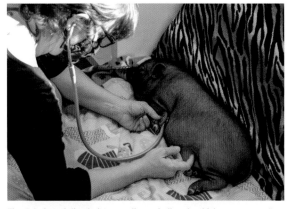

Fig. 5.1 A socialized pig may allow a belly rub which serves as a "restraint" for physical exam as well as subcutaneous injection (i.e., vaccination). This piglet is in a comfortable environment and is relaxed and quiet for auscultation. If additional restraint is necessary for a procedure, such as a hoof trim, the pig can be rolled onto the back from this position. A belly rub should be attempted first as the use of food motivators or more forceful methods will make the pig excitable. (Photo credit: Jennifer L. Davis.)

This method should be attempted first, as the introduction of food or use of more forcible methods, such as sorting panels, will make the pig excitable.

LAP

Small pigs may be comfortable when loosely held in the lap, especially in a calm, quiet environment, and maybe with the handler sitting on the floor (Fig. 5.2).

LIFT

Small pigs can be lifted and cradled against the body, held with one arm under the neck in front of the forelimbs and one arm under the rump (Fig. 5.3). Alternatively, a hand placed under the chest with the opposite arm pressed against the side (Edson 2018) also appears to be secure and comfortable for the pig. Expect loud squealing if the animal has not been

BOX 5.1 TIPS FOR MINIPIG RESTRAINT

- Start with the least amount of handling first. Routine examination and vaccination can readily be performed during a belly rub or by (loosely) confining the pig in a corner with sorting panels. Hoof or tusk trim, however, requires additional restraint in most animals (i.e., flipping, swine sling, and/or sedation).
- Secure footing is of utmost importance when working with pigs; slippery surfaces can almost guarantee a panicked patient before a procedure is even attempted. Rubber-backed rugs, yoga mats, or stall mats work well for this purpose.
- Have all supplies ready and in reach prior to restraint.
- A firm scratch to the rump in a standing pig will often render the animal immobile as they lift that hip and pause.

"Forking"—poking the pig with the tines of a fork—can have a similar effect. Video of the forking effect to "restrain" a pig for rectal temperature can be found at: https://open.lib. umn.edu/largeanimalsurgery/chapter/swine-sedation-and-anesthesia/.
- Keep treats on hand to facilitate handling as pigs are extremely food motivated. Use judiciously, however, as the presence of food causes excitability. Do not give food immediately prior to flipping due to risk of aspiration.
- Patience is key. Once panicked, a pig becomes unresponsive, with his sole purpose in life to escape the situation. If this occurs, stop and regroup until the pig calms down and/ or administer a sedative such as midazolam.

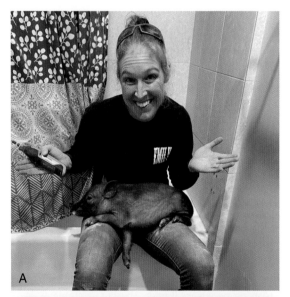

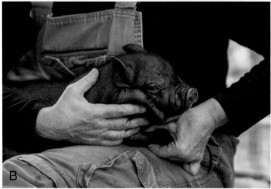

Fig. 5.2 Small pigs may be comfortable when held loosely in the lap. (A) A piglet held across the lap relaxes for a hoof trim. (B) A piglet held in the lap while handler sits on the floor relaxes for orthopedic examination. (A, Photo credit: Emily Mohring. B, Photo credit: Jennifer L. Davis.)

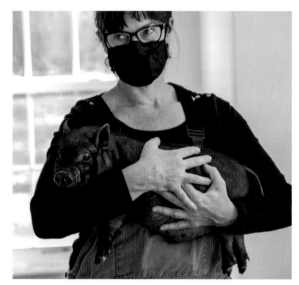

Fig. 5.3 Small pigs can be lifted and cradled against the body, held with one arm under the neck (in front of the forelimbs) and one arm under the rump. This position seems to be the most secure to the animal, and although squealing may occur initially, especially with young piglets, the animal usually calms over time. (Photo credit: Jennifer L. Davis.)

acclimated to this form of restraint, although many pigs will eventually quiet if properly held. Food distraction can sometimes help but take care to use options such as carrot sticks or peanut butter spread on a plate to avoid being accidentally bitten by an overly excited pig. Use your judgment, as food distraction can sometimes backfire by encouraging excitement rather than calm. There tends to be a "sweet spot" in terms of a small pig feeling secure when being lifted. If not level/horizontal, the pig struggles. If held too tightly, the pig struggles. If the handler is nervous, the pig struggles. Tynes 1999 also describes a 2-person "fireman's carry" for larger pigs.

SORTING PANELS

Sorting panels (a.k.a. crowd boards) are the number one specialized piece of equipment needed for minipig

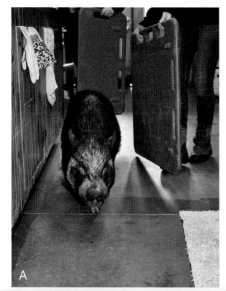

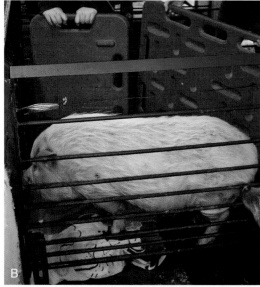

Fig. 5.4 Sorting panels are the number one piece of specialized equipment needed for minipig handling. (A) Two boards worked slightly behind the pig are used to direct forward movement along a wall. (B) Two boards are used to loosely confine a pig in a corner; from this position, physical exam or injection can be performed with little direct handling, or the pig can be flipped onto the back for procedures such as hoof and tusk trim.

handling. They are made of lightweight plastic and can be bought online at farm supply stores, come in different sizes, and cost about $20 to $50 USD each depending on size. A minimum of two is needed (Fig. 5.4). Pigs respond similarly to cattle, and general guidelines include: (1) work the boards slightly behind the pig to move the animal forward, (2) use a fence line or wall as a guide whenever possible, and (3) a board placed too far in front of the pig will result in movement backwards. Sorting panels are useful for directing movement of a pig or for cornering the animal as a means of restraint (i.e., to administer injections, perform physical exam, position for flipping).

CRATE/KENNEL

Solid plastic airline kennels (Fig. 5.5) are preferable to wire cages, as pigs frequently sustain hoof injuries in wire crates (not to mention pinched human fingers!). Additionally, wire cages are less sturdy for lifting with a heavy pig patient inside. Non-slip bathtub decals, a yoga mat, or a rug with rubber backing should be provided on the slippery plastic bottom. Owners can

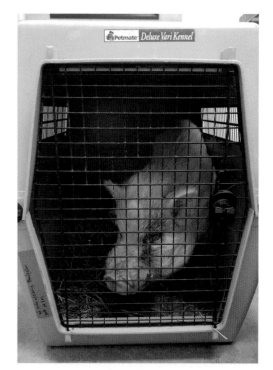

Fig. 5.5 A solid plastic airline kennel is the best means of transporting a pet pig; these are preferable to flimsy wire cages that cannot readily support the weight of a larger pig, and hoof injury is a risk as well.

use the crate as the pig's bed/den at home or easily train the pig to enter using food rewards. In this way, the pig becomes acclimated to the crate, and if/when the need arises for transport, there is no panic involved. Without acclimation, a pig can still be readily guided with sorting panels into a crate placed in a corner, against a wall. A crate can also be partially dismantled in the clinic and used as a corral for the patient. Crates are an excellent location for recovery from sedation as a confined area is preferred to prevent injury from the patient thrashing.

HARNESS

Pig-specific harnesses are available and have two separate clips for ease of use—one clip for the part that encircles the neck, and the other for the part that encircles the girth (Fig. 5.11). This is well worth the purchase and training effort and is a wonderful means of restraint for veterinary visits. Encourage owners to harness train!

Harness training tutorials can be found online (https://www.minipiginfo.com/mini-pig-harness-training.html),

but one technique involves clipping the neck portion and placing the pig's food bowl in the center of the loop at mealtimes. Once the pig is engaged in eating, gently lift the loop over the head. The pig will likely back away at first, but a hungry pig will return to the bowl and suffer this heinous offense once they realize that it is not painful and there is food to be had. After repeated placing of the neck loop over the head, the trainer can graduate to moving the harness over the pig's body, then eventually clipping the girth. Pigs do not take kindly to restraint and will buck and jump the first time a harness is successfully placed, but with food distraction, their minds are laser-focused, and this preoccupation relieves them of much of their fear. Take a week or two to train slowly and the pig will soon learn to stand for harnessing, especially if a snack is expected.

"PIG FLIP"

This technique uses leverage to prop a pig on the rump or on the back (Fig. 5.6) (Wilbers 2013) to allow basic procedures such as hoof trim, tusk trim, or blood draw

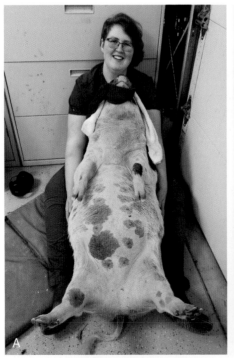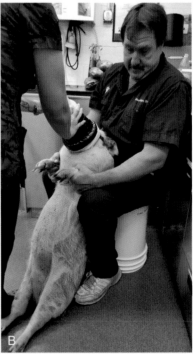

Fig. 5.6 Flipping a pig is one of the best means of restraint and allows hoof trim, tusk trim, blood draw, etc. to be performed without need of sedation. (A) This large pig is held in the lap and a soft bathrobe tie has been used as a makeshift muzzle to prevent open-mouthed screaming - the pig relaxed once screaming was prevented; (B) a pig flipped onto the haunches allows the handler to sit on an overturned bucket while gas sedation is administered;

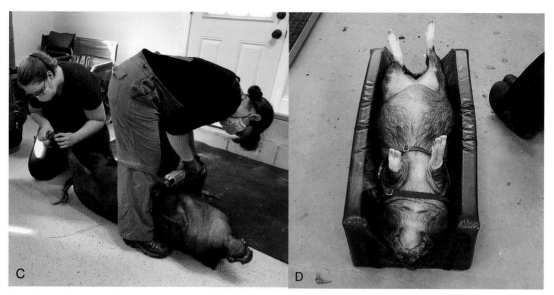

Fig. 5.6, cont'd (C) a pig flipped into dorsal recumbency and held on the back as multiple people attend to hooves; (D) young or thin animals may do best in a padded trough as they may not have enough of their own "padding" to remain comfortably positioned on a hard surface. (B, Photo credit: Ross Mill Farm.)

to be performed. Care should be taken with obese animals that may have difficulty breathing in this position or with elderly animals that may have significant spondylosis or arthritis of the spine. Young or thin animals may do best in a padded trough as they may not have enough of their own "padding" to remain comfortably positioned on a hard surface. Many larger pigs calm completely, or even fall asleep, when positioned in dorsal recumbency (Fig. 5.7).

There are several methods for flipping a pig. One technique starts with the pig facing away from the handler, maybe cornered with sorting panels to limit movement. Note: This is one instance in which food should NOT be offered due to risk of aspiration with vocalization. Grasp the pig behind the forelimbs (in the web of skin in the axillary region) and lift upward until the animal sits on the haunches. The handler can then sit on a stool or tall bucket if desired, holding the pig between the knees, or the pig can be lowered onto the back and straddled. Alternatively, the pig can rest in dorsal recumbency in the lap. The limit for single-handedly flipping pigs all of the way into dorsal recumbency using this method tends to be the height of the handler relative to the length of the pig (i.e., if the pig is long-bodied and hind limbs cannot clear the ground to swing forward as the pig is lifted, the animal will simply backpedal between the legs of the handler).

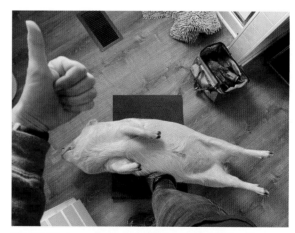

Fig. 5.7 Flipping a pig is one of the most effective handling techniques, and some pigs will ultimately fall asleep during restraint in dorsal recumbency—this pig is NOT sedated. (Photo credit: Emily Mohring.)

Another means of flipping is the "swipe." In this method, the handler squats close to the ground and grabs the *opposite* forelimb and hindlimb of the pig, using this leverage to push the animal off balance as it tries to escape, effectively rolling the pig onto the back. Note: The opposite leg is grasped because the near leg can easily be injured if yanked outward/laterally (i.e., muscle tears, dislocation of shoulder or hip joints). This technique requires a bit more skill and practice. When confined to a small area, the handler can squat, and the pig allowed to run past as often as is needed until caught. In a larger, open area, the technique becomes more difficult. This method is also more difficult for pigs that leap/jump to escape rather than try to run away.

A third method involves breaching the trust of your patient by offering a calming belly rub, then quickly grabbing both "down" limbs and rolling the pig onto the back. Of course, the pig has to be relaxed enough to roll over for a belly rub in the first place. With this technique, you only get one shot.

Once the pig is on its back, stabilize by tucking toes under the torso near the shoulders if straddling the animal, or by having the handler squeeze his/her/their legs along the sides of the pig—a wobbly pig that feels insecure or unstable will struggle. If the pig kicks while situated in the lap, do not grab the hind legs, as this usually intensifies struggles and risk of injury to the handler is high; instead, secure the rump to steady the animal until it calms. When straddling the pig, grasping one or both forelimb(s) is effective in maintaining

control until the pig calms, but do not maintain a tight hold on any limbs unless necessary as this may also result in greater struggle. Some pigs do best when held in the lap, others do best on the back. An aggressive pig at risk of biting is best restrained on the back.

SWINE SLING

Sling restraint (i.e., Panepinto Sling®) is commonly used in research, and pigs can be trained to tolerate this form of restraint for hours, without sedation (Fig. 5.8). It is a seemingly comfortable device for the animal which lifts the pig via a hammock with four leg holes ± a hole at the neck for cranial vena cava blood collection (Panepinto et al. 1983); the pressure on the belly seems to have a calming effect (Grandin 1986). Some versions are available for as little as $800 USD (https://www.lomir.com/slings/portable-panepinto-restraint-frame-3foot/) but require that the animal be lifted into the hammock, so use is limited to smaller individuals. The high $3000+ USD price tag of a version that includes a hand crank makes it impractical for many clinics.

CHEMICAL RESTRAINT

A variety of drugs can be used for minipig sedation (Box 5.2). Trazodone and gabapentin ± acepromazine

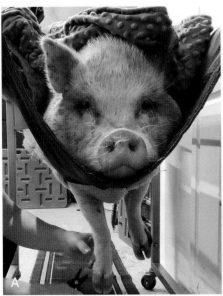
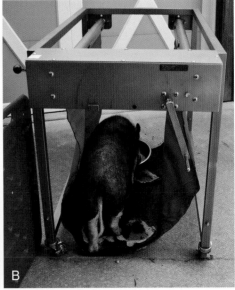

Fig. 5.8 A sling device (i.e., Panepinto Sling®; https://www.panepinto.com/) that restrains the pig via a hammock appears to be comfortable for the animal and is an excellent means of restraint (A). Some versions feature a cranking mechanism that allows larger animals to be lifted without manual effort. In this image (B), a sorting panel as well as a strategically placed bowl of food coaxes the pig to enter, and the crank is then used to hoist the animal. However, this version costs over $3000 USD, making it impractical for many clinics. (A, Photo credit: Swine Knot.)

BOX 5.2 CHEMICAL RESTRAINT OPTIONS FOR MINIPIGS

Chemical restraint options for non-painful, routine procedures that can be used alone or in combination include:

- Oral: Trazodone 10 mg/kg + Gabapentin 20 mg/kg ± Acepromazine 0.5–1 mg/kg given PO 2–3 h prior to appointment can significantly calm a pig without oversedation.
- Injectable:
  - Midazolam 0.1–0.5 mg/kg can be administered IM or intra-nasal to achieve the sedation needed to accomplish basic procedures. Reversal is possible but typically unnecessary.
  - Butorphanol 0.2–0.4 mg/kg + midazolam 0.1–0.3 mg/kg + dexmedetomidine 0.01–0.04 mg/kg [OR xylazine 1 mg/kg], combined in a single syringe and given IM, can provide anesthesia of about 30–40 min duration; atipamezole can be used to reverse the alpha-2 agonist to speed recovery, keeping in mind that this also reverses analgesic effects.
- Inhalant: Isoflurane or sevoflurane can be administered via face mask to achieve the desired level of sedation, with rapid recovery. This can sometimes be administered to an awake pig in a crate or cornered with sorting panels but may be easier if oral pre-medications have been given in advance.

or alprazolam given orally several hours prior to an appointment can calm a skittish animal. Midazolam given intra-pig (IM, SQ, intra-nasal, intra-rectal, intra-oral) can provide just enough sedation to allow routine procedures to proceed calmly and without struggle. If needed, deeper sedation is possible with a variety of drug combinations. Always consider recovery time, especially if the intended procedures are non-painful and/or short-lived; choosing drugs that can be reversed might be best in these situations (see also Chapter 8).

THE DON'TS

The more common methods of restraint used in commercial swine, including hog snares and lifting small pigs by the hind legs, are generally unsuitable for miniature pet pigs. At best, these techniques are disagreeable to owners or simply fail to restrain, and at worst, the pig can be injured. Catching and lifting a miniature pig by the leg may lead to joint dislocation or back injury (Braun and Casteel 1993; Jackson and Cockcroft 2007). And the response of the miniature pig to a hog snare is unpredictable. While larger commercial pigs pull away, pet pigs will often move forward or twist and turn, rendering the technique ineffective and more likely to result in injury (Woods et al. 2019).

BIBLIOGRAPHY

Braun WF, Casteel SW. Potbellied pigs: miniature porcine pets. *Vet Clin North Am Small Anim Pract.* 1993;23(6):1149–1177.

Edson M. *How to wrestle a mini-pig and win—basic procedures of miniature pigs.* 90th Annual Western Veterinary Conference Proceedings. Las Vegas, NV. 2018.

Grandin T. Minimizing stress in pig handling in the research lab. *Lab Animal.* 1986;15(3). https://www.grandin.com/references/minimizing.stress.in.pig.handling.html. Accessed February 2021.

Jackson PGG, Cockcroft PD. The pet pig. In: *Handbook of Pig Medicine.* Philadelphia, PA: Elsevier Ltd; 2007:215.

McCrackin MA, Swindle MM. Biology, handling, husbandry, and anatomy. In: Swindle MM, Smith AC, eds. *Swine in the Laboratory: Surgery, Anesthesia, Imaging, and Experimental Techniques.* 3rd ed. Boca Raton, FL: CRC Press; 2016:18–20.

Panepinto LM, Phillips RW, Norden S, et al. A comfortable, minimum stress method of restraint for Yucatan miniature swine. *Lab Anim Sci.* 1983;33(1):95–97.

Tynes VV. Preventive health care for pet potbellied pigs. *Vet Clin North Am Exot Anim Pract.* 1999;2(2):495–510.

Wilbers AM. Handling pet pigs as patients. North American Veterinary Conference Proceedings. Orlando, FL.: NAVCP; 2013.

Woods AL, Tynes VV, Mozzachio K. Special considerations for show and pet pigs. In: Zimmerman JJ, Karriker LA, Ramirez A, et al., eds. *Diseases of Swine.* 11th ed. Hoboken, NJ: John Wiley & Sons, Inc.; 2019:217–218.

Chapter 6

Physical Exam

Kristie Mozzachio

Overview

Physical examination of a miniature pig patient is performed as for any other species, with allowances made for their unique, often stubborn and vocal personalities, and the ability (or inability) to restrain. Yearly exam is recommended for otherwise healthy pet pigs. In geriatric patients, especially those receiving medications to address arthritis or suffering from other chronic illness, twice yearly minimum is suggested. See (Box 6.1) for tips on incorporating minipig patients into a practice.

After verifying signalment, including gender, obtaining a body weight is a great start to an exam, especially as it takes practice to be able to make an educated guess, and dosages of sedative agents, for example, rely on this measurement. The easiest in-clinic method is to weigh the pig in its crate then subtract the weight of the crate. Once the carrier is brought into an exam room, the pig can be released and allowed to explore. If the pig is harness–trained (see Fig. 3.11), it may walk onto a scale if led calmly and, maybe, treated along the way (Fig. 6.1). For uncrated animals, sorting panels are useful to guide—not force—the pig onto the scale and then into an exam room (see Fig. 5.4). For evaluation in the field, a portable livestock scale is ideal, but a hog weight tape is also an option. It should be noted, however, that weight tapes are intended for use in commercial swine and often overestimate the weight of a minipig, especially those with a short–bodied, short–legged conformation.

A thorough history should be taken during the initial visual evaluation and is of utmost importance given the often–limited hands–on exam of pig patients (Wilbers 2013). Questioning the owner on diet may result in a longer and longer list of foods as the exam proceeds, so ask this question first, especially if the

pet is overweight. Other important questions include where the pig was acquired, expectation of size, vaccination and deworming history, home environment, other pets in the household, and current issues/complaints/questions. For farm call visits, take note of the environment, housing, and bedding and look at the feed bag as well as measuring cups or scoops used to dispense, water source, other animals with which the pig has contact, and available shade (easy to forget about in winter), etc. A hand out providing basic information on veterinary care and reputable resources for further research is great for first–timers (whether a new pet pig owner or just new to the practice). An example can be found at: https://lafeber.com/vet/basic-miniature-pig-care/.

Visual examination can be performed as the pig is allowed to explore the exam room or other confined area—prior to a more hands-on approach—and should include observation of mentation, body condition, conformation, posture, gait, hair coat, skin health, hoof condition, ocular and nasal discharge, respiratory rate and character. After that, the fun begins.

In a calm environment, a well–socialized pig may succumb to a belly rub, allowing the opportunity for examination and auscultation (see Fig. 5.1). Many will even allow subcutaneous injection (i.e., vaccines). If not amenable to this, efforts can be made to examine while distracting with food. If necessary, restraint for physical examination is best performed using sorting panels to isolate the patient in a corner of the room or stall, without physical contact (see Fig. 5.4B). Then if further restraint is needed, the pig can be flipped onto the haunches or back (see Fig. 5.6). Sedation is also an option, and many pigs respond well to oral trazodone and gabapentin ± acepromazine pre-medication prior to the

BOX 6.1 TIPS FOR IN-CLINIC MINIATURE PIG APPOINTMENTS

- Schedule an appropriate amount of time for minipig appointments and, of course, charge accordingly (i.e., double the typical appointment time). These animals cannot be rushed and attempts to do so will frustrate veterinary staff, owner, and pig. If there is a space that lends better to a loudly protesting pig with the least disruption to the entire clinic, use it.
- Provide a calm, quiet environment (i.e., away from barking dogs, especially) and a non-slip surface with good traction (e.g., rubber gym or yoga mat, rubber–backed bathroom rugs, maybe a thick comforter to encourage the animal to lie down).
- Start with the least amount of physical handling possible. There is no need to flip a pig that will otherwise roll over for a belly rub or stand quietly while eating.
- If a pig might be amenable to a belly rub, try this first. The introduction of food or use of more forcible methods, such as sorting panels, will make the pig excitable and belly rub options will be off the table.

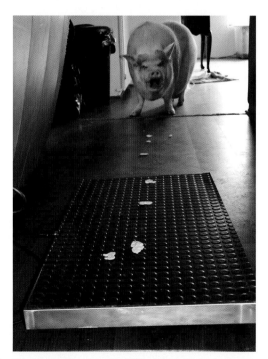

Fig. 6.1 A trail of treats and a little patience is the best means of stress–free weighing. A portable livestock scale can be used in the field; a hog weight tape is another, far less expensive, option though these were developed for commercial swine and tend to overestimate minipig weights.

visit to facilitate handling, although many injectable options exist for more immediate or profound sedation (see Box 5.2 and Chapter 8 for drug options and dosages). If a pig has been harness-trained (see Fig. 3.11), request that the owner have the pig harnessed prior to presentation; harnesses make excellent "pig handles."

Extrapolate from the species you are most comfortable with! Very few physical exam findings are unique to the pig, and any abnormalities identified will have a similar differential list to, say, a dog, even if the underlying etiology differs. Develop a systematic approach as for any species, even if parts of the exam cannot be completed. Record ALL exam findings, both positive and negative. While this is a good practice for any species, it becomes even more important for a minipig patient, as exam may be variably limited by difficulties unique to each animal. Unremarkable auscultation of the heart and lungs versus unable to auscultate (i.e., obese animal) versus auscultation not performed, for example, should be readily differentiated in the medical record.

THE VISUAL EXAMINATION

General Appearance

Step back and take a look at a distance to get an idea of overall appearance and symmetry.

Mentation

A normal, healthy pig will be bright and alert, on high alert, and ready to run if unsocialized or fearful. An unstressed pig will be curious and may explore the environment, while a well–socialized pig may approach strangers for interaction. However, an aggressive pig will also approach in a very "forward" manner with the intent to challenge or even attempt to bite (see Chapter 2). Lethargy or depression may be difficult to observe unless the pig is quite ill, as the stress/excitement of the clinical environment may override manifestation. Sick pigs observed in their home environment are more likely to demonstrate obvious lethargy.

Body Condition

A pig in acceptable body condition will have clearly visible eyes (even if deep–set, as seen with brachycephalic conformations), hip points just visible from the topline, palpable yet not visible ribs, no significant sagging of the belly when viewed from behind. In obese pigs, facial fat folds may render the pig blind, and fat accumulation may push the normally upright ears laterally, into a horizontal position on the head that seems to impair the ability to hear. See Chapter 3 for body condition scoring and detailed descriptions.

Posture

During evaluation, a pig will likely stand upright, with its head held high. Dog-sitting is uncommon unless the pig is performing a trick, so this warrants further investigation. A hunched posture (Fig. 6.2) may indicate spondylosis of the spine, arthritis, abdominal pain, or generalized weakness. Pigs do not generally lower the head to explore as a dog might (unless there is a suspicion of food on the ground); remember, they are a prey animal and on constant alert for any threat.

Gait

The pig should be able to ambulate without issue if provided with adequate traction. Painful pigs will stop and kneel frequently, possibly moving about on the "knees" rather than fully extending the forelimbs (Fig. 6.3). An obvious limp may be observed, most commonly a forelimb lameness. Ataxia may indicate a musculoskeletal or neurologic issue.

Musculoskeletal

Congenital abnormalities may be noted and are especially common in pets bred to be very small. These animals may have an exceedingly large head relative to body size, may be "cow-hocked" in the hind, or may have defects of the phalanges that result in abnormal weight-bearing and hoof growth. Both syndactyly (mulefoot) and polydactyly are common (Fig. 6.4). Valgus deformity of the forelimbs can be seen with obesity or arthritis, and bony enlargement of the elbows is another chronic arthritic change.

Skin

Many pet pigs develop dry, flaky skin that worsens with age and is especially prevalent in light-colored animals. Sun exposure can exacerbate the condition. A variety of features may be observed, ranging from

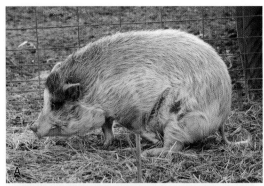
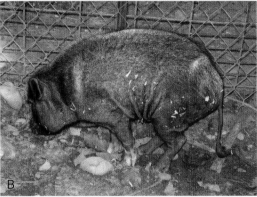

Fig. 6.2 A hunched posture may indicate spondylosis of the spine, arthritis, abdominal pain, or generalized weakness. (A) This pig is severely arthritic; the left forelimb is locked into a straight position and moved from the shoulder as the elbow joint is "frozen," while the right forelimb exhibits valgus deformity distal to the carpus. (B) The hunched posture of this animal is associated with weakness from starvation.

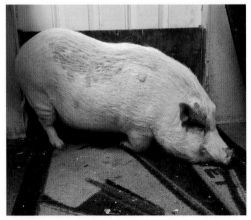

Fig. 6.3 While this pig was observed to ambulate without apparent difficulty, she frequently stopped to rest in a "kneeling" position. This is abnormal and most indicative of musculoskeletal pain (e.g., arthritis, traumatic injury).

slight scaling to hyperkeratosis to plate–like ichthyosis (Fig. 6.5A). Sunburn is common, especially in lightly–pigmented animals, and presents as one would expect—erythema over exposed areas such as the dorsum and ears. With chronic sun exposure, crusts may form, especially over the dorsal pinnae (Fig. 6.5B), and neoplasia such as squamous cell carcinoma may develop. Excoriations, alopecia, and erythema in an intensely pruritic pig (Fig. 6.5C) likely indicate sarcoptic mange, although other differentials including louse infestation, pyoderma, or a combination of these must be considered. Pigs exhibiting small brown crusts centered over hair follicle openings and giving the pig a "rusty" color (Fig. 6.5D) may result from fungal (yeast) infection; a condition which is not pruritic and appears to cause no significant issues for the animal, while aesthetically displeasing to the owner. Raised, round, red papules on the ventrum may result from insect bite hypersensitivity, although contact allergy is also possible (Fig. 6.5E). Cutaneous nodules or masses may be noted (Fig. 6.5F), and benign melanocytoma and cutaneous mast cell tumor are common. See Chapter 10 for more information.

Hair Coat

Pigs have true hair, not fur, and the texture becomes increasingly more stiff/wiry with age. Some animals have a glossy hair coat, especially at a young age, but dry brittle hair is much more common. The amount of hair varies with breed, age, environment, and disease. Minipigs shed seasonally (Fig. 6.6), once or twice a year, and hair loss patterns vary. As the shedding cycle does not typically begin until 2 to 3 years of age, the first shed may cause concern for owners. Some pigs also shed abnormally (defluvium or "blown coat") when fearful or physiologically stressed from lactation, illness, etc. (Lawhorn 1993). Hair easily epilates during shedding (Fig. 6.6C), and the pig may seem slightly pruritic. Aged pigs often develop regional, permanent alopecia (e.g., over the rump).

Hooves

The pig should be able to stand with the hoof flat on the ground and the limb situated in a linear fashion above the foot (Fig. 6.7A). The bottom of the hoof (sole) should be flat and the toe short enough to prevent "rocking back" onto the fleshy pad (heel);

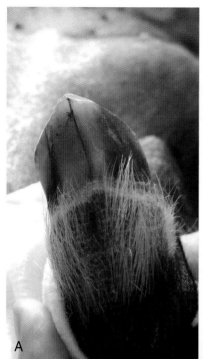

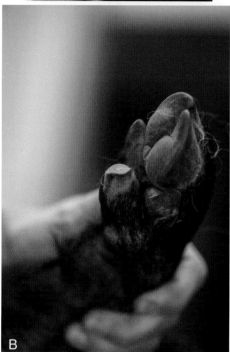

Fig. 6.4 Common congenital musculoskeletal abnormalities include **(A) syndactyly (mulefoot) and (B) polydactyly.** (Photo credit: Jennifer L. Davis.)

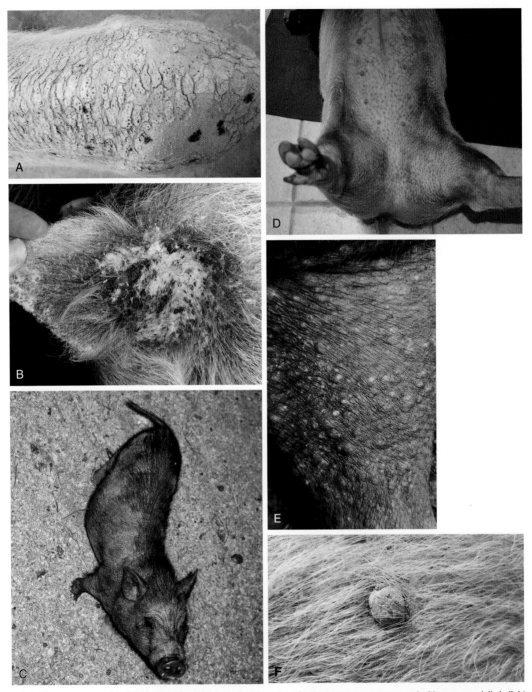

Fig. 6.5 Skin lesions are common in miniature pet pigs. (A) Hyperkeratosis and scaling becomes more pronounced with age, especially in light-colored animals, sometimes progressing to plate–like thickenings (ichthyosis). (B) Sunburn acutely presents as warm, erythematous lesions over exposed areas of the body but progresses to crusting and is especially common on the poorly haired dorsal pinnae of white pigs. (C) This piglet suffers from sarcoptic mange and exhibits erythema, excoriations, and hair loss over the flanks due to self–trauma associated with intense pruritis. (D) Small brown crusts centered over hair follicle openings and giving the pig a "rusty" color may be due to fungal (yeast) infection and is commonly observed in axillary and inguinal regions. (E) Raised papules on the ventrum and/or medial aspect of the limbs may be indicative of insect bite hypersensitivity; in this case, the pig laid near an ant hill. (F) Cutaneous masses may be noted, with mast cell tumor (pictured) one of the most common.

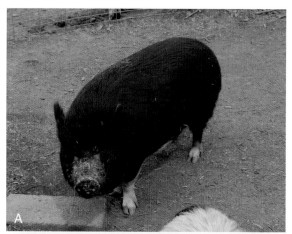

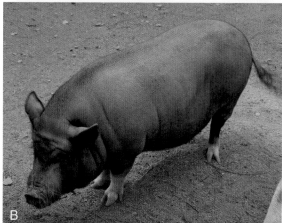

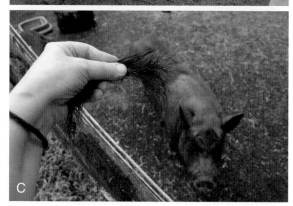

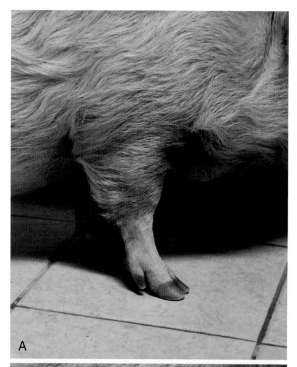

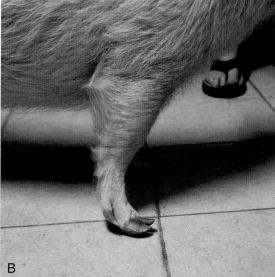

Fig. 6.6 Seasonal shedding is normal in pigs (A, before; B, after) but may not begin until 2+ years of age; (C) hair easily epilates, and the animal may be slightly pruritic. (Photo credit: A, B, Ross Mill Farm.)

Fig. 6.7 (A) A pig with good conformation versus (B) one in which laxity at the carpus forces weight towards the heel, allowing the toes to lift off the ground and the dew claws to wear along the caudal aspect due to ground contact during ambulation. This can be conformational (as in this animal) but can also be the result of extreme hoof overgrowth, in which case corrective hoof trim can overcome the problem.

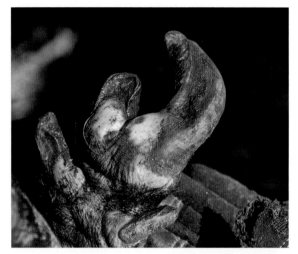

Fig. 6.8 Laminitis can cause extreme, thick hoof overgrowth and one claw (pictured) or multiple claws can be affected. (Photo credit: Jennifer L. Davis.)

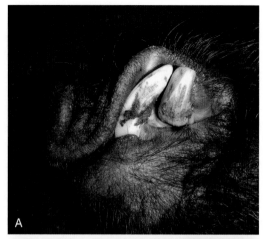

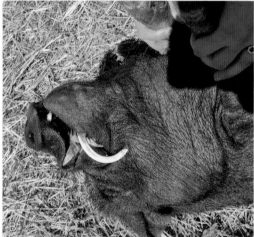

the dew claws should not touch the ground, unless they are overgrown or the pig displays joint laxity (Fig. 6.7B). Laminitis produces hard, thick, nearly tubular growth and a single toe or multiple claws may be affected, with overgrowth often significantly greater than that of unaffected claws (Fig. 6.8).

Tusks

Both males and females have tusks (upper and lower canines), although tusk growth ceases in the female at about 2 years of age, while growth in males continues throughout life (Dyce et al. 2018). Tusks may naturally project from the mouth in males, but this fact alone should not prompt automatic trim. For tusk trim indications and procedural details, see Chapter 7. Given that miniature pigs are proportionate dwarves and skeletal abnormalities common (i.e., narrowed mandible, shortened maxilla), tusks should be checked for proper occlusion/angle of growth to ensure that lower tusks do not damage soft tissues or interfere with opening and closing of the mouth (Fig. 6.9).

Ocular Discharge

Ocular secretions are very common (Fig. 6.10), become more pronounced as the pig ages, and are more apparent in light–colored animals. Discharge is typically dark

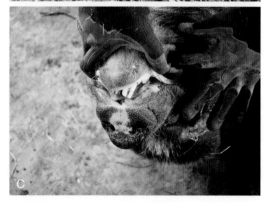

Fig. 6.9 Tusks in the male should be evaluated for overgrowth or abnormal positioning. (A) Normal relative positions of upper and lower tusks, with the expected outpouching of the upper lip to accommodate growth; (B) overgrown tusk penetrating into the face; (C) abnormally angled tusk growing in a caudal direction, situating the canine tooth on the inside of the cheek.

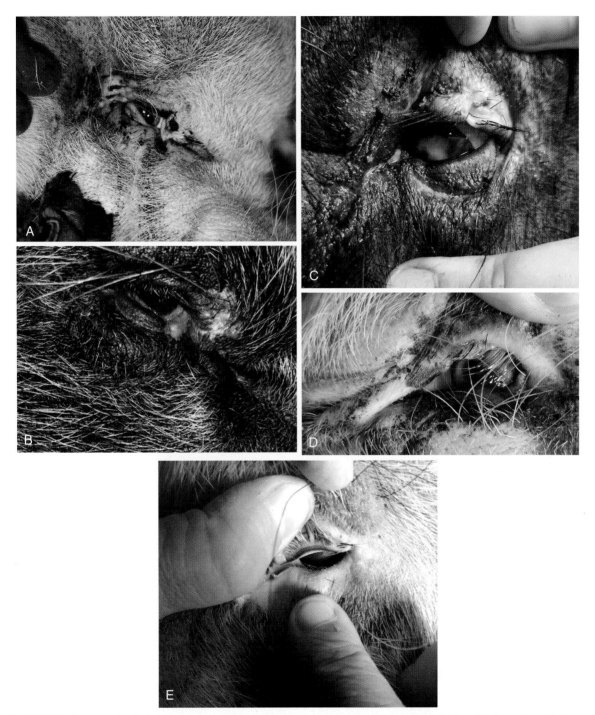

Fig. 6.10 (A) Red-brown ocular discharge is common and thick crusts may accumulate and irritate the skin; underlying etiologies such as entropion or foreign body should be ruled out, but frequently, the cause remains undetermined. Regular, gentle cleaning is recommended. (B) Abnormal tan, mucoid ocular discharge as well as slight chemosis are present in this pig; the white area near the medial canthus is due to self-trauma, indicating a pruritic condition. Note: Bulging of the conjunctiva is sometimes seen on the lateral aspect of the lower eyelid and may be a normal finding related to periocular fat distribution (Ehall 2012); however, concurrent findings in this animal are indicative of a problem. (C) Cataract in an elderly minipig. (D) Entropion is common and upper eyelids are usually affected as periocular fat accumulation leads to inward rolling; (E) entropion of the lower lid is possible but uncommon.

red–brown and may stain the face along "tear tracks" (Tynes 1999); thick crusts can build up over time and irritate underlying skin. In Göttingen minipigs, discharge has been postulated to represent a courtship signal given onset at sexual maturity and prevalence in boars (Ehall 2012), but pet minipigs of either gender can be affected including neutered animals. Underlying etiologies such as entropion or foreign body should be ruled out; allergies may play a role. A history of sudden intense tearing, especially if the animal is squinting or holding the eye closed, warrants further investigation as this may indicate the presence of an irritating foreign body and possible corneal ulcer.

Nasal Discharge

A small amount of serous nasal discharge may be seen in stressed or overheated animals, but most healthy pigs have no drainage from the nares. Mucoid discharge may indicate irritating foreign material within the nasal passages, allergies, or upper respiratory tract infection.

Respiration

While respiration rate may be slightly elevated during the stress of a veterinary visit, a pig should be eupneic, showing no obvious effort, with no abdominal component. However, even pigs with severe pneumonia rarely exhibit dyspnea that is as obvious as in other species. Open–mouth breathing is rare and should be considered an emergency.

Reproductive

Verify gender and ensure both testicles are in a scrotal location in intact males as cryptorchidism is common. Evaluate for penile prolapse (paraphimosis) due to trauma from excessive or inappropriate "humping" (see Fig. 4.16)—the penis should not be visible unless the pig is actively mounting, masturbating, or mating; the penis should never be visible in a castrated male. Evaluate the female for swelling of the vulva ± mucoid discharge that might indicate estrus (Fig. 4.1); check for abnormal discharge or mating trauma. Note: Male characteristics, such as thick shoulder plates and scrotal hyperkeratosis (see Fig. 4.12), recede post–castration. If these are present in a supposedly castrated male, it is likely that a testicle remains. This

may be more likely with breeder castrations, but some veterinarians will remove the descended testicle without removing the undescended testis.

Appetite

While history plays a significant role in assessing appetite, this can also be assessed during exam by offering food/treats to evaluate desire to eat as well as ability to prehend and chew food. This may also allow brief oral examination as many pigs open widely if a treat is held over the head (Fig. 6.11). This may be best reserved for the end of the appointment since the introduction of food tends to make pigs excitable.

Feces

Owners should be asked to provide a fresh fecal sample. However, although pigs do not commonly defecate during in–clinic exam, they frequently do so during transport. With rump scratch or "forking" (see Box 5.1), many pigs do not mind a rectal exam, and feces are nearly always available from this source. During field evaluation, several discrete toileting areas may be noted, although the pig will move to other areas if the preferred spot is too soiled. Although pasture pigs may toilet over a wide area, a normal, healthy pig will not defecate in or near the sleeping area. Normal feces are formed and tend to occur in discrete balls that stick together. Overly moist feces may be more tubular in form to cow patty–like and might occur with excessive grazing or with illness. Obese pigs tend to have abnormally small, firm fecal pellets that lack enough moisture to stick together. Excessively hard fecal balls of any size may indicate dehydration or too little dietary fiber. Normal fecal color is brown, but diet may alter color. Excessive acorn ingestion, for example, may yield a black color (Fig. 6.12A) while beets yield purple poop. Yellowish feces are abnormal and may be due to bile pigment (Fig. 6.12B).

Urine

Both males and females should produce a steady stream of clear yellow urine, and frequency is typically 1 to 3 times a day for adults, 6 to 8 times daily for piglets less than 6 months of age; however, pigs can

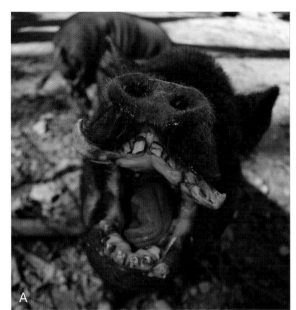

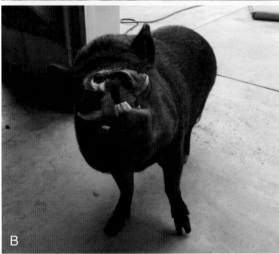

Fig. 6.11 Many pigs open widely in anticipation of a food treat to allow brief oral examination. (A) Older male with worn incisors that are separated from one another by marked gingival proliferation; (B) cleft palate.

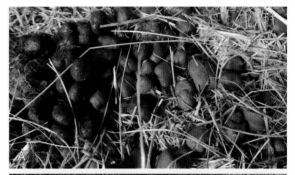

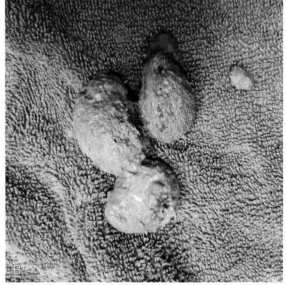

Fig. 6.12 Normal feces are produced as clusters of formed fecal balls and color/consistency can be affected by diet, medication, or illness. (A) Feces are commonly brown, but acorn ingestion can lead to black coloration. (B) Poorly formed, wet, yellow fecal material produced by a sick pig suffering from hepatic abscesses and biliary obstruction secondary to pancreatitis. (Photo credit: A, Penny Jeffrey. B, Ross Mill Farm.)

hold their urine for an extended period of time (sometimes days) and will resist eliminating outdoors in cold or wet weather or will resist getting up to eliminate with painful conditions such as arthritis. Male pigs can take an exceedingly long time to complete urination. Crystalline debris is common and may collect on the long hairs at the preputial orifice of the male or, less commonly, around the vulva of the female (Fig. 6.13); in the female especially, white sludge may appear at the end of the urine stream. Presence of a white granular material warrants further investigation (i.e., urinalysis, imaging). Frequent urination of small volumes may indicate urinary tract infection but may also be observed in females in estrus. Frequent

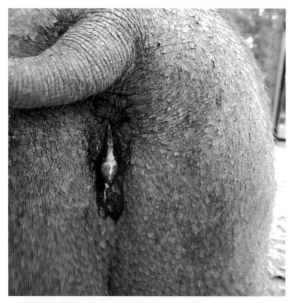

Fig. 6.13 White crystalline material seen around the vulva (or attached to preputial hairs in the male) warrants further investigation such as urinalysis and/or imaging, but crystalluria is common and may be identified in clinically normal animals. (Photo credit: Swine Knot.)

TABLE 6.1 Normal Biological and Physiological Parameters for Miniature Pigs.	
Parameter	**Range[a]**
Temperature	37.6–39°C (99.7–102.2°F)*
Pulse	70–100 beats/min (up to ~200 for newborns)
Respiration	12–24 breaths/min (up to ~40 for piglets)
Body condition	Minipig body condition score (BCS) is based on the 5-point scale used in commercial swine, with 3 or slightly under considered ideal. Both written and pictorial descriptions can be found at the following link: https://www.minipiginfo.com/mini-pig-body-scoring.html.
Full growth	3–5 years
Average size	75–200 lb (34–91 kg)
Life expectancy	14–22 years (average 15–18)
Reproductive	—
Puberty	2–6 months
Estrus cycle	21 days (range 18–24 days)
Gestation	114 days (range 113–115)
Litter size	6–8 average (range 1–15)

[a]Derived from Mozzachio and Asseo; Burlatschenko (Chapter 4); Mozzachio personal observation.

*In my experience, rectal temperatures as low as 96°F (36°C) are not uncommon.

posturing with only drips or squirts rather than a steady stream may be due to crystalluria or urolithiasis; in males, this warrants immediate investigation as the issue is urgent if not emergent.

If urinalysis is desired, the owner should be asked to collect a fresh urine sample near the time of appointment, although this is easier said than done. However, as difficult as it may be for the owner to catch a sample, it is nearly impossible for a stranger (e.g., veterinary staff) to approach a pig during urination. Cystocentesis can be performed but requires restraint, possibly sedation, and is technically more difficult than in the dog or cat given inability to palpate the bladder, especially in an obese animal. Ultrasound guidance may be helpful. See Chapter 7 for more tips on urine collection.

THE HANDS–ON EXAMINATION
Vital Signs

Temperature, pulse, and respiration can be measured in tractable patients; otherwise, respiration rate (prior to handling) and rectal temperature can be obtained at a minimum. Normal biological and physiological parameters for miniature pigs are listed in Table 6.1.

Auscultation

Heart, lung, and gut sounds can be auscultated in less vocal patients; obesity can interfere, but a pulse oximeter probe placed on the pinna (also vulva or wattle, if present) may allow at least heart rate determination.

Eyes

Complete ophthalmologic exam may not be feasible or is limited, unless the animal is small enough to be held in the arms or is restrained in a sling to limit movement. Additionally, pigs have tight eyelids and abundant periocular fat that inhibits access, especially in brachycephalic conformations with deep-set eyes. At a minimum, eyelids, conjunctiva, cornea, and lens can be examined to evaluate for obvious abnormalities such as entropion or cataract (Fig. 6.10). Bulging of the conjunctiva is sometimes seen on the lateral aspect of the lower eyelid and may be a normal finding related to periocular fat distribution and should not be confused with chemosis or edema (Ehall 2012).

Ears

A copious amount of dark brown, typically greasy, ear wax is normal in minipigs (Fig. 6.14) and resembles ear mite infestation in dogs/cats, but although reported in the miniature pet pig (Reeves 1991), this is extremely rare. The external ear canal may be cleaned with moistened gauze or cotton ball if desired but should never be cleaned by putting fluid directly into the ear canal (i.e., do *not* clean like a dog/cat as trapping of fluid frequently causes head tilt); pet grooming wipes also work well. Do not insert swabs into the canal as the anatomy of the pig lends to pushing wax deeper rather than removing it. Luckily, ear problems are relatively uncommon, with head tilt or shaking the most common manifestation (Tynes 1999). Cytologic evaluation of aural secretions typically reveals numerous yeast, which must be interpreted in light of clinical signs as this may be considered within normal limits for a pig.

Oral Cavity

Care should be taken around the mouth of the pig— their strong bite is crushing, and even well–socialized

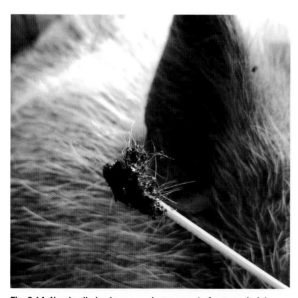

Fig. 6.14 Nearly all pigs bear a copious amount of greasy, dark brown ear wax, which resembles ear mite infestation in the dog or cat, but this is rarely (if ever) diagnosed in the minipig. Cleaning is not necessary but may be preferred by the owner and can be accomplished with a moistened cotton ball or pet grooming wipes. Fluid should never be placed directly into the ear as is done for dogs/cats.

animals presume any approach to be presentation of a snack and may accidentally bite. The mouth cannot be forced open for examination so is best evaluated while feeding a treat (Fig. 6.11) or while flipped and vocalizing. Sedation is necessary for complete oral exam.

Palpation

Palpation of the body, skin, and limbs is possible and may be necessary to verify body condition in hairy pigs (i.e., a thick hair coat can disguise a thin body condition). Abdominal palpation is generally unrewarding in an awake patient; in a sedated patient, abdominal palpation may be hampered by the feces– filled, mass–like spiral colon. Peripheral lymph nodes are not typically palpable in pigs.

Congenital Conditions

Piglets should be examined for patency of the anus as atresia ani is a common birth defect and may not be evident to owners until weaning. The testicles of intact males can be palpated to ensure scrotal location (if not readily apparent on visual exam) and checked for scrotal hernia.

Normal Anatomic Structures

Mental Gland. The mental gland appears as a round midline "lump" on the ventral aspect of the chin and has both scent–marking and tactile functions (Fig. 6.15A).

Carpal Glands. Carpal glands are scent marking glands found on the medial aspect of the forelimbs, forming a linear arrangement parallel to the limb (Fig. 6.15B). White to brown, pasty debris can sometimes be expressed from the glands and inspissation of secretion is common.

Preputial Diverticulum. The preputial diverticulum is a butterfly–shaped sac that surrounds the preputial opening on the mid-abdomen (Fig. 6.15C). It fills with foul-smelling smegma in intact males, and although the odor is less pungent and the sac less likely to fill in castrated males, it is still possible. This sac can become quite large and prominent and should not be confused with an umbilical hernia. Surgical removal is possible (Lawhorn et al. 1994) but generally unnecessary. The preputial diverticulum often

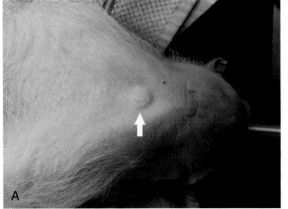

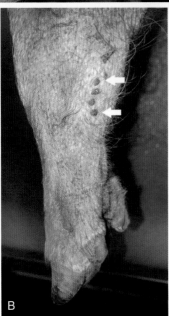

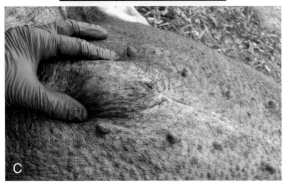

Fig. 6.15 Normal anatomical structures in the miniature pig include: (A) mental gland, (B) carpal glands, (C) preputial diverticulum.

swells dramatically immediately post-castration and may cause concern for owners.

THE SICK PIG

Although some signs (e.g., limping, coughing, diarrhea) may be obvious and similar to those observed in other species. Pigs are stoic and while they may not be actively hiding illness, clinical signs can be subtle and difficult to recognize (Mozzachio and Tynes 2014). Additionally, when on high alert during examination, clinical signs may disappear in the face of adrenalin.

Activity

A sick pig will be less active, although this may be ascertained more from history than from direct evaluation. Most pigs rise to meet a stranger and will not lie down in an unfamiliar environment, so a pig that remains recumbent on initial approach is likely ill.

Appetite

A pig that does not readily eat his normal pelleted feed is ill, even if eating other foods. Older pigs with neoplasia or organ failure, for example, stop eating their normal pelleted ration but are willing to eat a variety of other foods offered. They often accept one type of food only to refuse after a few days and move on to a different food item. Owners frequently disregard this behavior as long as the pig is eating something, but a finicky appetite is a sign of illness.

A pig fed an appropriate amount should eat all feed offered. Pigs with dental issues may gingerly prehend harder foods such as carrots or apples or begin to refuse these altogether. Dental problems may cause the pig to demonstrate an unusual/atypical chewing pattern (using only one side of the mouth or dropping food) or may cause the animal to shake or tilt the head when eating. Offering a food item as part of the evaluation may help differentiate desire to eat versus difficulty in prehension, chewing, or swallowing. A nauseous pig may show initial interest in a novel food item then turn the head away and refuse, may salivate excessively, smack the lips, or stand with the snout held against the ground.

Vocalizations

Pigs are vocal animals and produce a wide variety of sounds requiring some practice to distinguish and interpret. High–pitched vocalizations can indicate pain and are of a different character than those made when the pig is simply annoyed. Vocalizations made during a bout of Dippity Pig (see Chapter 10), for example, can be found in online videos and are representative of the kind of squeal made when a pig is experiencing intense pain.

Lip Smacking/Teeth Grinding

Repeated smacking of the lips or grinding of the teeth can indicate nausea or pain, especially of the gastrointestinal tract. However, these behaviors must be interpreted in light of the complete physical examination, as lip smacking can be a challenge from an aggressive pig while teeth grinding might be due to dental issues, stress, or boredom.

Abnormal Postures

A pig that is hunched may be experiencing active pain, including abdominal or musculoskeletal pain. However, an aged arthritic pig can also have severe bridging spondylosis that simply limits mobility of the spine but does not cause overt pain. A hunched posture is most often interpreted as constipation; however, this is an infrequent issue in my experience and other potential causes should be investigated.

A male pig that appears dull yet agitated, moving around then repeatedly stopping with the tail raised, may be suffering from urinary tract obstruction. There is often abdominal pushing, which may expel a few dry fecal balls. This is frequently interpreted as constipation by both owner and veterinarian, but the urinary tract should also be evaluated as blockage constitutes an emergency. See Urinary Tract Obstruction; Urolithiasis in Chapter 10 for more detailed information.

Pigs do not typically dog–sit, especially in an unfamiliar environment or in the presence of a stranger, so this posture warrants further investigation (Fig. 6.16). A dog–sitting pig hanging the head may be orthopneic, with the animal sitting in the

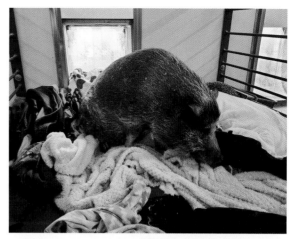

Fig. 6.16 Pigs will not normally maintain a sitting position in an unfamiliar environment or in the presence of a stranger, so this posture is generally considered to be abnormal, especially given the lowered head in this animal. This pig presented for lethargy and inappetence, and although respiration rate was slightly elevated, dyspnea was not observed and auscultation was unremarkable. In this case, the abnormal position was considered due to orthopnea as the pig died a few days later of severe pneumonia.

most comfortable position to breathe, even in the absence of tachypnea or dyspnea. Severe abdominal pain, such as that which might occur with intestinal volvulus, may present similarly. Imaging, including radiographs or ultrasound, may be indicated in these animals.

An animal that shifts position frequently or repeatedly lies down then rises again is likely in pain. Visceral pain is most likely; musculoskeletal pain does not tend to result in constant repositioning as pain is alleviated with immobility.

Floppy Ears

The normally upright pinnae may lose turgor and become floppy or begin to curl in a sick animal (Fig. 6.17). This is a non-specific finding but seems to be an indicator of severe illness in miniature pigs, although etiology is unknown. Thorough evaluation, possible hospitalization, is indicated as this finding is a poor prognostic indicator in my experience.

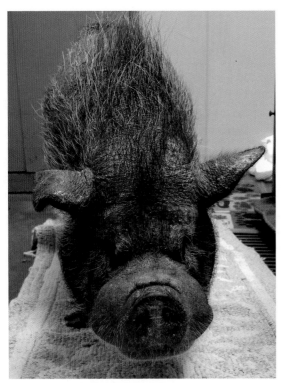

Fig. 6.17 The normally upright ears of a miniature pig may lose turgor and begin to flop over in extremely sick animals; this finding is non-specific and etiology is unknown. Blood work revealed this pig to be in renal failure.

BIBLIOGRAPHY

Dyce KM, Sack WO, Wensing CJG. The head and ventral neck of the pig. In: Singh B, ed. *Dyce, Sack and Wensing's Textbook of Veterinary Anatomy.* St. Louis, MI: Elsevier Inc; 2018:741–743. 5th ed.

Ehall H. Ocular examination and background observations. In: McAnulty PA, Dayan AD, Hastings K, Ganderup N, eds, et al. *The Minipig in Biomedical Research.* Boca Raton, FL: CRC Press; 2012:293–303.

Jackson PGG, Cockcroft PD. The pet pig. In: *Handbook of Pig Medicine.* Philadelphia, PA: Elsevier Ltd; 2007:212–219.

Lawhorn B. Defluvium in pot-bellied pigs. *Texas Veterinarian.* 1993:17.

Lawhorn BL, Jarrett PD, Lackey GF, et al. Removal of the preputial diverticulum in swine. *J Am Vet Med Assoc.* 1994;205:92–96.

Mozzachio K, Asseo L. Miniature pigs. In: Carpenter JW, ed. *Exotic Animal Formulary.* 6th ed. In press.

Mozzachio K, Tynes VV. Recognition and treatment of pain in pet pigs. In: Egger CM, Love L, Doherty T, eds. *Pain Management in Veterinary Practice.* Ames, IA: John Wiley & Sons, Inc.; 2014:383–389.

Reeves DE. Parasite control in miniature pet pigs. In: Reeves DE, ed. *Guidelines for the Veterinary Practitioner: Care and Management of Miniature Pet Pigs.* Santa Barbara, CA: Brillig Hill, Inc.; 1991:101.

Scott DW. Porcine. In: *Color Atlas of Farm Animal Dermatology.* 2nd ed. Hoboken, NJ: John Wiley & Sons, Inc.; 2018:235–292.

Tynes VV. Preventive health care for pet potbellied pigs. *Vet Clin North Am Exot Anim Pract.* 1999;2(2):495–510.

Wilbers AM. Handling pet pigs as patients. Presentation at: North American Veterinary Conference. Orlando, FL.: NAVC; 2013: 333–335.

Chapter 7

Routine Procedures

Kristie Mozzachio

Overview

Routine maintenance care of the miniature pet pig includes physical examination (see Chapter 6), vaccination, deworming, hoof trim, tusk trim, and clinical pathology evaluation such as complete blood count (CBC), chemistry, and urinalysis (UA); spay or castration is recommended for all pets and is covered in Chapter 9. Yearly physical exam is recommended for otherwise healthy animals, most vaccinations are boostered yearly, and hoof and tusk trim are performed as needed. Hoof trim is commonly performed every 6 to 8 months but may be necessary as often as every 2 to 3 months in some pigs. Tusk trim may be needed every 6 months (intact) to every 1 to 5 years (castrated) but may not be necessary in all males; females do not typically require tusk trim. Fecal flotation can be performed yearly in most pets and a deworming protocol determined from results. In "open" herds with constant influx of new animals, fecal monitoring can be increased to every 4 to 6 months and suitable antiparasitic medications used in rotation to help diminish parasite burden. Extrapolating from general guidelines for the dog and cat, surveillance CBC, chemistry, and UA diagnostic testing should be performed at a young age (1 to 6 years) to establish a baseline, every 1 to 2 years for mature adults (6 to 12 years), and yearly to twice yearly for senior animals (12+ years).

Vaccination

There is no single widely accepted vaccination protocol for miniature pet pigs, but suggestions can be found in Table 7.1. The veterinarian must assess risk based on age, environment, breeding status, and geographical location to determine likelihood of exposure; zoning regulations may also require certain vaccinations. Commercially available vaccines are manufactured for farmed swine and labeled as such. Many are available as combination products and 1 to 2 cc doses are common. However, 5 cc doses are occasionally listed, and although this volume is large for small minipigs, efficacy is not guaranteed if label instructions are not followed; given the numerous options available, products specifying smaller dose volumes may be more practical for miniature pet pigs. Severe reactions are rare but lethargy, anorexia, and slight elevation in body temperature may be observed for 12 to 24 hours post-vaccination (Tynes 1999). Larger dose volumes have anecdotally been associated with a higher incidence of adverse reactions, and leptospirosis vaccination, in particular, is also more likely to cause a reaction (Lawhorn 2013). Premedication with diphenhydramine (Benadryl®) or post-vaccination treatment with an oral non-steroidal antiinflammatory drug (NSAID) can ameliorate these effects.

There is also variability in vaccination intervals for the porcine pet population. Industry practice may necessitate vaccination of swine as early as a few weeks of age; however, maternal antibody can interfere with piglet response (Chase and Lunney 2019), so delaying initial vaccination in pets may be beneficial. Guidelines extrapolated from dogs and cats are acceptable (AAHA 2021), with initial dose(s) given as early as 6 to 8 weeks of age, then boostered in 2 to 4 weeks and yearly thereafter; rabies vaccination should be administered at or after 12 weeks of age, boostered yearly, and is considered off–label.

The most commonly used vaccines in miniature pet pigs in the United States include those for rabies, erysipelas, leptospirosis, and tetanus. Parvovirus vaccine should be considered for breeding animals as this is a reproductive disease in pigs, not diarrheal as in the canine. In larger groups such as breeding or rescue herds, respiratory issues or diarrhea outbreaks may

TABLE 7.1 Miniature Pig Vaccination Protocol		
The following are suggested vaccinations for pet miniature pigs in the United States. Age, environment, breeding status, and geographical location should be considered to determine risk level and vaccinations added or deleted as warranted.		
Disease	**Frequency**	**Comment**
Rabies	yearly	Off–label use of either small or large animal products, but recommended due to fatality rate and zoonotic potential
Erysipelas	every 6–12 months	Carried by healthy pigs as well as other animals and present in the environment; zoonotic potential
Leptospirosis	yearly	Zoonotic potential; vaccine more likely to cause mild adverse reaction
Tetanus	prn (i.e., with surgical procedures), maybe yearly	Control primarily through prevention of wound contamination via good sanitation practices and wound cleansing

warrant future vaccination if the causative agent can be definitively identified. Interaction of commercial hogs and miniature pigs or residence outside of North America may warrant further investigation into common diseases for which pet pigs may be at risk.

ADMINISTRATION

Vaccines are labeled for either intramuscular (IM) and/or subcutaneous (SQ) administration. A 1- to 1.5-in, 20- to 22-gauge needle is recommended.

Intramuscular

IM administration can be performed in the lateral neck region behind the ear (Fig. 7.1) while the pig is distracted with food. One well–tolerated technique involves firm scratching of the area prior to rapid needle placement, and once the pig recovers from insertion, the syringe can be attached and the neck continuously scratched during injection. Another technique uses "a slapping motion to instill a butterfly catheter" followed by injection of medication while the pig moves about the area (McCrackin and Swindle 2016). Pigs tend to react less to injections into the neck muscle versus injections into the hind leg; however, increased fat deposition may dictate alternate IM access in certain individuals, and the semimembranosus or semitendinosus muscles have less fat cover and are readily accessible. While adults often have little reaction to injection if otherwise occupied (i.e., with food or belly rub), young pigs tend to be overly dramatic and will likely require some form of physical

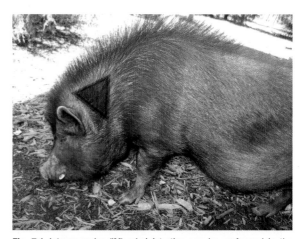

Fig. 7.1 Intramuscular (IM) administration can be performed in the lateral neck region, behind the ear (darkened triangle), and is less sensitive than injections into the hind leg. However, fat deposition may render this site inappropriate for IM access in overconditioned pets. This region on the left side (pictured) is also the preferred site for microchip placement.

restraint. Restraint can be minimal for simple injection (i.e., holding a small piglet or cornering a larger animal with sorting panels). See Chapter 5 for more information on restraint methods.

Subcutaneous

SQ injections can be given while the pig is standing and distracted with food or can be given during a belly rub in socialized pets. Skin is tightly adhered over most of the body and the subcutis only readily accessible in the folds of the axilla and inguinal areas

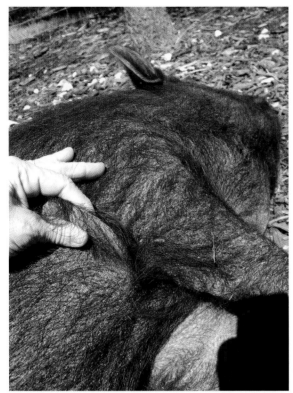

Fig. 7.2 Pig skin is tightly adhered over most of the body and the subcutis only readily accessible in the folds of the axilla (shown) and inguinal areas.

(Fig. 7.2). SQ vaccination commonly results in the formation of local nodules that may persist for several weeks, and owners should be forewarned.

VACCINATION OPTIONS

Rabies

Although reported cases in the United States are rare, pigs can contract rabies (de Macedo Pessoa et al. 2011; DuVernoy et al. 2008), and given the fatality rate and zoonotic potential, vaccination is recommended for at–risk animals. Both small animal and large animal products have been used at either the labeled 1 or 2 cc doses; boosters must be given yearly. This is considered an off-label use, but the vaccine is efficacious in all species tested and is expected to be effective in pigs as well. Titers performed in individual pet pigs support the presumption that the vaccine is efficacious in the porcine. For more information, see Chapter 10.

Erysipelas

Erysipelas is a disease caused by the organism, *Erysipelothrix rhusiopathiae*, and can cause acute or subacute septicemia, arthritis, or endocarditis, as well as result in abortion. Although it is a ubiquitous organism that can be carried in the tonsils of healthy animals, it can also be present in the environment, affects multiple species, and has zoonotic potential. Vaccination is effective against acute disease but may not be as effective in preventing chronic forms. Immunity lasts 6 to 12 months, and biannual to yearly boosters are recommended for pet pigs. Both oral and injectable forms of the vaccine exist. For more information, see Chapter 10.

Leptospirosis

Vaccination against leptospirosis is primarily recommended for breeding herds in the commercial industry to avoid reproductive losses, but individual non-breeding pet pigs can suffer clinical disease as in any other small animal species, plus zoonotic potential must be considered. In endemic areas (i.e., Hawaii), vaccination may be prudent. Anecdotally, the leptospirosis vaccine is more likely to cause mild adverse reactions.

Tetanus

Tetanus has been reported only rarely in miniature pigs, likely due to limited exposure, as most infections in swine occur through castration incisions or umbilical infections in a soiled environment (Uzal and Songer 2019). The extremely low incidence of reported disease in pets is unusual, though, given common wounding through pig-to-pig aggression or dog attack as well as the common practice of field surgery. The susceptibility of pigs to the tetanus toxin has not been reported as is the case for other animal species (Popoff 2016), but my personal suspicion is that pigs are relatively resistant. If exposure is likely, vaccination is recommended, particularly following castration or other field surgical procedures; however, the primary means of control is through prevention of wound contamination via good sanitation practices and wound cleansing.

Bordetella/Pasteurella

Bordetella bronchiseptica and *Pasteurella multicoda* are respiratory pathogens associated with atrophic rhinitis. Disease is characterized by mild upper respiratory signs such as sneezing, coughing, and excessive lacrimation, but toxigenic strains can cause abnormal turbinate development in young, growing animals that may permanently distort the snout. Vaccination is recommended for pregnant sows at about 4 and 2 weeks prior to farrowing and at 1 and 4 weeks of age for piglets from unvaccinated dams; the need for vaccination of older pets is questionable as the most significant effects occur in growing animals (Register and Brockmeier 2019). This disease has not been a major issue in the miniature pig population, although vaccination may be given as part of a combination product such as Rhini Shield® TX4; a commonly used product that also protects against erysipelas.

Parvovirus

Parvovirus is a reproductive disease in the pig, resulting in stillbirths, mummification, embryonic death, and infertility (SMEDI syndrome). It is a ubiquitous virus and immunity can be achieved through vaccination as well as through field exposure. Current literature suggests that immunity may be short lived and revaccination of breeding sows every 4 to 6 months is recommended (Truyen and Streck 2019). However, infectious reproductive disease is uncommon in miniature pigs.

Diarrheal and Respiratory Disease

Diarrhea and pneumonia are common causes of morbidity and mortality in commercial swine operations, and vaccination protocols often cover a number of potential agents such as *Escherichia coli*, rotavirus, and transmissible gastroenteritis virus (TGE) for diarrhea or *Mycoplasma hyopneumoniae*, swine influenza virus, and *Actinobacillus pleuropneumonia* for respiratory disease. Individual pet pigs are typically at low risk for exposure to infectious agents and are often symptomatically treated when ill, regardless of underlying etiology, so preventative vaccination may be unnecessary. In herd outbreaks (e.g., rescue or breeding herd), identification of the etiologic agent is necessary to determine vaccination(s) most likely to provide control. In some instances, antemortem diagnostic options may be available (i.e., Iowa State University offers a host of tests including ELISA, PCR, and culture; https://vetmed.iastate.edu/vdl/laboratories/phast/pdf-forms),

but most infectious agents are identified at necropsy. If disease is severe enough to cause death, necropsy is warranted, and this can then dictate vaccination protocol for the rest of the herd.

Porcine Reproductive and Respiratory Syndrome Virus

Porcine Reproductive and Respiratory Syndrome Virus is mentioned only because it is so common in commercial swine. However, routine postmortem screening by diagnostic laboratories has not revealed this to be an important pathogen in the miniature pig. If there is interaction between farm swine and miniature pigs, vaccination should be considered as the organism is ubiquitous in the former, while the latter may be naive and subject to more intense disease as a result.

Parasite Control

The majority of pet miniature pigs in North America, excluding high volume operations such as a breeder or rescue, have little issue with internal parasites. The one exception in my personal experience might be the Kunekune breed. These pigs may harbor parasites routinely, even in pet households, although they still do not typically develop associated clinical illness. Healthy pigs should be dewormed at a young age or when newly acquired then monitored through regularly scheduled fecal flotation (i.e., yearly for individual pet households, every 4 to 6 months for larger herds). If a pig is sick, by all means, test and treat for internal parasites as needed but continue to look for other underlying illness. Gastrointestinal parasites infrequently cause major disease, much different from commercial swine counterparts or other livestock species. External parasitism, the most common of which is sarcoptic mange, is more likely to cause clinical illness but is readily treated.

DIAGNOSIS

Fecal flotation is performed as for other small animal species, such as a dog or cat, and ova are similar in appearance. Fresh feces are preferably sampled immediately from an observed defecation or from the rectum and can be stored in a refrigerator (approximately 39°F, 4°C) for more than 3 weeks without significant changes in egg counts (Roepstorff and Nansen 1998).

TABLE 7.2 Miniature Pig Antiparasitic Medications[a]

Agent	Dose/Route	Frequency	Effective Against	Comment
Internal Parasites[b]				
Avermectins (ivermectin, doramectin)	0.3 mg/kg IM, SQ, or PO	Once for prevention; repeat in 14 days for a minimum of 2 doses for treatment	Roundworm, stomach worm, nodular worm, lungworm, kidney worm, threadworm	Also effective against mange mites, lice and larval flies; doramectin activity persists longer than ivermectin (Arends et al. 1999) and redosing interval can be as long as 3 weeks
Fenbendazole	9 mg/kg PO	Once for prevention; give in divided doses over 3–12 days for treatment	Roundworm, stomach worm, nodular worm, whipworm, lungworm, kidney worm	One of the few agents effective against whipworms
Piperazine	275–440 mg/kg PO	Once	Roundworm, nodular worm	
Pyrantel	22 mg/kg PO	Once for prevention; give for 3 consecutive days to remove adults; administer continuously to address larval forms	Roundworm, nodular worm	
External Parasites				
Coumaphos (Co-Ral®, Bayer)	Topical dust or spray	Treat once, reapply if needed no sooner than 10 days	Lice	Product label instructions for mixing and/or application should be followed[c]
Fipronil (Frontline® Spray, Boehringer Ingelheim)	Topical spray	Treat once, reapply if needed no sooner than 30 days	Ticks (off-label use in pigs)	
Permethrin (Permectrin™, Bayer)	Topical powder, spray, pour-on	Treat once, reapply if needed no sooner than 2 weeks	Mites, lice, ticks, flies, mosquitos	
Phosmet (Prolate/Lintox HD™, Central Life Sciences)	Topical spray	Treat once, reapply if needed in 14 days	Mites, lice	

[a]Jacela et al. 2009; Mozzachio and Asseo, in press; swine product labels.
[b]Nematodes are the primary internal parasites affecting miniature pet pigs, although clinical illness is rather uncommon; protozoa, cestodes and trematodes rarely cause disease and are not typically treated. Sanitation (i.e., removal of feces, pen rotation) is necessary to prevent reinfection.
[c]Pet pigs often react unfavorably to topical liquids, so powder/dust may be preferable for ease of application.

Skin scrape is warranted if mange is suspected and performed as for a dog or cat. Collection of material from the ear often gives a higher parasite yield with *Sarcoptes* infection (Brewer and Greve 2019).

TREATMENT

Treatment (Table 7.2) involves deworming with an appropriate antiparasitic medication on a schedule that accounts for the prepatent period in order to address emerging larvae (i.e., repeat dosing prior to the minimum prepatent period to kill adult forms and prevent laying of eggs); reduction of environmental contamination (i.e., poop scooping or pasture rotation) is indicated to prevent reinfection. A preventative deworming schedule can be developed for "open" herds such as breeding or rescue facilities and can be monitored through fecal flotation. Regular deworming with a broad spectrum anthelmintic such as ivermectin ± fenbendazole can be performed every 4 to 6 months in well-controlled herds, although medication choice and frequency should be adjusted as needed based on fecal evaluations. Open herds should also have good sanitation practices as well as quarantine to keep parasites (and other contagious disease) in check.

Administration Tips

Oral medication is often preferred due to ease of administration, and many pigs readily accept flavored preparations or those mixed with yogurt, apple sauce, or bread/cake. Note: Flavored horse dewormers are usually palatable to pigs, but liquid formulations are preferred as pastes are difficult to dispense at the doses needed for pet pigs.

Medicated feeds are commercially available (e.g., Safe-Guard® [fenbendazole] is available as a feed pellet). This is an option if pigs are fed separately, and it can be assured that the entire dose is ingested. Otherwise, oral administration of a concentrated injectable form (such as ivermectin) in a treat that will be readily and quickly consumed is suggested. Medications for commercial swine also include those added to the water; however, this is not recommended in pet pigs as altered taste may reduce water intake.

Internal Parasites

The following provides a brief overview of internal parasites known to affect swine. However, most are uncommon in the US pet pig population, with *Ascaris suum* most frequently identified. Strongyle–type ova are also common in low numbers, but larval examination is needed for speciation and is not typically performed. The majority of internal parasites are transmitted through ingestion of the infective form, and sometimes an intermediate host is involved. Detection is generally via fecal flotation, although urine evaluation is necessary to detect the kidney worm.

HELMINTHS

Ascaris suum (Large Roundworm)

The largest of the intestinal nematodes, up to 40 cm long, inhabits the small bowel. Large numbers of

intermittently shed eggs pass in the feces and develop into an infective form in the environment within 3 to 4 weeks. Eggs are resistant to chemical treatment and can survive in the environment for over 10 years, although heat, direct sunlight, or low moisture significantly reduce survival. The life cycle is direct and ingested eggs hatch in the intestine to release larvae that penetrate the intestinal wall and migrate to the liver and lungs; while migrating forms can cause significant clinical disease in commercial swine including respiratory signs and generalized unthriftiness, this is rare in the pet population. The prepatent period is 6 to 8 weeks. A number of antiparasitic agents are effective against ascarids, including palatable oral forms that a pet pig may readily ingest. Expect large white worms in the feces post-treatment (Fig. 7.3). Previously exposed pigs mount an immune response that limits clinical signs, although adult pigs may still be carriers that contribute to environmental contamination (Brewer and Greve 2019).

Hyostrongylus rubidus (Red Stomach Worm)

These tiny red blood-sucking worms, less than 10 mm long and the width of a hair, live in the stomach and tend to be clinically insignificant (Brewer and Greve

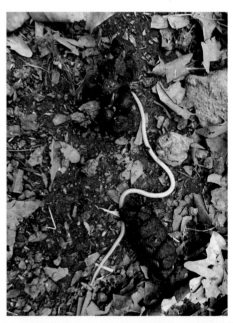

Fig. 7.3 Large white *Ascaris suum* worm expelled with feces following deworming.

2019; Reeves 1991). Eggs pass in the feces and hatch to an infective larval form in the environment. The life cycle is direct and ingested larvae enter gastric gland pits to develop for approximately 2 weeks before emerging into the stomach lumen, although larvae can remain in the mucosa in a hypobiotic (arrested) state for several months; the prepatent period is 3 weeks. Ova cannot be distinguished from *Oesophagostomum* spp. as both are typical strongyle–type eggs.

Macracanthorhynchus hirudinaceus (Thorny–Headed Worm)

This large worm inhabits the small intestine and is grossly similar to *Ascaris suum,* with the exception of a spiny proboscis used to firmly attach to the intestinal wall. Although small granulomas develop at the site of attachment, clinical signs are usually absent. Ante-mortem diagnosis can be difficult as the eggs may not float, so sedimentation may be necessary to confirm infection. The life cycle is indirect, and the intermediate host is the beetle.

Metastrongylus spp. (Lungworm)

As indicated by the common name, these worms live within bronchi and bronchioles of the lungs. Eggs are coughed up, swallowed, then passed in the feces; the earthworm is the intermediate host, and pigs become infected through earthworm ingestion. Larvae penetrate the small intestinal wall and are transported via the lymphatic system through the heart to the lungs. The prepatent period is about 30 days. Cough is the primary clinical sign. Confirmation of infection through fecal flotation may be problematic as ova do not reliably float.

Oesophagostomum spp. (Nodular Worm)

This small slender worm inhabits the large intestine, with larval forms responsible for the characteristic nodules. Eggs pass in the feces and infective larvae develop in the environment. Ingested larvae burrow into cecal and colonic mucosa and later emerge into the lumen, with a prepatent period of about 3 to 6 weeks. Non-specific clinical signs of depression, anorexia, or diarrhea are often related to secondary infection associated with intestinal damage by larval forms, but most infections are asymptomatic. Eggs are strongyle-type and may be difficult to differentiate from similar ova.

Stephanurus dentatus (Kidney Worm)

Large, robust, adults up to 5 cm long are found in the perirenal fat within cysts that open into ureters or kidneys via a fistula. Strongyle-type eggs pass in the urine and infective larvae develop in the environment where they are either ingested or penetrate the skin. Larvae migrate from intestine or skin to mesenteric lymph nodes and liver, then migrate through the body cavity to reach the perirenal area. The prepatent period can be as long as a year, therefore infection is not seen in young piglets. Aggressive larval migration can cause lesions observed at necropsy but not necessarily attributed to clinical disease; reduced growth is the most common finding in infected swine.

Strongyloides ransomi (Threadworm)

The threadworm is a tiny, thin worm, just 3 to 5 mm long, and only the parthenogenetic female is parasitic. Embryonated eggs are passed in the feces and hatch directly into infective female larvae or can produce free-living male and female larvae that then propagate in the environment. Infection occurs through penetration of skin or oral mucosa, through colostrum, or can occur in utero, and larvae are carried by the bloodstream to the lungs where they are coughed up and swallowed. The prepatent period is 4 to 9 days. Adults are found in the small intestine and non-specific clinical signs may include diarrhea and stunted growth.

Trichuris suis (Whipworm)

Similar to whipworms in other species, the swine version lives in the cecum and colon, with the proximal two-thirds of its whiplike body buried within the mucosa. Sporadically shed, lemon-shaped (double-operculated) eggs pass in the feces and infective larvae develop within the egg until ingested by a pig. Eggs are resistant to chemical treatment—though susceptible to desiccation—and can remain viable in the environment for 3 to 4 years. After ingestion, migrating larvae penetrate cecal and colonic mucosa and clinical disease commonly occurs before adults are present. Low numbers of sporadically shed eggs and the long 6- to 8-week prepatent period may lead to false negatives on fecal flotation. Light infection is typically subclinical, but a heavy worm burden can cause mucoid to bloody diarrhea and intestinal damage may lead to secondary bacterial infection.

PROTOZOA

Protozoan parasites including coccidia, *Cryptosporidium*, and *Giardia* infrequently cause clinical disease, usually limited to diarrhea in young piglets (Grand 2012), and detection of these parasites on routine fecal evaluation should be interpreted in light of this. Treatment is rarely warranted and limited by a lack of approved or effective drugs. For example, toltrazuril is the primary medication used to treat neonatal coccidiosis but is not available in the United States; there are no known effective treatments for *Cryptosporidium* (Lindsay et al. 2019). In commercial operations, improved sanitation is the primary means of control and miniature pet pigs are usually maintained in a clean environment.

CESTODES

Unlike a dog or cat, pigs are not generally a definitive host for adult tapeworms. However, swine can be intermediate hosts for *Taenia* and *Echinococcus* species. These can be important in terms of public health but involve ingestion of porcine tissue and are typically diagnosed at necropsy.

TREMATODES

Both *Paragonimus kellicotti* (lung fluke) and *Fasciola hepatica* (liver fluke) infect a variety of species, including swine, and transmission requires a snail and/or crayfish intermediate host. Clinical signs are uncommon and non-specific. Antemortem diagnosis requires a sedimentation technique as ova do not readily float.

External Parasites

Unlike infection with internal parasites, external parasitism often manifests clinically and sarcoptic mange is most common. Louse infestation is occasionally noted; ear mites have been reported (Reeves 1991) but infestation is extremely rare. Although pet pigs can be bitten by fleas, they are not a definitive host and individual treatment is usually unnecessary (although other pets in the household may require treatment if fleas are identified).

DEMODEX PHYLLOIDES

Demodecosis is not reported to be clinically relevant in pigs, although low numbers of mites may be identified

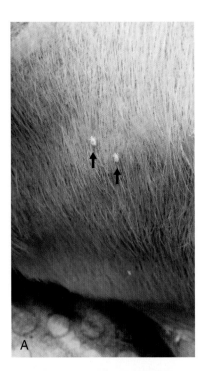

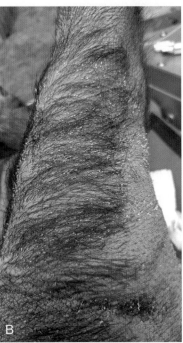

Fig. 7.4 (A) *Hematopinus suis* is a large bloodsucking louse, readily visible and highlighted by permethrin dust treatment in this image (*arrows*). (B) Nits attach to the base of the hair shafts (vs. blow fly eggs which are more diffusely distributed).

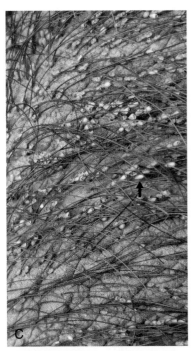

Fig. 7.4, cont'd (C) Viable nits have a smooth pearly white appearance (*arrow*), while dead or hatched nits are tan and irregular.

Swine lice are vectors of swine pox and associated lesions may be observed, although this disease is uncommon in the pet population. Affected pigs can be treated topically with dusts, sprays, or pour-ons, and cleaning/treatment of the environment is also recommended. Systemic treatment is also effective as nymphs and adults are bloodsucking rather than chewing.

SARCOPTES SCABIEI VAR. *SUIS* (MANGE MITE)

The pig mange mite is host specific, and infestation is through direct contact with other pigs as survival in the environment is only about 3 days. As with mange mites in other species, the adult lives within the epidermis and is not visible to the naked eye. Eggs laid by burrowing females hatch and mature to egg–laying adults in 10 to 25 days (Brewer and Greve 2019). Clinical signs in acute disease include intense pruritis, excoriation/abrasion from self–trauma, erythema, hair loss, papules, and hyperkeratotic crusting (Fig. 7.5). Chronic disease is

on deep skin scrapings as they are thought to be part of the normal flora of mammals (Brewer and Greve 2019).

HAEMATOPINUS SUIS (PIG LOUSE)

Lice are species–specific and the pig louse is the largest (5 to 6 mm), easily visible to the naked eye. The adult louse is long and flat–bodied, gray-brown in color, and can be seen crawling over the body (Fig. 7.4A). Small white to tan nits are cemented to the lower part of hair shafts (to differentiate from blow fly eggs which are more diffusely distributed); nits hatch in 12 to 20 days (Fig. 7.4B & C) (Brewer and Greve 2019). Spread is via direct contact as adults have limited survival in the environment (2 to 3 days). The swine louse is blood–sucking and severe infestation can cause anemia and related signs such as pallor, weakness, and lethargy, especially in small pigs. Pruritis and associated self–trauma are more typical clinical signs, although some pigs seem unaffected, with infestation noted incidentally on routine exam.

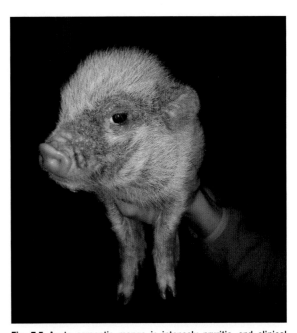

Fig. 7.5 Acute sarcoptic mange is intensely pruritic, and clinical signs include excoriation/abrasion from self–trauma, erythema, hair loss, papules, and hyperkeratotic crusting. As acute disease involves a hypersensitivity reaction, few mites may be present which can hinder definitive diagnosis. However, clinical signs warrant treatment regardless.

asymptomatic and manifests only as isolated areas of hyperkeratosis, but these pigs can serve as reservoirs for infection of naive animals. Diagnosis is confirmed through visualization of adults or ova on skin scrape, and crusts from the inner surface of the pinnae and outer ear canal are often high yield. The acute form involves a hypersensitivity reaction so few mites may be present and, thus, hinder definitive diagnosis; mites are numerous in the chronic form. Treatment options include ivermectin 300 mcg/kg SQ repeated in 2 weeks or doramectin 300 mcg/kg IM repeated in 3 weeks (Lawhorn 2013). Differential diagnoses for the aforementioned skin lesions include exudative epidermitis (greasy pig disease), dermatomycosis, swine pox, sunburn, parakeratosis, photosensitization, niacin and biotin deficiencies (Brewer and Greve 2019) as well as cutaneous lymphoma, although sarcoptic mange is by far the most common of these in the pet pig population. Humans in close contact with affected pigs may develop a temporary dermatitis.

OTHER EXTERNAL PARASITES

Fleas, mosquitoes, flies, fire ants, ticks, etc. are not host–specific and will bite pigs, although serious issues are uncommon. Pigs often react strongly to insect bites and develop large, erythematous papules typically over the ventrum, axilla and inguinal areas, and behind the ears where skin is thinnest and/or ground contact more likely. Treatment is generally unnecessary, although environmental modification may be warranted (i.e., improved sanitation if flies are an issue, removal of leaf litter with ticks, restriction of access to ant mounds).

Hoof Care

Pigs have a pair of principal digits (weight–bearing claws) and a pair of accessory digits (dew claws) per leg. Common genetic anomalies include syndactyly (mulefoot) as well as polydactyly (Fig. 7.6), the latter especially common in dew claws. The anatomy of the hoof is similar to that of the bovine, but in terms of care might be better likened to the horse as regular hoof care is critical and sensitive laminae comprise the inner layers. As a result, the "quick" stays fixed and will not extend with overgrowth and recede with regular trimming as in the canine, and damage to the laminae during trim is not only painful but can have lingering effects on hoof wall growth. Non-veterinary

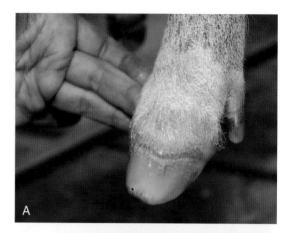

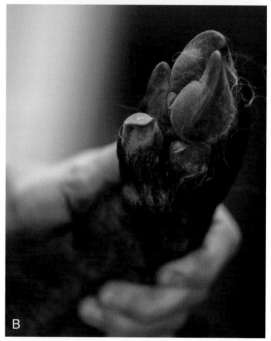

Fig. 7.6 Common congenital defects include (A) syndactyly (mulefoot) as well as (B) polydactyly. (B, Photo credit: Jennifer L. Davis.)

BOX 7.1 MINIPIG FARRIERS

Regular hoof care is a primary need of the pet pig and while veterinarians are often tasked to do this, there are several traveling "minipig farriers" available, offering services in all 50 US states and several foreign countries. See the following link for more information on one such service: https://www.mohrmethodgroup.com/. More options can be found at: https://www.facebook.com/groups/pigvetsandfarriers/about.

options for hoof care are available from a number of sources (Box 7.1).

FREQUENCY

Hoof trim frequency depends on several factors including genetics, age, diet, environment, disease, and ability of the owner to provide home hoof care. In general, a normal, healthy pig will require a hoof trim every 6 to 8 months, often beginning at about 10 to 12 months of age. Frequency may increase with hoof deformities, imbalance, cracking, laminitis, or with the development of arthritis. Extreme hoof overgrowth is common in pigs that spend a large amount of time indoors, and these animals may require a maintenance trim as often as every 2 to 3 months.

RESTRAINT

A hoof trim can be performed with or without chemical restraint. Oral trazodone and gabapentin ± acepromazine, administered approximately 2 to 3 hours prior to the appointment, can reduce struggling and stress without excessive sedation; midazolam administered intra-pig (SQ, IM, intra-nasal, orally, rectally) is quite effective, safe, and does not cause excessive sedation for this short, non-painful procedure. See Box 5.2 for drug doses. Of course, deeper sedation can be achieved with a variety of drugs when needed; see Chapter 8 for drug options and doses. Many pigs tolerate a sling device (if available) and will readily allow a hoof trim while receiving food treats or scratches. Some smaller pigs can be held across the lap while the trim is performed (Fig. 5.2A). The "flip" technique that positions the animal on its haunches or in dorsal recumbency is an excellent means of restraint (Fig. 5.6) and is safe and effective for most mini-pig patients. Further details can be found in Chapter 5.

HOOF TRIM TECHNIQUE

The goal of the porcine hoof trim is to return the hooves to normal shape and length and balance weight distribution – a bit more involved than simply chopping off excess length. Using appropriate trimmers/nippers, excess length should be removed from the main claws and dew claws to create short, rounded toes balanced over weight–bearing surfaces (Fig. 7.7). For more severe hoof overgrowth (Fig. 7.8), pony nippers may be necessary as overgrowth of this magnitude is extremely hard and

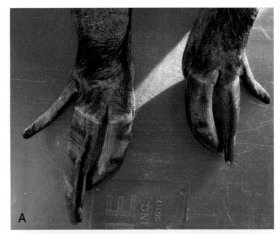

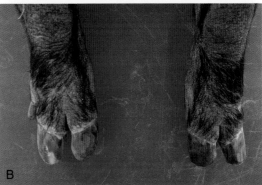

Fig. 7.7 The "quick" of a pig hoof is fixed and does not grow with the nail then recede with trimming as in a dog. Overgrowth should be trimmed with nippers and/or a grinding tool such as a rotary Dremel® to create short, rounded toes balanced along weight–bearing surfaces. Breaching of sensitive laminae can cause bleeding, pain, and lead to growth abnormalities. (A) Before trim. (B) After trim.

impossible to penetrate with smaller nippers. Care must be taken to avoid damage to the sensitive laminae, which is not only painful but can lead to growth abnormalities. Visualization of the "quick" can sometimes be enhanced by wetting the claw and backlighting with a light source, especially in darkly pigmented hooves (Fig. 7.9). Balancing can be performed and rough edges filed smooth with a grinding tool such as a Dremel® rotary tool or the Hoof Boss. Equipment needed for trim of hooves and tusks and sources to purchase such equipment are shown in Fig. 7.10.

A pig hoof should be trimmed for function over form. For example, if the distal phalanx is rotated, as might happen with arthritis or some congenital conditions, the

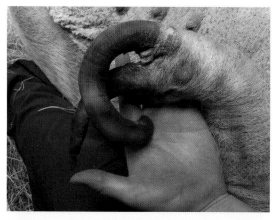

Fig. 7.8 Hoof overgrowth can be extreme, interfering greatly with ambulation and causing intense pressure on misaligned joints. Growth of such severity as that pictured is especially common in pets that spend a large amount of time indoors.

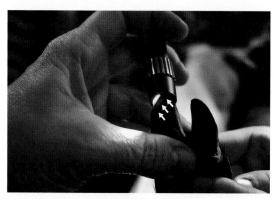

Fig. 7.9 Visualization of the "quick" can sometimes be enhanced by wetting the claw and backlighting with a light source. In this image, the blood supply *(arrows)* is dark relative to adjacent hoof wall along the tip and outside edge.

position of the laminae will be altered relative to the (abnormal) weight–bearing surface. This means that it may not be possible to level the bottom of the hoof proper as laminae will be exposed, causing bleeding and pain. Basically, try to create a short, rounded, functional toe within the limitations of each pig's anatomy and avoid "quicking."

Dentition

Pigs have the most complete dentition of the domestic mammals, with a total of 32 deciduous and 44 permanent

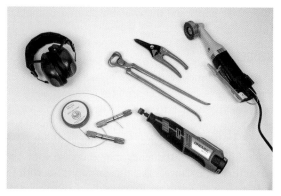

Fig. 7.10 Equipment needed for hoof and tusk trim includes hearing protection, large (pony) and small (goat) nippers, Hoof Boss and/or rotary tool such as a Dremel®, obstetric saw (gigli) wire, and saw wire handles. Options for purchase include: Small hoof trimmers – https://rossmillfarmstore.com/collections/grooming/products/hoof-trimmer; Rotary tool - https://us.dremel.com/en_US/products/-/show-product/tools/8220-12vmax-high-performance-cordless; Hoof Boss grinding tool - https://mybosstools.com/product/complete-pig-hoof-care-trimmer-set/. (Photo credit: Jennifer L. Davis.)

teeth. However, there are discrepancies in the literature over the dental formula. The most widely recognized formula for permanent dentition is 2x (I 3/3, C 1/1, P 4/4, M 3/3). The first premolar (P1) is a variable tooth that, when present, has been purported to be either a persistent deciduous tooth with no successor or a permanent tooth with no temporary precursor (Weaver et al. 1969). It has been reported that there are no deciduous precursors for any of the veterinary species that retain P1 (Smallwood 1992), so it stands to reason that this tooth in the pig would best be described as permanent. Yet there are histologic studies as far back as 1899 that describe the structure to be most like that of other deciduous teeth (Weaver et al. 1966). In 1966, Weaver et al. were the first to describe the deciduous dentition in miniature pigs of the Pitman–Moore strain, and at the time, there was controversy over whether the dentition included three or four molars. (Note: Teeth now considered to be deciduous premolars were originally classified as molars). The authors chose to designate the first tooth caudal to the canine as the first molar (m1), rather than designate it a premolar, followed by m2 to m4. Over the years, however, this tooth became more widely classified as the first premolar, and recent literature generally agrees that there are no more than three molars, all of them permanent.

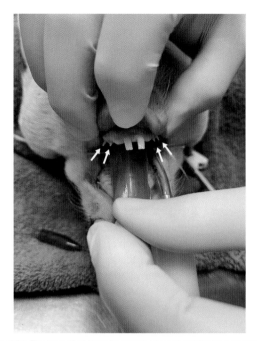

Fig. 7.11 The so-called "needle teeth" present at birth represent the deciduous upper and lower third incisors and canines *(arrows).* Although these teeth are often clipped in commercial piglets, clipping is unnecessary and not typically performed in miniature pet pigs.

TABLE 7.3 Porcine Dental Formula and Eruption Times

Porcine dental formula[a]: 2 (I 1–3/3, C 1/1, P 3–4/3–4, M 3/3) = 40–44 total teeth
Eruption sequence of permanent teeth[a,b]: (P1), M1, C, I3, M2, P3, P4, I1, P2, I2, M3 (maxilla)
(P1), M1, I3, C, M2, I1, P4, P3, P2, I2, M3 (mandible)

Tooth	Deciduous[c]	Permanent[c]
Incisor 1	1–4 weeks	12–16 months
Incisor 2	6–12 weeks	16–20 months
Incisor 3	Present at birth	8–12 months
Canine	Present at birth	8–12 months
Premolar 1[d]	—	4–24 months
Premolar 2	7–10 weeks	12–15 months
Premolar 3	1–5 weeks	12–15 months
Premolar 4	1–7 weeks	12–15 months
Molar 1	—	4–6 months
Molar 2	—	8–12 months
Molar 3	—	18–28 months

[a]Weaver et al. (1969).
[b]Herring et al. (2012).
[c]Eruption times are derived from Li (1993), Fails and Magee (2018), and Herring et al. 2012 but should be considered generalities as there is quite a bit of variation in reported eruption times in the porcine.
[d]There is controversy over the classification of the variable first premolar as deciduous or permanent; this tooth is more commonly present in the maxillary arch and frequently absent in the mandibular arch.

The majority of pig teeth are diphyodont and brachydont, except for the canines which are continuously growing aradicular hypsodont teeth (a.k.a. "open rooted" teeth [also called elodont]) (Fecchio et al. 2019; Lennox and Yasutsugu 2016; Smith et al. 2021). However, the canine teeth or tusks exhibit sexual dimorphism, and the root ultimately closes and tooth growth ceases in the female (Mayer and Brisbin 1988; Dyce 2018). The so-called "needle teeth" present at birth represent the deciduous upper and lower third incisors and canines (Fig. 7.11). These teeth are often clipped at birth in the commercial industry as the sharp points can damage the teats of the sow; however, clipping is not typically performed in miniature pet pigs nor is it recommended; it's simply unnecessary and has the potential to cause traumatic damage to the piglet. Deciduous teeth continue to erupt over the next several months and are fully erupted at 3 months of age (Herring et al. 2012; Li 1993), and permanent teeth erupt from about 4 months to 2 years of age (Li 1993; Weaver et al. 1969); see Table 7.3 for sequence and timing of eruption. Given this overlap, there is a prolonged period in which mixed dentition is present, one of the features making the porcine model well suited to research of human conditions. Beyond the eruption of the permanent teeth, there is no means to definitively determine the age of a pig using dentition. Thick tusks in males and mild to moderate calculus build-up can roughly point towards an age of 3 to 5+ years and multiple missing teeth perhaps an age of 8 to 10+ years, but these are generalities.

Pig teeth are suited to their omnivorous diet. Short upper incisors curve toward one another and meet the long, forward–projecting lower incisors to allow grasping, while upper and lower cheek teeth (premolars and molars) occlude along wide, convoluted surfaces to allow crushing and grinding. The cheek teeth also progressively increase in size moving caudally—a consideration for extraction as these teeth are difficult to access given narrow gape. There may be several

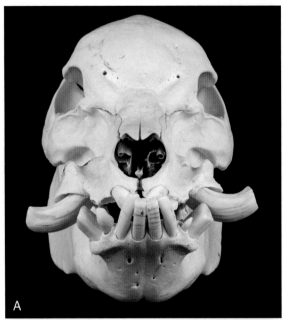

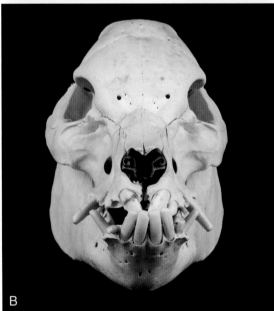

Fig. 7.12 The canine teeth or tusks grow throughout life in the male, while growth ceases at around 2 years of age in the female. In the male (A), tusks become thicker with age and the upper curves outward and upward and bears longitudinal grooves over the ventral aspect, while in the female (B), upper tusks extend in a lateral direction only, and grooves are absent. Note the horizontal lines on the crowns of the lower incisors in this male. These teeth are often cleanly broken off along these lines (in either sex), although associated clinical signs are uncommon. (Photo credit: Jennifer L. Davis.)

diastemata or gaps, including those associated with the upper and lower third incisors, upper and lower canines, and lower first premolars when present but there is considerable variability among individual miniature pigs; the interdental space caudal to the lower canine is the largest of these (Feldhamer and McCann 2004; Harvey and Penny 1985; Lennox and Yasutsugu 2016; Mozzachio, personal observation). The upper and lower canine teeth or tusks are so-called "open rooted" (aka "rootless") teeth that grow continuously in the male, while in the female the open root closes at approximately 2 years of age and growth ceases (Dyce 2018). A number of other differences are noted between male and female tusks (Fig. 7.12) including: the root of the lower tusk is longer in the male, extending through the body of the mandible to the level of M1–2, whereas that of the female extends only to the level of P1–3; the cross–sectional shape of both upper and lower tusks remains consistent over the entire length in the male but tapers to a point in the female; upper tusks in the male have longitudinal grooves along the ventral aspect that are absent in the female; upper tusks in the male curve outward and upward while those of the female extend in a lateral direction only; and males have enamel covering the crown and root while enamel is limited to the crown in the female, with a distinct enamocementum junction line (Mayer and Brisbin 1988).

Abnormalities of dentition are common in miniature pigs. The maxilla is frequently shortened such that upper and lower incisors no longer occlude; crowding of teeth is possible within the shortened jaws of these proportionate dwarves, and the caudal molars may not fully erupt (Fig. 7.13). Oligodonty is common as permanent teeth may fail to develop, and although polydonty should not be expected given that additional teeth would represent a number greater than that of the primitive eutherian number (Feldhamer and McCann 2004), supernumerary teeth have been identified in the species (Eubanks 2013; Malmsten et al. 2015).

Regardless of deviations, pet pigs have a lot of teeth with the potential for disease including periodontitis, caries, mobile or fractured teeth, malocclusion, and so on. To complicate matters, the pig also has a narrow gape; the mouth cannot be opened wide enough to readily evaluate the caudal oral cavity, let alone provide treatment in the far reaches of the mouth. In an

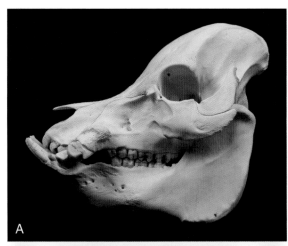

A

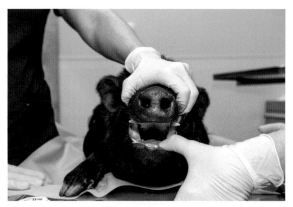

Fig. 7.14 As part of a routine health evaluation, thorough oral exam and regular dental prophylaxis is recommended for the pet pig, just as for a dog or cat. However, although technique is similar, dental care can be technically challenging given intubation difficulties and anatomical features such as narrow gape (pictured) which limits oral cavity access. (Photo credit: Jennifer L. Davis.)

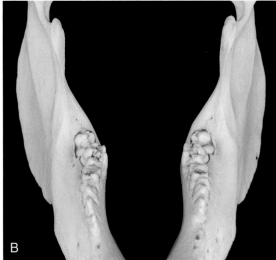

B

Fig. 7.13 Abnormalities of dentition are common in miniature pigs. **(A)** The maxilla is frequently shortened such that upper and lower incisors no longer occlude. **(B)** Crowding of teeth is common within the shortened jaws of these proportionate dwarves, and the caudal molars may not fully erupt, especially in the mandible. (Photo credit: Jennifer L. Davis.)

animal restrained by flipping (see Chapter 5), a limited examination of the oral cavity can be performed, made all the easier if the pig is vocalizing. More thorough evaluation requires anesthesia.

DENTAL PROCEDURES

A complete oral exam is not feasible in most (if not all) pig patients during a routine, non-sedated health evaluation; although pet pigs suffer from the same dental pathology as dogs or cats, with gingivitis and periodontitis reported as early as 6 months of age and becoming serious by 16 months (Wang et al. 2007), relatively few practices offer dental care for this species. A thorough oral exam and regular prophylactic scaling and polishing is recommended, with removal of grossly diseased teeth at a minimum; intraoral radiographs are ideal. However, although techniques are the same as those used in other species, intubation is required and narrow gape limits access to the oral cavity (Fig. 7.14), making the procedure technically challenging.

Dental pathology (Fig. 7.15) can be severe, with only subtle clinical signs that require an astute owner to recognize. Alteration of chewing patterns, eating more slowly, or refusing hard/crunchy food items are a few of the more obvious signs. A bad odor emanating from the mouth may indicate infection or may simply be entrapped food material, particularly in the lip pockets around upper tusks. Teeth grinding is a common behavior that may signal dental issues such as eruption pain in piglets or painfully diseased teeth in adults but may also be a behavioral habit; grinding may also be indicative of gastrointestinal pain. Draining tracts (Fig. 7.15C) are a dead giveaway, yet they may not be noticed by an owner as the pig is low to the ground and the lesions on the ventral chin are not readily visible. Excess salivation is difficult to interpret as pigs tend to salivate profusely in anticipation of

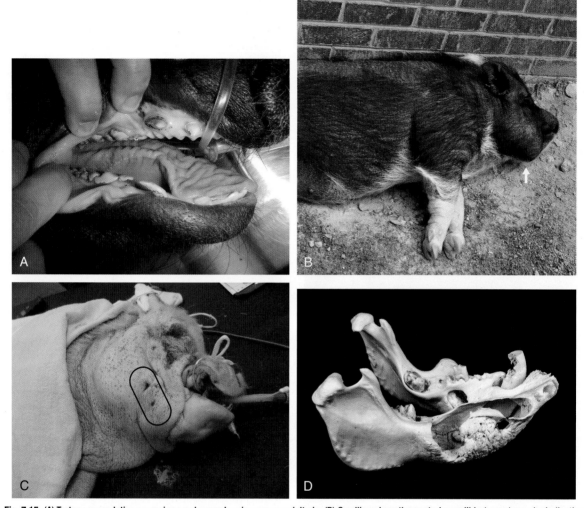

Fig. 7.15 (A) Tartar accumulation on canines and premolars in a young adult pig. (B) Swelling along the ventral mandible (*arrow*) may be indicative of abscessation with tusk infection, a common issue in males. (C) Chronic tusk infection may present as a draining tract along the ventrolateral mandible (*circled*) and many pigs exhibit no associated clinical signs despite extensive, frequently bilateral, bony involvement (D). (B, Photo credit: Leanne Jones. D, Photo credit: Jennifer L. Davis.)

food; however, profuse salivation leading to dampening of bedding during sleep is abnormal. Pigs suffering from tusk root abscesses often present with a facial abscess (Fig. 7.14B) and no other clinical signs of pain despite extensive infection and bony involvement (Fig. 7.14D). Standard radiographic imaging is helpful, but more advanced imaging such as computed tomography (CT) or magnetic resonance imaging (MRI) may be necessary and is ideal if surgical extraction of the canine(s) is intended.

In my personal experience, the majority of miniature pigs over the age of 8 to 10 years have markedly severe dental disease, with many teeth held in place only by accumulation of calculus; some have significant malocclusion and associated "wave mouth" with sharp points that damage soft tissues. Ideally, these older pigs should be anesthetized every few years to at least do a thorough oral exam and extract severely diseased teeth, if nothing else. Sharp points may be lightly filed as is done in humans to improve bite, but pig teeth cannot be floated as in the horse or smoothed and reshaped as in the rabbit (remember, these teeth are brachydont in the pig, not hypsodont). Gingival proliferation should be biopsied and submitted for histopathological evaluation as oral squamous cell carcinoma is common and may not be grossly distinguishable from benign hyperplasia.

Points to consider for tooth extraction:

- The roots of the lower incisors are at least as long as the (intact) crowns (in other words, very long). The crowns bear regular horizontal lines (Fig. 7.12A) and are frequently broken off cleanly along these; the majority of pigs will eventually fracture all of the lower incisors or, at the very least, wear them down to the gumline. Extraction is not commonly performed. Although many pigs do not seem to have any associated clinical issues, extraction or root canal should be performed if the patient seems painful (i.e., refusal of certain crunchy foods like carrots, gingerly eating, salivating excessively).
- Premolars have two to four roots and molars four to six roots (Fig. 7.16); roots may be thinly tapered (see Eubanks, 2013, and Ide et al. 2013, for imaging photos), some may be fused or overlapping, and with disease the tooth may ankylose to the alveolar bone.
- Lower canines/tusks in the male have roots as thick as the crown extending through the jaw to the level of M1–2 and are typically semicircular in shape,

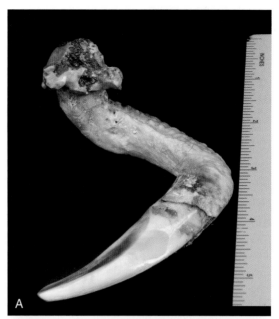

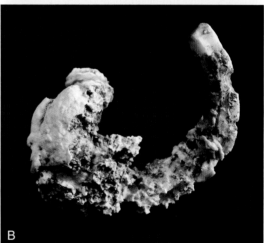

Fig. 7.17 Mandibular tusk abscess is common in the male, but this large tooth is typically curved in a C-shape, sometimes spiraling at the caudal end, and extraction is extremely difficult. (A) Minor irregular remodeling of the tooth can progress to (B) severe proliferation that further complicates extraction. (A, Photo credit: Jennifer L. Davis.)

sometimes spiraling at the caudal end (Fig. 7.17A). When diseased, the tusk may be markedly remodeled and irregular (Fig. 7.17B) and mandibular bone severely compromised (Fig. 7.15D), and the tusk may be the primary stabilizer of the jaw. Given the open root, there is no obvious delineation at the

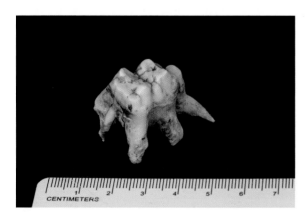

Fig. 7.16 Pig molars are large teeth with 4 to 6 roots that may be thinly tapered, fused or overlapping, and with disease, may ankylose to the alveolar bone. (Photo credit: Jennifer L. Davis.)

caudal end, making complete removal of germinal tissue difficult unless infection has caused death of the entire tooth (and, likely, a good portion of the mandibular bone as well). While radiographs are helpful, CT or MRI is recommended prior to extraction.

- Strong snout attachments place extreme tension on soft tissues along the rostral portion of the upper arcade. This may limit the ability to maintain gingival closure post-extraction in this region.

DENTAL PATHOLOGY

Smith et al. (2021) describe oral pathology of miniature pet pigs with missing teeth, periodontal disease, partially erupted or unerupted teeth, open apices, supernumerary roots, and persistent deciduous teeth being the most common abnormalities identified. See Chapter 10 for more information on common dental/oral issues under the headings of dental disease; tusk abscessation; tusk overgrowth; mass/swelling, facial; and neoplasia—squamous cell carcinoma.

Tusk Care

Both males and females have tusks, but these teeth exhibit sexual dimorphism, as mentioned above. Most importantly, the canines grow throughout life in males (intact or castrated) while the root closes at about 2 years of age in females, so trim is generally unnecessary in females. Growth of the lower canines exceeds that of the upper tusks as the upper serve to sharpen the lower for defense. Tusk root abscesses are a common issue in older males (see Chapter 10), and the mandibular canines are most commonly affected. The pulp cavity of the tusk may extend above the gumline, and it has been reported that innervation extends even further, into nonvascularized areas. For these reasons, tusk trim should be performed only as needed and trimmed at least 1 in (2.5 cm) above the gumline (Bovey et al. 2008).

TUSK TRIM

Reasons for tusk trim in males include the following.
- **Excessive Length:** Mandibular tusks can grow quite long in the male, and while some break off naturally, others continue to grow and may

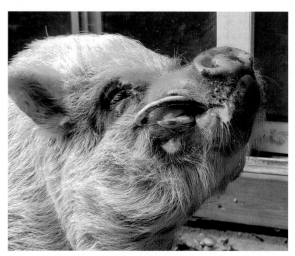

Fig. 7.18 This lower tusk has grown into the face; however, penetrating injury is chronic, and treatment typically only involves trim to remove the inciting cause. Note that the upper and lower tusks have no contact, and this malocclusion likely contributed to the problem.

penetrate through the soft tissues of the cheek (Fig. 7.18). The wounds created are like healing piercings, well granulated but oozing from constant trauma. The wounds don't typically require treatment other than to trim the tusks and remove the inciting agent.
- **Razor–Sharp Points:** Lower tusks can be sharp even without excess length, and upper tusks should be closely evaluated as well. Although excess length is not typically a concern for the maxillary canines, these tusks can be sharp and must be filed smooth to prevent damage to the soft tissues of the overlying lip or to other animals or people. Sharp lower tusks pose a risk to people and other animals, as accidental injury can occur even with friendly, well socialized pets (Fig. 10.66).
- **Catching:** For all of their intelligence, a pig catching a tusk on a fence will panic and scream. Pigs stuck on fencing often remain so until either the tusk or fence is cut, despite the fact that a step forward to release tension may be all that is needed to unhook the offending tooth. Knowledgeable pig owners always have bolt cutters on hand to clip fencing, or better yet, gigli wire to take advantage of the restraint provided to perform a tusk trim. To prevent future entrapment,

regular tusk trims may be necessary for certain individuals, although some animals manage to catch even short tusks. Another option is to attach small–gauge chicken wire or a solid surface such as wood over the fence to prevent a tooth from catching at all.

- **Malocclusion:** Occasionally, the position of the tusks relative to one another causes friction on opening and closing of the mouth, sometimes altering alignment between upper and lower arcades, sometimes placing excessive pressure on the temporomandibular joint; this can cause difficulty eating or discomfort, and trim is warranted in this instance.
- **Hooking:** Upper tusks may hook upward at such a steep angle that a tight pocket is created between the tusk and maxillary gingiva, causing food, hair, dirt, and debris to become entrapped, which can painfully traumatize the gingiva and result in gingivitis and periodontal disease.

FREQUENCY

The tusks in intact males grow quickly and trim may be needed as often as every 6 months for any of the aforementioned indications. Tusks grow more slowly in castrated males and trim frequency is variable. Overweight pigs may be in danger of tusks penetrating flesh due to large jowls encroaching on otherwise normal (not overly long) tusks, and trim may be indicated every 1 to 2 years. Some develop sharp edges only every 4 or 5 years. Some pigs never require tusk trim. Growth often slows or ceases in older males and trim may not be necessary beyond a certain age (about 10+ years). As the tusks are not continuously growing in females, regular trim is unnecessary, although some animals may require a single trim to reduce length and remove sharp edges.

EQUIPMENT

Obstetric (OB) or dehorning saw wire (a.k.a. gigli wire) is best for trimming excess length; tools such as nippers or bolt cutters should not be used, as the crushing force may crack or shatter the tooth, causing pain or leading to infection. A rotary tool with a grinding head attachment is excellent for blunting sharp points. Take care not to damage the soft tissues; gigli wire gets extremely hot during use and a rotary tool runs at a high speed. If anesthetized in a hospital setting, a high–speed dental drill with a long straight cutting bit (701L) can be used to accomplish tusk trim (Eubanks 2013; Asseo, personal communication).

TUSK TRIM TECHNIQUE

Tusk trim can be performed on a properly restrained, awake animal, or sedation can be used (see Box 5.2 for drug options and doses). Flipping the pig onto the haunches or the back (see Chapter 5) allows access to the tusks, especially if the pig is vocalizing. A length of gigli wire is cut with wire snips and attached to saw wire handles. (Tip: Cut a length of about 24 in [60 cm], long enough to make long sawing strokes that speed the trim and short enough to easily control, and replace the wire between pigs. After each use, the wire becomes increasingly curled and more difficult to maneuver so I don't reuse for more than one or two animals.)

The wire is looped around the tusk, well above the gingiva and angled along the natural slope of the tooth (Fig. 7.19). Take care to note gingival attachment at the base of the tusk. Gingiva may extend quite far onto one aspect of the tusk, and proper sedation including local anesthetic may be needed to surgically remove gingival attachments prior to trim in these pigs. The lower tusk should be trimmed at the level of contact with the upper tusk to maintain alignment unless malocclusion warrants otherwise. Saw wire handles are held close together and short, quick, sawing movements are made to create a groove in which the gigli wire becomes seated. Once seated (you can feel the wire grip into the tooth), sawing movements should become long and fast, still holding the handles close together.

Ideally, the pig's lips should be held away from the moving wire as enough heat can build to painfully burn the tissue. Some people have an assistant drip water from a syringe over the moving gigli wire to prevent it from becoming heated. Use judgment here, as some unsedated pigs may react negatively to this, and of course, the application of water drops must not cause choking; use of cooling water may be best reserved for fully sedated patients and has been described in the literature (Eubanks and Gilbo 2005). If the pig is held on the haunches in an upright position, take care that the tusk tip does not enter the pig's mouth when trim is complete. Tusk tips may

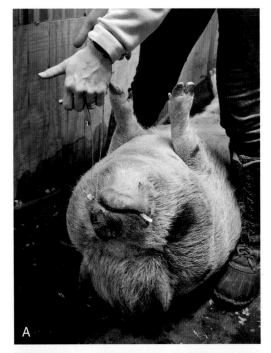

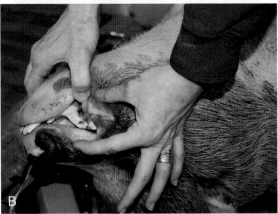

Fig. 7.19 Regular tusk trim may be required in the male and should be performed with gigli wire, as bolt cutters or other crushing instruments may crack the tooth, leading to pain and possible infection. (A) Gigli wire is looped around the tusk along the natural slope of the tooth. (B) The lower tusk should be trimmed well above the gumline, at the level of contact with the upper tusk to maintain alignment.

become lodged in the throat and create a choking hazard that can lead to death.

A dental bur on a high–speed handpiece can also be used in the clinic to cut through the tusk then round off sharp edges (Eubanks 2013). Placement of a tongue depressor behind the tooth can protect soft tissues, and angling the snout in a downward direction, with water flow reduced just enough to allow cooling of the drill and tooth during trim, minimizes risk of aspiration (Asseo, personal communication).

Microchipping

Microchipping can be done as in a dog or cat, with the current convention to place it in the lateral neck behind the left ear where skin is relatively pliable and thin (Fig. 7.1). As pet pigs are considered livestock, interstate movement requires a certificate of veterinary inspection (CVI, a.k.a. health certificate) which, in turn, always requires some form of permanent identification. Ear notching or placement of an official ear tag are legally acceptable and common in domestic swine but unpalatable to pet pig owners. Many states simply list "official individual identification" as a requirement but do not specify whether a microchip is acceptable; others, such as California, specifically require "840 Electronic Implants or microchips that are ISO 11784/85 compliant." It is always a good idea to directly contact the state veterinary office to verify acceptability of a microchip in a minipig to be imported.

In addition to CVI requirements for interstate transport, microchipping is recommended to track pets that may have been lost or stolen, and rescue organizations frequently chip pigs to ensure traceability of adopted animals.

Clinical Pathology Evaluation

Analysis of blood and urine may be desired as part of a screening health check, pre-surgical evaluation, or necessary for an ill patient. Most laboratories will run porcine samples, and as instrumentation, reagents, and methods affect results, reference values are unique to each (Thorn 2010). However, results should be interpreted in light of the fact that normal ranges for miniature pet pigs are not well established.

Brockus et al. (2005) published hematologic and serum biochemical reference intervals for Vietnamese potbellied pigs using a cohort of 100 animals, but values have not been recently updated. Although numerous published values exist for research miniature pig breeds, these are typically separated by breed, weight, age, gender, and pregnancy status and are too detailed for easy reference (Swindle and Smith 2016); additionally, breed differences have been reported so values may not directly apply to the pet population. However, data available for research animals can provide basic guidelines, and values in the miniature pet pig do not differ significantly from those of domestic swine either (Clark and Coffer 2008). Tables 7.4 and 7.5 list hematologic and serum biochemical reference intervals for domestic swine and potbellied pigs.

In general, reference ranges for most parameters are comparable to those in more familiar companion animal species, such as the dog, and interpretation is also similar. For example, white blood cells (WBCs) increase in response to bacterial infection, with neutrophilia and, typically, a left shift observed (Clark and Coffer 2008); blood urea nitrogen (BUN) and creatinine might increase with pre-renal, renal, or post-renal issues; and so on. Interpret in light of clinical signs and physical examination. For example, alkaline

TABLE 7.4 Hematologic Reference Intervals

Parameter	Unit	Domestic Pig[a]	Vietnamese Potbellied Pig[b]
PCV	%	32–50	22–50
Hemoglobin	g/dL	10.0–16.0	7.8–16.2
RBC	$\times10^6/\mu$L	5.0–8.0	3.6–7.8
Reticulocytes	%	0–1.0	–
RBC lifespan	Days	86	–
MCV	fL	50–68	55–71
MCH	Pg	17–21	18–24
MCHC	%	30–34	31–36
Platelets	$\times10^3/\mu$L	200–500	204–518
MPV	fL	–	8.4–12.4
WBC	$\times10^3/\mu$L	11–22	5.2–17.9
Neutrophils, segs	%	28–47	–
	$\times10^3/\mu$L	2–15	0–11.4
Neutrophils, bands	%	0–4	–
	$\times10^3/\mu$L	0–0.8	0–0.19
Lymphocytes	%	39–62	–
	$\times10^3/\mu$L	3.8–16.5	0.8–9.8
Monocytes	%	2–10	–
	$\times10^3/\mu$L	0–1	0–0.67
Eosinophils	%	0.5–11	–
	$\times10^3/\mu$L	0–1.5	0–0.73
Basophils	%	0–2	–
	$\times10^3/\mu$L	0–0.5	0–0.61
Fibrinogen	mg/dL	100–500	100–400

[a]Taken from Fielder SE. Hematologic reference ranges. In: *Merck Veterinary Manual*. www.merckvetmanual.com/special-subjects/reference-guides/hematologic-reference-ranges, and Thorn CE. Hematology of the pig. In: Weiss DJ, Wardrop KJ, eds. *Schalm's Veterinary Hematology*. 6th ed. Ames, IA: Blackwell Publishing, Ltd.; 2010:843–851.
[b]Taken from Brockus CW, Mahaffey EA, Bush SE, et al. Hematologic and serum biochemical reference intervals for Vietnamese potbellied pigs (*Sus scrofa*). *Comp Clin Path*. 2005;13:162–165.

TABLE 7.5 Serum Biochemical Reference Intervals

Parameter	Unit	Domestic Pig[a]	Vietnamese Potbellied Pig[b]
ALT	U/L	31–58	10.9–95.1
Alk phos	U/L	118–395	27–160
AST	U/L	32–84	16.0–64.0
Creatine kinase (CK)	U/L	2.4–22.5	212.5–2851.5
GGT	U/L	10–60	14.5–56.2
LDH	U/L	380–634	–
SDH	U/L	1.0–5.8	–
Bicarbonate (TCO2)	mmol/L	18–27	8.0–31.0
Bilirubin	mg/dL	0–1.0	0.2–0.45
Calcium	mg/dL	7.1–11.6	–
Chloride	mmol/L	94–106	106–113
Cholesterol	mg/dL	36–54	–
Creatinine	mg/dL	1.0–2.7	1.0–2.3
Glucose	mg/dL	85–150	59.8–175.2
Magnesium	mg/dL	2.7–3.7	–
Phosphorus	mg/dL	5.3–9.6	–
Potassium	mmol/L	4.4–6.7	3.7–5.0
Protein	g/dL	7.9–8.9	6.6–8.9
Albumin	g/dL	1.9–3.9	3.6–5.0
Globulin	g/dL	5.3–6.4	–
Sodium	mmol/L	135–150	139–148.8
Urea nitrogen (BUN)	mg/dL	10–30	4.2–15.1

[a]Taken from Kaneko JJ, Harvey JW, Bruss ML. *Clinical Biochemistry of Domestic Animals*. 6th ed. Burlington, MA: Academic Press; 2008:882–900. www.merckvetmanual.com/special-subjects/reference-guides/serum-biochemical-reference-ranges.
[b]Taken from Brockus CW, Mahaffey EA, Bush SE, et al. Hematologic and serum biochemical reference intervals for Vietnamese potbellied pigs (*Sus scrofa*). *Comp Clin Path*. 2005;13:162–165.

phosphatase (ALP) is often reported as low by reference laboratories based on their reference ranges, but this value is typically lower in the pig and may fall within published ranges. Regardless, would a very low ALP have meaning clinically?

Some notable points:

- The stress response develops within 2 minutes and can rapidly alter the leukogram, with white blood cell (WBC) and neutrophil counts increasing 2 to 3× (Thorn 2010), and physiologic leukocytosis can reach as high as 22,000 cells/μL (Clark and Coffer 2008).
- With a stress response, elevations can be seen in hemoglobin (Hgb) concentration, hematocrit, and RBC sedimentation rate, while decreased hematocrit and Hgb concentration have been reported with inflammatory processes (Thorn 2010).
- Creatine kinase (CK) can be quite elevated depending on restraint method.
- WBCs decline with viral disease (Clark and Coffer 2008).
- Lymphocyte count is comparatively high in the pig, and lymphocyte numbers may be higher than neutrophils.

If urinalysis is desired, the owner should be asked to collect a fresh urine sample near the time of appointment, although this is easier said than done. However, as difficult as it may be for the owner to catch a sample, it is nearly impossible for a stranger (e.g., veterinary staff) to approach a pig during urination. Two newer collection methods for female swine—the tampon and Whirl-Pak® techniques—have recently been reported and may prove applicable to minipigs as well. For the first method, an unscented tampon is inserted into the vestibule using its plastic applicator, and the attached string secured to the outside of the animal with tape; the Whirl-Pak® method involves securing the bag around the vulva with elastic tape. The tampon or bag contents are then transferred to a urine cup. Success rates for adequate sample collection were 89% and 59%, respectively, and urinalysis results were comparable to free–catch collection. Cystocentesis can be performed but requires restraint, possibly sedation, and is technically more difficult than in a dog or cat given inability to palpate the bladder, especially in an obese animal. Ultrasound guidance may be helpful.

Minipig urine, as expected, is typically yellow to amber in color although diet and, especially, supplements (e.g., vitamins) may alter color. The mean specific gravity of adult swine is around 1.020, one of the lowest found in domestic animals, and is even lower in young pigs; range is 1.010 to 1.030, and pH is typically 5.5 to 7.5 and is influenced by diet (Drolet 2006; Kaneko et al. 2008). Amorphous sediment is common and may collect around the vulva (Fig. 6.13) or on the hairs at the preputial orifice; this warrants investigation, especially in the male, as urinary tract obstruction is a common issue that can be caused by sediment as well as discrete calculi. Amorphous magnesium calcium phosphate uroliths, a possible precursor to struvite, are reportedly the most common type in the potbellied pig, although calculi composed of struvite, calcium oxalate, and calcium carbonate have also been reported (Chigerwe et al. 2013).

Venipuncture

Venous access in the minipig is limited, to say the least, and as proper restraint and positioning is necessary for "blind sticks," blood collection may be more easily performed under sedation. However, sampling from the radial vein or jugular vein is possible in a properly restrained (flipped) conscious patient (see Chapter 5). Peripheral veins are often neither visible nor palpable, and pig blood clots unusually fast. Options for blood sampling include:

AURICULAR VEIN

The ear vein is the most obvious in the porcine patient, easily accessible, visible, and palpable (Fig. 7.20). However, ear veins are of small caliber and easily collapsible, so despite appearances to the contrary, they are rarely suitable for withdrawal of blood unless only a very small quantity is needed. If catheterization is expected, these veins should be preserved due to otherwise severely limited access for an indwelling catheter.

CRANIAL VENA CAVA

As it is not recommended to snare miniature pigs as a form of restraint, the cranial vena cava is accessed in a dorsally recumbent animal, as in a commercial swine piglet. With the animal restrained on its back with the head and neck extended and the forelimbs pulled caudally, a needle is inserted into the right jugular of the way from the sternum to the jaw (Dyce et al. 1996). This vein is more superficial than the cranial vena cava but still cannot be visualized or palpated. Although the vein is relatively large, access is hampered by the thick neck, overlying cutaneous colli muscle, large salivary glands, and in some animals, excessive adipose.

ORBITAL SINUS

A venous sinus is present near the medial canthus of the eye and can be accessed using a 20-gauge, 1-in needle in a standing or ventrally recumbent animal. Application of topical 0.5% proparacaine hydrochloride ophthalmic solution may be helpful in an awake animal (Dove and Alworth 2015). The site is accessed with a needle placed just inside the nictitating membrane, advancing medially and slightly cranioventral until the sinus is punctured; the blood is then allowed to drip out of the needle into a collection tube (Dewey and Straw 2006). This location is more commonly used in laboratory animals as proximity to the eye and post-collection bleeding may make owners (and unfamiliar veterinarians) a bit squeamish. Both Dove and Alworth (2015) and Huhn et al. (1969) describe sample collection from this location in conscious pigs held in dorsal recumbency, a reportedly easy, non-invasive technique that may be useful if other sites are unrewarding.

RADIAL VEIN

The radial vein is my go-to for miniature pig blood collection. It lies along the medial aspect of the forelimb, parallel to the long bones, and is a straight, relatively superficial vessel that can be accessed just cranial to the accessory carpal bone, in the region of the carpal glands (Fig. 7.21A). Skin in this region is relatively thin and hairless such that the vein may be palpable. This site is readily accessed in a "flipped" pig (or a pig restrained in a sling) and access does not require sedation (Fig. 7.21B).

SAPHENOUS VEINS

The medial and lateral saphenous veins are similar to those of a dog, and the skin over the medial thigh is relatively thin and poorly haired such that the vein may be visible and palpable, especially in young animals. The lateral saphenous vein is accessed more

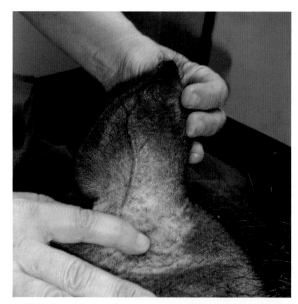

Fig. 7.20 The auricular vein is the most obvious in the porcine patient, easily accessible, visible, and palpable. However, ear veins are fragile, of small caliber, and easily collapsible, so despite appearances to the contrary, they are generally not suitable for withdrawal of blood and should be reserved for catheterization.

furrow at the thoracic inlet, cranial to the sternum and just lateral to midline. The needle is directed towards the opposite (left) shoulder at a 30- to 45-degree angle (McCrackin and Swindle 2016). A 20 gauge, 1.5- to 2.5-in needle is recommended, with needle length dependent on the size of the pig; a vacutainer may facilitate sampling. Note: The right jugular furrow is preferred over the left to avoid the vagus nerve which, if punctured, can lead to signs of dyspnea, cyanosis, and convulsions as it innervates the heart and diaphragm (Dewey and Straw 2006; Dyce et al. 1996).

CEPHALIC VEIN

The cephalic vein is similar in location to that of a dog but cannot be seen or palpated as the skin over the dorsal aspect of the forelimb is extremely thick and difficult to penetrate with a needle, except in very young animals. Nicking with a scalpel can aid access but use of this site is impractical given other available options.

JUGULAR VEIN

The external jugular vein can be accessed cranial to the location used for the vena cava, about one-third

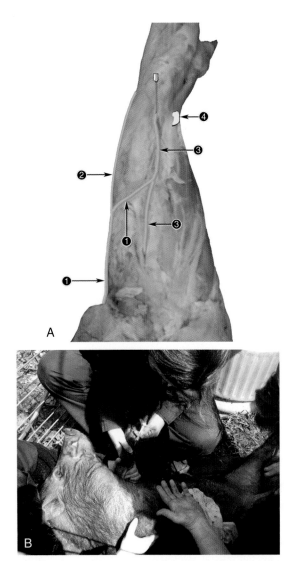

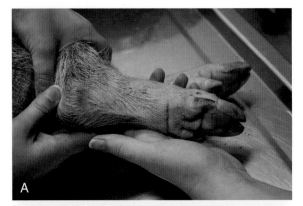

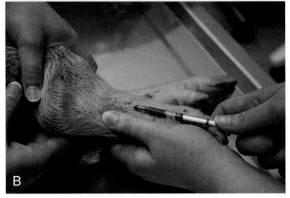

Fig. 7.22 The lateral saphenous vein is accessed more distally than in a dog, below the tarsus/hock (A, B), and is frequently palpable. It is useful for collecting approximately 1 to 3 cc of blood.

Fig. 7.21 (A) The radial vein *(3)* is located on the medial aspect of the forelimb, parallel to the long bones, and extending cranial to the palpable carpal bone *(4)* in the region of the grossly visible carpal glands; the cephalic vein *(1)* and accessory cephalic vein *(2)* are also identified. (B). This site is readily accessed in a "flipped" pig and does not require sedation. (A, Photo credit: James E. Smallwood.)

distally than is done in a dog, below the tarsus/hock, along the caudolateral aspect of the limb (Fig. 7.22; Zeltner 2019); this vein is frequently palpable.

SUBCUTANEOUS ABDOMINAL VEIN

The subcutaneous abdominal vein or "milk vein" lies lateral to the mammary chain bilaterally, and "firm

pressure applied directly behind the elbow joint, along the thorax, will allow the vein to fill" so it can be readily visualized as well as palpated (Snook 2001); a 22- to 20-gauge needle is used, although the relatively large vessel size may allow use of an 18-gauge needle. At least 10 mL of blood can be readily collected from this site. These vessels often become distended in abdominal pathology (Fig. 7.23) and can be readily accessed (but be ready for a "rolling" target).

TAIL VEIN

The coccygeal or tail vein is accessed by lifting the tail and inserting a small 20- to 21-gauge, 1-in needle along ventral midline close to the tail base (Fig. 7.24); the vein is superficial, and it is recommended to hold the tail almost horizontal and insert

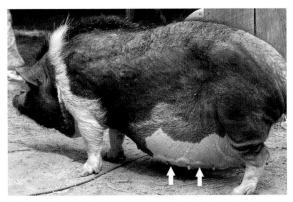

Fig. 7.23 The subcutaneous abdominal vein lies lateral to the mammary chain bilaterally and is easily accessed to collect up to approximately 10 cc of blood; it is also a well–tolerated site for catheterization (Snook 2001). These vessels often become distended in abdominal pathology *(arrows)*—in this case, uterine tumor.

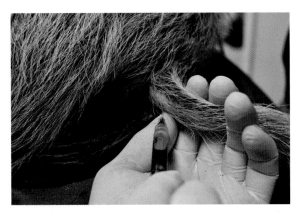

Fig. 7.24 The coccygeal or tail vein is a superficial vessel accessed by lifting the tail and inserting a needle along ventral midline close to the tail base. It is useful for collecting about 1 to 3 cc of blood.

the needle at a 45 degree angle to nearly parallel. This site is useful for collection amounts of approximately 1 to 3 cc.

Catheterization

As previously mentioned, venous access is extremely limited in the minipig as most peripheral veins are neither visible nor palpable, and pig blood clots unusually fast. Catheterization is best performed in a sedated animal unless the patient is extremely ill

and unlikely to struggle. Options for catheterization include:

AURICULAR VEIN

The ear veins are the most accessible and may be the only vessels readily visualized and palpated in the miniature pig. They generally run along the lateral margin or, less commonly, through the middle of the dorsal aspect of the pinnae (Fig. 7.20). Veins are of small caliber and easily collapsible, so despite appearances to the contrary, they are not suitable for withdrawal of blood. However, they are ideal for catheterization (Fig. 7.25A). A 1-in, 20 to 22 gauge, over-the-needle catheter is suggested and can be secured as

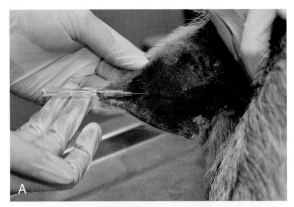

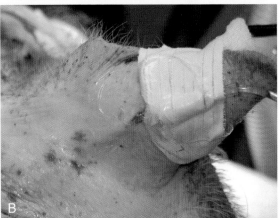

Fig. 7.25 (A) The auricular or ear veins are easily accessible, visible, and palpable, making them ideal for catheterization; however, they are fragile, small–caliber vessels, so unsuitable for rapid (bolus) administration. (B) A gauze roll has been placed on the inside of the pinna to create a "strut" support that allows the catheter to be more easily secured with tape. A Tegaderm patch has also been applied in this animal to help secure the site.

with a dog forelimb. A gauze roll or other suitably shaped "strut" can be placed inside the ear to create a more cylindrical shape for ease of securing in place (Fig. 7.25B). The fluid line can be looped and taped to the base of the ear and, for more active patients, secured to the hair over the dorsum. Due to rapid clotting, a slow fluid drip should be maintained to keep the catheter patent. If flow stops, the catheter can lose patency within about 10 to 15 minutes. Twice daily flushing with heparinized saline will also help maintain the catheter, typically for up to 3 days (VA Tech 2017). One limitation of this site is that the small–caliber, fragile vessel does not allow rapid bolus administration.

CEPHALIC VEIN

The cephalic vein is similar in location to that of a dog but cannot be seen or palpated as the skin over the dorsal aspect of the forelimb is extremely thick and difficult to penetrate with a needle, except in very young animals. Nicking with a scalpel can aid access but use of this site is impractical given other available options. Given the short limbs of the minipig, a 1-in catheter is suggested, and 22 or 20 gauge is suitable.

FEMORAL ARTERY AND VEIN

A step-by-step technique for catheterization of the femoral artery and vein is described, with accompanying video, by Ettrup et al. (2011).

JUGULAR VEIN

Unlike a dog or cat, the jugular vein is situated deep within dense soft tissues of the neck and can neither be visualized nor palpated. A rapid, non-surgical technique for jugular catheterization in conscious pigs has been described (Matte 1999); however, catheterization typically requires anesthesia and aseptic preparation. One non-surgical option involves percutaneous placement ("floating") of the catheter into place (Gade et al. 2013) but requires a certain level of training/practice; ultrasound guidance may aid this "blind" procedure. Access otherwise requires surgical "cut down" in order to visualize the vein and properly secure the catheter (Meyers Jr. et al. 2016). In a research setting, placement may include a vascular port to allow repeated access for blood collection or drug administration. Catheterization of the jugular vein might be a consideration for repeat administration of intravenous drugs

or in a critically ill hospitalized patient, perhaps, but would not be routinely performed in a general practice setting. Indwelling jugular catheters must be carefully measured as those long enough to enter into the chambers of the heart create substantial risk for thrombosis and possible endocarditis.

SAPHENOUS VEINS

Medial and lateral saphenous veins are similar in location and relative size to those of a dog or cat. While the skin over the medial thigh is relatively thin and poorly haired such that the vein may be visible and palpable, especially in young animals, securing a catheter on the proximal limb is difficult in a pig. The lateral saphenous vein can be accessed along the caudolateral aspect of the limb, below the tarsus/hock (Zeltner 2019), and may be better suited to catheterization. Access in these locations requires sedation in most cases.

SUBCUTANEOUS ABDOMINAL VEIN

The subcutaneous abdominal vein lies lateral to the mammary chain bilaterally, and "firm pressure applied directly behind the elbow joint, along the thorax, will allow the vein to fill" so it can be readily visualized as well as palpated (Snook 2001). Snook describes successful catheter placement at this site "when conducted in a manner similar to placement of a lateral thoracic vein catheter in horses." Pigs tolerated the catheter sutured into place and did not attempt to dislodge it. Due to larger vessel size, this site may allow repeated blood sampling as well as bolus fluid administration and may remain patent for as long as 7 days.

INTRAOSSEOUS

If vascular access is vital but IV catheterization not possible or unsuccessful (e.g., tiny piglet), intramedullary cannulation can be performed by inserting an 18-gauge cannula into the greater tubercle of the humerus (Anderson and Mulon 2019) using techniques similar to the dog (Gunn–Moore 2006). Use of the trochanteric fossa of the proximal femur has also been described but heavy muscle covering makes access more difficult than in the canine. The distal femur and proximal tibia are additional possibilities for intraosseous (IO) catheterization, albeit yielding a slower flow rate as compared to the humerus (Lairet et al. 2013). Fluid administration is more successful in immature animals as the marrow composition of fat and connective tissue limits administration rate in older individuals (Anderson and Mulon 2019).

Further detail on specific techniques for blood collection and catheterization, including images (Framstad et al. 2021; McCrackin and Swindle 2016; Zeltner 2019) as well as video (Ettrup et al. 2011; Framstad et al. 2021), can be found in the listed references.

BIBLIOGRAPHY

American Animal Hospital Association (AAHA). Vaccination recommendations for general practice. https://www.aaha.org/aaha-guidelines/vaccination-canineconfiguration/vaccination-recommendations-for-general-practice/.Copyright 2021. Accessed October 17, 2021.

Anderson DE, Mulon PY. Anesthesia and surgical procedures in swine. In: Zimmeran JJ, Karriker LA, Ramirez A, et al., eds. *Diseases of Swine*. 11th ed. Hoboken, NJ: John Wiley & Sons, Inc.; 2019:173.

Arends JJ, Skogerboe TL, Ritzhaupt LK. Persistent efficacy of doramectin and ivermectin against experimental infestations of *Sarcoptes scabiei* var. *suis* in swine. *Vet Parasitol*. 1999;82(1):71–79.

Asseo L, personal communication.

Boldrick L. *Veterinary Care of Pot-Bellied Pet Pigs*. Orange, CA: All Publishing Company; 1993.

Bovey K, DeLay J, Widowski T. *Trim Boar Tusks with Care*. https://www.nationalhogfarmer.com/behavior-welfare/trim-boar-tusks-with-care, Published 2008. Accessed February 2021.

Brewer MT, Greve JH. External parasites. In: Zimmeran JJ, Karriker LA, Ramirez A, et al., eds. *Diseases of Swine*. 11th ed. Hoboken, NJ: John Wiley & Sons, Inc.; 2019:1005–1014.

Brewer MT, Greve JH. Internal parasites. In: Zimmeran JJ, Karriker LA, Ramirez A, et al., eds. *Diseases of Swine*. 11th ed. Hoboken, NJ: John Wiley & Sons, Inc.; 2019:1028–1040.

Brockus CW, Mahaffey EA, Bush SE, et al. Hematologic and serum biochemical reference intervals for Vietnamese potbellied pigs (*Sus scrofa*). *Comp Clin Path*. 2005;13:162–165.

Chase C, Lunney JK. Immune system. In: Zimmerman JJ, Karriker LA, Ramirez A, et al., eds. *Diseases of Swine*. 11th ed. Hoboken, NJ: John Wiley & Sons, Inc.; 2019:284–288.

Chigerwe M, Shiraki R, Olstad EC, et al. Mineral composition of urinary calculi from potbellied pigs with urolithiasis: 50 cases (1982–2012). *J Am Vet Med Assoc*. 2013;243(3):389–393.

Clark SG, Coffer N. Normal hematology and hematologic disorders in potbellied pigs. *Vet Clin North Am Exot Anim Pract*. 2008; 11(3):569–582.

Dewey CE, Straw BE. Herd examination. In: Straw BE, Zimmerman JJ, D'Allaire S, et al., eds. *Diseases of Swine*. 9th ed. Ames, IA: Blackwell Publishing; 2006:12–13.

Dove CR, Alworth LC. Blood collection from the orbital sinus of swine. *Lab Animal*. 2015;44(10):383–384.

Drolet R. Urinary system. In: Straw BE, Zimmerman JJ, D'Allaire S, et al., eds. *Diseases of Swine*. 9th ed. Ames, IA: Blackwell Publishing; 2006:409.

DuVernoy TS, Mitchell KC, Myers RA, et al. The first laboratory confirmed rabid pig in Maryland, 2003. *Zoonoses Public Health*. 2008;55(8–10):431–435.

Dyce KM, Sack WO, Wensing CJG. The head and neck of the pig. In: *Textbook of Veterinary Anatomy*. 2nd ed. Philadelphia, PA: WB Saunders; 1996:777–778.

Ettrup KS, Glud AN, Orlowski D, et al. Basic surgical techniques in the Göttingen minipig: intubation, bladder catheterization, femoral vessel catheterization, and transcardial perfusion. *J Vis Exp*. 2011;26(52):2652.

Eubanks DL. Dental anatomy, radiography, and extraction of mandibular premolar teeth in Yucatan minipigs. *J Vet Dent*. 2013; 30(2):96–98.

Eubanks DL, Gilbo K. Trimming tusks in the Yucatan minipig. *Lab Anim*. 2005;34(9):35–38.

Fails AD, Magee C. Anatomy of the Digestive System. *Anatomy and Physiology of Farm Animals*. 8th ed. Hoboken, NJ: John Wiley & Sons, Inc.; 2018:373.

Fecchio R, Gioso MA, Bannon K. Exotic animals oral and dental diseases. In: Lobprise HB, Dodd JR, eds. *Wiggs's Veterinary Dentistry: Principles and Practice*. 2nd ed. Hoboken, NJ: John Wiley & Sons, Inc.; 2019:481–499.

Feldhamer GA, McCann BE. Dental anomalies in wild and domestic Sus scrofa in Illinois. *Acta Theriologica*. 2004;49(1):139–143.

Fernandez Sanchez JM, del Campo Velasco M, Garcia M, et al. Morphology of the dental arcade in adult pigs (*Sus scrofa domesticus*). Poster presented at: *2003 at European Veterinary Dental Society*; Madrid, Spain; http://cvrioduero.com/ArticulosPublicados.

Fielder SE. Hematologic reference ranges. In: *Merck Veterinary Manual*. https://www.merckvetmanual.com/special-subjects/reference-guides/hematologic-reference-ranges, Revised October 2015. Accessed October 2021.

Framstad T, Sjaastad Ø, Aass RA. Bleeding and intravenous techniques in pigs. Updated January 2021. https://norecopa.no/education-training/other-teaching-materials/pig-bleeding. Accessed February 2021.

Gade LP, Ludvigsen TP, Zeltner A. Repeated jugular catheterization of Göttingen minipigs using ultrasound. Poster presented at: *2013 FELASA/SECAL Congress*; 2013; Barcelona, Spain.

Grand N. Diseases of minipigs. In: McAnulty PA, Dayan AD, Ganderup N, Hastings K, eds. *The Minipig in Biomedical Research*. Boca Raton, FL: CRC Press; 2012:56–60.

Gunn-Moore D. How to perform intraosseous fluid administration in neonates. In: *2006 World Small Animal Veterinary Association World Congress Proceedings*. https://www.vin.com/apputil/content/defaultadv1.aspx?id=3859265&pid=11223&print=1. Accessed February 2021.

Harvey CE, Penny RHC. Oral and dental disease in pigs. In: *Veterinary Dentistry*. Philadelphia, PA: WB Saunders; 1985:272–280.

Herring SW, Li Y, Liu Y, et al. Oral biology and dental models. In: McAnulty PA, Dayan AD, Ganderup N, et al., eds. *The Minipig in Biomedical Research*. Boca Raton, FL: CRC Press; 2012:492–495.

Holtgrew-Bohling K. Porcine clinical procedures. In: *Large Animal Clinical Procedures for Veterinary Technicians*. 4th ed. St. Louis, MI: Elsevier, Inc; 2020:619–630.

Huhn RG, Osweiler GD, Switzer WP. Application of the orbital sinus bleeding technique to swine. *Lab Anim Care*. 1969;19(3): 403–405.

Iowa State University College of Veterinary Medicine. Anthelmintics and parasiticides for swine. https://vetmed.iastate.edu/vdpam/FSVD/swine/index-diseases/anthelmintics-parasiticides-swine. Accessed October 13, 2021.

Iowa State University College of Veterinary Medicine. Diarrheal diseases. https://vetmed.iastate.edu/vdpam/FSVD/swine/index-diseases/diarrheal-diseases. Accessed October 13, 2021.

Iowa State University College of Veterinary Medicine. Respiratory diseases https://vetmed.iastate.edu/vdpam/FSVD/swine/index-diseases/respiratory-diseases. Accessed October 13, 2021.

Ide Y, Nakahara T, Nasu M, et al. Postnatal mandibular cheek tooth development in the miniature pig based on two-dimensional and three-dimensional X-ray analyses. *Anat Rec*. 2013;296(8):1247–1254.

Jacela JY, DeRouchey JM, Tokach MD, et al. Feed additives for swine: Fact sheets—carcass modifiers, carbohydrate-degrading enzymes and proteases, and anthelmintics. *J Swine Health Prod.* 2009;17(6):325–332.

Kaneko JJ, Harvey JW, Bruss ML eds. *Appendix VIII Blood Analyte Reference Values in Large Animals. Clinical Biochemistry of Domestic Animals.* 6th ed. Burlington, MA: Academic Press; 2008:882–888.

Kaneko JJ, Harvey JW, Bruss ML, eds. Appendix XII Urine Analyte Reference Values in Animals. *Clinical Biochemistry of Domestic Animals.* Burlington, MA: Academic Press; 2008:900. 6th ed.

Lairet J, Bebarta V, Lairet K, et al. A comparison of proximal tibia, distal femur, and proximal humerus infusion rates using the EZ-IO intraosseous device on the adult swine (*Sus scrofa*) model. *Prehosp Emerg Care.* 2013;17(2):280–284.

Lawhorn DB. *Diseases of potbellied pigs.* Merck Veterinary Manual; Revised June 2013. https://www.merckvetmanual.com/exotic-and-laboratory-animals/potbellied-pigs/diseases-of-potbellied-pigs. Accessed February 2021.

Lawhorn DB. *Management of potbellied pigs.* Merck Veterinary Manual; Revised June 2013. https://www.merckvetmanual.com/exotic-and-laboratory-animals/potbellied-pigs/management-of-potbellied-pigs#v3306168. Accessed February 2021.

Lennox AM, Yasutsugu M. Anatomy and disorders of the oral cavity of miscellaneous exotic companion mammals. *Vet Clin North Am Exot Anim Pract.* 2016;19(3):929–945.

Li YJ. The characters of the dental system in Chinese minipig. *Zhonghua Kou Qiang Yi Xue Za Zhi.* 1993; 28: 234–236 (in Chinese). Cited in: Wang S, Liu Y, Fang D, et al. The miniature pig: a useful large animal model for dental and orofacial research. *Oral Dis.* 2007;13(6):530–537.

Lindsay DS, Dubey JP, Santin-Duran M. Coccidia and other protozoa. In: Zimmeran JJ, Karriker LA, Ramirez A, et al., eds. *Diseases of Swine.* 11th ed. Hoboken, NJ: John Wiley & Sons, Inc.; 2019:1015–1027.

de Macedo Pessoa CR, Cristiny Rodrigues Silva ML, de Barros Gomes AA, et al. Paralytic rabies in Swine. *Braz J Microbiol.* 2011;42(1):298–302.

Malmsten A, Dalin AM, Pettersson A. Caries, periodontal disease, supernumerary teeth and other dental disorders in Swedish wild boar (*Sus scrofa*). *J Comp Path.* 2015;153:50–57.

Matlock S. Microchipping Guidelines. https://americanminipigrescue.com/rescue-101/adoption/microchipping/. Published October 2015. Accessed October 13, 2021.

Matte JJ. A rapid and non-surgical procedure for jugular catheterization of pigs. *Lab Anim.* 1999;33(3):258–264.

Mayer JJ, Brisbin Jr IL. Sex identification of Sus scrofa based on canine morphology. *J Mammal.* 1988;69(2):408–412.

McCrackin MA, Swindle MM. Biology, handling, husbandry, and anatomy. In: Swindle MM, Smith AC, eds. *Swine in the Laboratory: Surgery, Anesthesia, Imaging, and Experimental Techniques.* 3rd ed. Boca Raton, FL: CRC Press; 2016:20–29.

Meyers Jr DD, Diaz JA, Conte ML, et al. Cardiothoracic and vascular surgery/chronic intravascular catheterization. In: Swindle MM, Smith AC, eds. *Swine in the Laboratory: Surgery, Anesthesia, Imaging, and Experimental Techniques.* 3rd ed. Boca Raton, FL: CRC Press; 2016:236–253.

Mozzachio K. Radial vein blood collection in the miniature pig. Poster presented at: *2012 Minipig Research Forum;* November 26–27, 2012; Frankfurt, Germany.

Mozzachio K, Asseo L. Miniature pigs. In: Carpenter JW, ed. *Exotic Animal Formulary.* Elsevier. 6th ed. In press.

Nickel M, Skoland K, Forseth A, et al. In: American Association of Swine Veterinarians, ed. Metting. Curran Associates, Inc.; 2017:63–64. Accessed February 2021.

Popoff MR. *Clostridium botulinum and Clostridium tetani neurotoxins.* In: Uzal FA, Songer JG, Prescott JF, Popoff MR, eds. Clostridial Diseases of Animals. Ames, IA: John Wiley & Sons, Inc; 2016: 71–106.

Reeves DE. Parasite control in miniature pet pigs. In: Reeves DE, ed. *Guidelines for the Veterinary Practitioner: Care and Management of Miniature Pet Pigs.* Santa Barbara, CA: Brillig Hill, Inc.; 1991:101–107.

Register KB, Brockmeier SL. *Diseases of Swine. Hoboken, NJ: John Wiley & Sons, Inc.; 2019:884-897. 11th ed.* In: Zimmeran JJ, Karriker LA, Ramirez A, eds, et al. Pasteurellosis. Hoboken, NJ: John Wiley & Sons, Inc.; 2019:884–897. 11th ed.

Roepstorff A, Nansen P. Faecal examinations for parasites. In: *Epidemiology, Diagnosis and Control of Helminth Parasites of Swine.* Rome: Food and Agriculture Organization of the United Nations; 1998:37.

Sawyer B. Should I microchip my pig? https://www.minipiginfo.com/microchipping-mini-pigs.html. Accessed October 13, 2021. (website copyright 2020).

Singh B, ed. *Dyce, Sack and Wensing's Textbook of Veterinary Anatomy.* 5th ed. St. Louis, MO: Elsevier; 2018:372, 502, 643–644, 741–744.

Smallwood J. The Forelimb. In: *A Guided Tour of Veterinary Anatomy.* Raleigh, NC: Millenium Print Group; 2010:319–320.

Smallwood JE. The head. In: Mills LE, ed. *A Guided Tour of Veterinary Anatomy.* Philadelphia, PA: WB Saunders; 1992:324.

Smith MA, Rao S, Rawlinson JE. Dental pathology of the domestic pig (*Sus Scrofa Domesticus*). *J Vet Dent.* 2021. doi:10.1177/0898756421989097.

Snook CS. Use of the subcutaneous abdominal vein for blood sampling and intravenous catheterization in potbellied pigs. *J Am Vet Med Assoc.* 2001;219(6):809–810.

Swindle MM, Smith AC. *Swine in the Laboratory: Surgery, Anesthesia, Imaging, and Experimental Techniques.* Appendix: Section II Hematology and Serum Chemistry. Boca Raton, FL: CRC Press; 2016:543–555. 3rd ed.

Thorn CE. Hematology of the pig. In: Weiss DJ, Wardrop KJ, eds. *Schalm's Veterinary Hematology.* 6th ed. Ames, IA: Blackwell Publishing, Ltd.; 2010:843–851.

Truyen U, Streck AF. Paroviruses. In: Zimmerman JJ, ed, et al. *Diseases of Swine.* Hoboken, NJ: John Wiley & Sons, Iinc.; 2019:611–621. 11th ed.

Tynes VV. Preventive health care for pet potbellied pigs. *Vet Clin North Am Exot Anim Pract.* 1999;2(2):495–510.

Uzal FA, Songer JG. Clostridial diseases. In: Zimmeran JJ, Karriker LA, Ramirez A, et al., eds. *Diseases of Swine.* 11th ed. Hoboken, NJ: John Wiley & Sons, Inc.; 2019:792–806.

Vaccination recommendations for general practice, 2021. [Accessed 17 October 2021].

Virginia Tech. SOP: *Swine Intravenous Catheterization.* Published December 12, 2017. https://ouv.vt.edu/content/dam/ouv_vt_edu/sops/large-animal/sop-swine-intravenous-catheterization.pdf. Accessed February 2021.

Wang S, Liu Y, Fang D, Shi S. The miniature pig: a useful large animal model for dental and orofacial research. *Oral Dis.* 2007; 13(6):530–537.

Weaver ME, Jump EB, McKean CF. The eruption pattern of deciduous teeth in miniature swine. *Anat Rec.* 1966;154:81–86.

Weaver ME, Jump EB, McKean CF. The eruption pattern of permanent teeth in miniature swine. *Arch Oral Biol.* 1969;14:323–331.

Zeltner A. Catheters for vascular access and the Göttingen minipig. *Ellegaard Göttingen Minipigs.* https://minipigs.dk/fileadmin/_migrated/content_uploads/Catheters_for_Vascular_Access_and_the_Goettingen_Minipig.pdf. Accessed February 2021.

Chapter 8

Sedation and Anesthesia

Lysa Pam Posner

Anesthesia Considerations Specific for Minipigs

ENVIRONMENTAL CONSIDERATIONS

Most of the drugs used for sedation and/or anesthesia interrupt thermoregulation, thus it is important to consider the location in which you will be working: inside or outside, with or without shade, ambient temperature, etc. Similarly, it is important to consider the logistics of that location with respect to where and how you will restrain the minipig including: size of the work area, whether wire fence or walls will be used for sorting, if other animals are present, etc. A quiet, enclosed, climate-controlled area or one outside with shade is preferable. The area should be small enough to prevent having to chase the minipig, with sturdy walls to aid in restraint and prevent escape. Good flooring with adequate traction can prevent injury during induction and facilitate a good recovery from anesthesia. Chapter 5 details proper restraint techniques.

AIRWAY CONSIDERATIONS

Before anesthetizing a minipig, the practitioner should consider the anatomic differences of minipigs and the often specialized equipment that is necessary to properly anesthetize, monitor, and recover them. Minipigs, like large pigs, have a small gape (the distance the maxilla and mandible can extend from each other), which makes visualization of the larynx difficult. Additionally, minipigs are proportionate dwarves and often have skeletal abnormalities such as a narrowed mandible and shortened maxilla, which further limits visualization and access to the oral cavity and larynx. All pigs have a **pharyngeal diverticulum** located in the caudodorsal pharynx (Fig. 8.1). When placing an endotracheal (ET) tube, it is easy for the ET tube to be inadvertently directed into this diverticulum, preventing proper intubation (Fig. 8.2). Repeated ET placement into the diverticulum can cause tissue damage, bleeding, and pharyngeal edema, which can further complicate intubation and lead to airway obstruction (Fig. 8.3). Proper placement of an ET tube through the larynx can be seen in Fig. 8.4. Minipigs have a tracheal bronchus located just cranial to the carina, which can lead to inadvertent bronchial intubation. Intubating the bronchus of one lung lobe can lead to hypoxemia and inadequate anesthetic uptake. A review of ET tube intubation in minipigs is described below.

MALIGNANT HYPERTHERMIA/PORCINE STRESS SYNDROME

Porcine stress syndrome (PSS) is a relatively uncommon genetic disease of pigs that can cause malignant hyperthermia (MH). PSS is an autosomal recessive genetic mutation of the ryanodine receptors (RyR-1) in skeletal muscle, which causes excessive calcium release from the sarcoplasmic reticulum that leads to sustained muscle contraction. Muscle tetany leads to hyperthermia, muscle damage, increased carbon dioxide production, acidemia, and death. Triggers for the development of MH include exposure to anesthetic inhalants, stress (handling, transport, fighting), and high environmental temperature. While MH is less commonly seen in minipigs, the genetic defect has been identified in Göttingen minipigs and was suspected following isoflurane anesthesia in a potbellied pig (Claxton-Gill et al. 1993). Since some minipigs have genetic ties to breeds with a higher risk of MH (e.g., Landrace pigs), there may be some risk of MH when anesthetizing minipigs. Minipigs can be tested for the RyR-1 mutation.

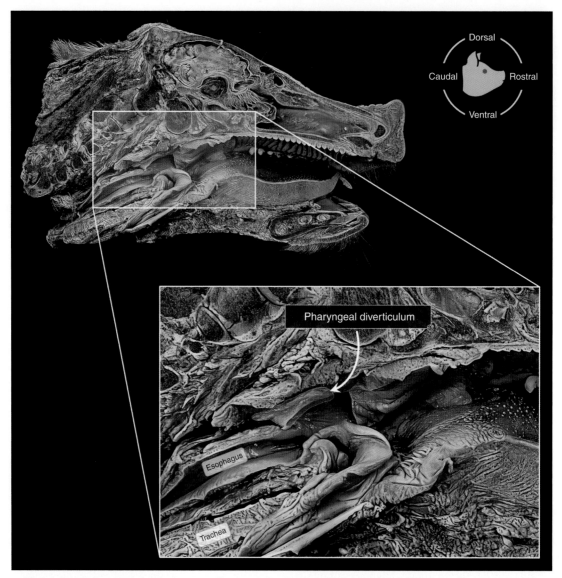

Fig. 8.1 Dorsal pharyngeal diverticulum. Inset: Pharyngeal diverticulum is highlighted in blue. (Photo credit: Christopher S. Walker.)

CONSIDERATIONS FOR DRUG ADMINISTRATION

Although minipigs have been bred to be smaller than traditional pigs, many are large enough that it is important to consider proper restraint for drug administration (see Chapter 5). Minipigs are smart, difficult to restrain by hand, and are quite vocal with their displeasure, which can be distressing for owners. If the minipig is food motivated, sedatives (e.g., trazodone, gabapentin) can be administered by mouth before the veterinary appointment, which will decrease the stress of any other procedures (e.g., physical exam, IM sedation, etc.).

Intramuscular drug administration can be performed in the muscle of the lateral neck region behind the ear (Fig. 7.1), epaxial, semimembranosus/semitendinosus, or triceps/biceps muscles. When choosing

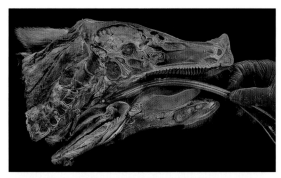

Fig. 8.2 Dorsal pharyngeal diverticulum identified by green pin. The endotracheal tube can easily be advanced into the diverticulum (rather than the trachea). (Photo credit: Christopher S. Walker.)

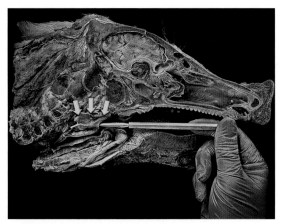

Fig. 8.3 Speculum advanced into the pharyngeal diverticulum *(arrows)* shows ruptured diverticulum at the caudal aspect. (Photo credit: Christopher S. Walker.)

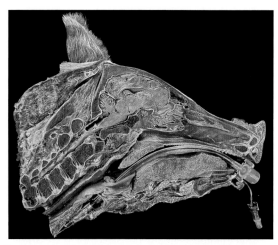

Fig. 8.4 Proper placement of endotracheal tube through the larynx into the trachea. Pharyngeal diverticulum identified by blue pin. (Photo credit: Christopher S. Walker.)

the muscle site, it is important to consider the body condition of the pig as well as what muscle will be available with proper restraint. In minipigs with a large fat component, some muscles (e.g., lateral neck) might be covered in inches of fat that can result in drugs being deposited into the fat, which slows systemic absorption. Access to muscles can also be limited by restraint method; for example, use of a press board may limit access to the triceps or biceps muscles. Injections can be facilitated by distracting the pig, for example, with firm scratching. Alternatively, in minipigs that object to restraint, some will tolerate the insertion of a butterfly catheter into a muscle, which allows for injection while the pig is free to move around. With this method, the minipig needs to be in

a confined area because the injection takes longer, and the operator must follow the pig around. Pigs tend to react less to injections into the neck muscle versus injections into the hind leg. Intramuscular injections should be made with a long large-gauge needle to allow rapid administration and at a sufficient depth to reach muscle (versus fat), such as a 1 to 1.5 inch, 20 to 22 gauge needle. A larger gauge, stronger needle (e.g., 18 gauge) may be necessary for bigger, more rambunctious patients.

Pre-Sedation/Pre-Anesthesia Assessment for the Minipig

As with other species, it is important to obtain a good history and complete a full physical exam before deciding to proceed with sedation and anesthesia (see Chapter 6). The physical exam should include (if possible) temperature, pulse and respiration (TPR), auscultation of lungs/heart, and assessment of possible IV access sites. Assessing packed cell volume (PCV) and total protein (TP) provides valuable information but is not always possible before sedation. Normal values for TPR and PCV/TP are in Tables 6.1 and 7.4 or 7.5, respectively. The decision to proceed with sedation and anesthesia should be based on the compilation of history, physical exam, blood work, any comorbidities, and the owner's comfort with anesthetic risks.

Accurate dosing of sedative and anesthetic drugs requires knowing the body weight of the patient. Ideally, the pig should be weighed directly; otherwise, it can be weighed indirectly in the transport crate. Estimating the weight of a minipig is often inaccurate but can be done with hog-specific weight tapes or equations using the heart girth and body length. However, weight tapes and published mathematical formulas are intended for use in commercial swine and often overestimate the weight of a minipig, especially those with a short-bodied, short-legged conformation. Since many minipigs are overweight, consideration should be given to estimating lean body weight for drug calculations.

Adult minipigs should be fasted for 6 to 8 hours before sedation or anesthesia to decrease the risk of vomiting and aspiration. Water should not be restricted. Piglet fasting time should be adjusted based on diet (weaned or not) and risk of hypoglycemia. In general, nursing piglets do not need to be fasted and should not be fasted longer than 1 to 2 hours. Younger and thinner piglets are at more risk for hypoglycemia than older, fatter piglets.

Prior to the administration of drugs, it is important to consider available equipment (see below) and what might be needed, particularly if there are complications. For example, do you have the equipment necessary to intubate a minipig, or do you have oxygen available if the patient becomes hypoxemic, or do you have physiologic monitoring equipment? The decision to proceed should be based on those criteria as well as the owner's expectations.

Another important consideration is that although minipigs are primarily kept as pets, they are classified as food animals and, therefore, must follow the rules for drug restrictions and withdrawal times as a food animal. Table 8.1 lists withdrawal time recommendations for selected sedative and anesthetic drugs. Additional information regarding the Animal Medicinal Drug Use Clarification Act (AMDUCA) list of prohibited and restricted drugs in food animals can be found at www.farad.org (FARAD 2021).

EQUIPMENT CHECKLIST

- Weight tape/scale
- Long needles for IM injection (1 to 1.5 inches, 20 to 22 gauge)
- Sedative/anesthetic drugs
- Reversal agents
- Stethoscope/monitoring equipment
- Restraint device
- Eye lubricant and towel to protect eyes
- ET tubes of various sizes (5 to 10 mm ID)
- Laryngoscope with a long blade (300 to 350 mm/12 to 14 inches)
- Long-length (> 600 mm/24 inches) smooth-edged stylet
- Anesthetic machine (with inhalant and oxygen supplies)
- Facemask for connection to an anesthesia machine

Sedative and Anesthetic Drugs in the Minipig

Minipigs often require sedation or anesthesia due to limited restraint options, their vocal nature, and the inconsistent ability to obtain IV access in a non-sedated animal. However, with planning (e.g., oral sedation), patience, and good handling, most procedures can be accomplished in these often unruly patients. For minipigs that will be anesthetized, moderate to profound sedation permits general anesthesia to be produced via mask induction with inhalant anesthetics. If general anesthesia is not required, then following sedation, the minipig can either recover with time or administration of antagonist drugs. In general, minipigs require greater dosages (mg/kg) of drugs to produce sedation compared with other domestic animals.

ORAL AND INTRANASAL ADMINISTRATION OF SEDATIVES

Pre-emptively administering sedatives before veterinary care can significantly decrease stress for the minipig, the owner, and the veterinarian. Drugs can be mixed with sweet juice, jam, maple syrup, molasses, or similar, which many pigs will willingly swallow. Depending on the temperament of the pig, drugs can be administered a few hours prior to the appointment or the night before and morning of the appointment. This approach has been very beneficial to facilitate good medical care in minipigs. Intranasal midazolam has good bioavailability (~64%) and efficacy in pigs

TABLE 8.1 Summary of Sedative and Anesthetic Drugs Commonly used in Minipigs

Drug	Mechanism of Action	Metabolism	Analgesia	Reversible	Side Effects	Miscellaneous	Farad Recommended Withdrawal Times	Controlled Drug Schedule
Acepromazine	Dopamine (D2) antagonist	Liver	None	No	Long lasting Vasodilation	Alters thermoregulation	7 days	Non-scheduled
Alfaxalone	Gamma aminobutyric acid (GABA) agonist	Liver	None	No		Can be administered IM	None listed	Schedule IV
Azaperone (Stresnil)	Dopamine (D2) antagonist	Liver	None	No	Long lasting Vasodilation	FDA (Food and Drug Administration) approved for use in pigs; alters thermoregulation; can cause dysphoria	None listed	Non-scheduled
Butorphanol	Kappa opioid agonists	Liver	Yes	Limited, Naloxone	Decreased GI motility; bradycardia; hypoventilation		None listed	Schedule IV
Dexmedetomidine	Alpha-2 agonist	Liver	Yes	Atipamezole; yohimbine	Vasoconstriction; bradycardia	$\alpha2$:$\alpha1$ ratio- ~1600:1	None listed	Non-scheduled
Fentanyl	Mu opioid agonists	Liver	Yes	Naloxone; naltrexone	Decreased GI motility; bradycardia; respiratory depression	Transdermal patches available	None listed	Schedule II
Gabapentin	Calcium channels	Unknown	Yes	No	Sedation		None listed	Non-scheduled
Hydromorphone	Mu opioid agonists	Liver	Yes	Naloxone; naltrexone	Decreased GI motility; bradycardia; hypoventilation		None listed	Schedule II

Continued

Drug	Mechanism of Action	Metabolism	Analgesia	Reversible	Side Effects	Miscellaneous	Farad Recommended Withdrawal Times	Controlled Drug Schedule
Ketamine	N-methyl-D-aspartate (NMDA) antagonist	Liver	Yes	No	Tachycardia; increased intracranial pressure; increased intraocular pressure	Minimal muscle relaxation	2 days	Schedule III
Midazolam/Diazepam	GABA agonist	Liver	None	Flumazenil			None listed	Schedule IV
Propofol	GABA agonist	Extrahepatic metabolism	None	No	Respiratory depression	IV only administration	None listed	Schedule IV
Telazol (zolazepam + tiletamine)	GABA agonist/NMDA antagonist	Liver	Yes	Flumazenil for zolazepam		Slow recovery in pigs	None listed	Schedule III
Tramadol	Mu opioid agonist; serotonin antagonist/reuptake inhibitor	Liver	Yes	No			None listed	Schedule IV
Trazodone	Serotonin antagonist/reuptake inhibitor	Liver	No	No			None listed	Non-scheduled
Xylazine	Alpha-2 agonist	Liver	Yes	Yohimbine; atipamezole	Vasoconstriction; bradycardia	α2: α1 ratio- ~160:1	None listed	Non-scheduled
Zolazepam	GABA agonist	Liver	None	Flumazenil		Only available as part of Telazol	None listed	Schedule IV

TABLE 8.1 Summary of Sedative and Anesthetic Drugs Commonly used in Minipigs—cont'd

(Lacoste 2000). Unfortunately, many pigs object to this form of administration. Refer to "Sedation/Anesthesia Protocols for Minipigs" section for oral and intranasal sedative drug and dosage recommendations.

SEDATIVE AND ANALGESIC DRUGS USED IN MINIPIGS

Choosing proper sedative drugs requires assessing the temperament of the pig, the duration of sedation required, how painful the procedure will be, and knowledge of sedative drugs. The following section reviews the use of these drugs in minipigs, whereas Table 8.1 provides a pharmacologic summary, including withdrawal times and controlled drug scheduling. Additional information can be found in the Exotic Animal Formulary (Mozzachio, in press).

Acepromazine

Acepromazine is a commonly used tranquilizer in veterinary medicine. In minipigs, acepromazine produces mild to moderate sedation but is often insufficient for frightened or aggressive pigs. In general, acepromazine is more effective when combined with other sedatives (e.g., trazodone, gabapentin). Acepromazine is long acting and requires liver metabolism, so it should be used with caution in minipigs with hepatic dysfunction. Acepromazine can alter thermoregulation centrally in the hypothalamus and peripherally via vasodilation. Following administration, patients should be protected from extreme temperature fluctuations (heat or cold).

Alfaxalone

In the United States, alfaxalone is approved for IV use in dogs and cats; however, it is labeled for IM use in other countries. Intramuscular alfaxalone produced deep sedation when administered to pigs in conjunction with other anesthetic agents (Bigby et al. 2017). In pigs, alfaxalone produces less respiratory depression compared with propofol (Lervik et al. 2020), which is favorable in species like minipigs where intubation can be more difficult and therefore might take longer to accomplish.

Alpha-2 Adrenergic Agonists (e.g., xylazine, dexmedetomidine)

Alpha-2 adrenergic agonists (α2 agonists) are commonly used in veterinary medicine because they produce reliable sedation, muscle relaxation, and analgesia in addition to being reversible. All α2 agonist drugs activate both the α2 and α1 receptors. However, it is the α2 activation that produces sedation and analgesia. The primary difference between xylazine and dexmedetomidine is their α2:α1 ratios. Drugs that are more specific for the α2 receptor will have a high ratio, and drugs that are less specific for the α2 receptor will have a lower ratio. Dexmedetomidine is the most specific (α2:α1 ratio ~1600:1) and xylazine is the least specific (α2:α1 ratio ~160:1). The increased specificity of dexmedetomidine means that it is more potent (lower dosage needed) and likely produces more sedation and analgesia. Not surprisingly, dexmedetomidine is more expensive than xylazine. Thermoregulation can be affected by α2 agonists, so care must be taken during the recovery phase to prevent both hypothermia and overheating. All α2 agonists can be reversed with α2 antagonists such as yohimbine or atipamezole. As with the agonist drugs, the reversal drugs have different specificity for α2 and α1 receptors. Atipamezole is more specific for antagonizing the α2 receptor, so the reversal of sedation (and analgesia) will be accomplished with a lower dosage compared with yohimbine.

Azaperone

Azaperone is a butyrophenone, a class of drugs used as antipsychotic agents in human medicine. It is FDA approved for use in pigs (Stresnil); however, that product is not marketed in the United States. Azaperone is available in Canada and is also sold as part of a combination product BAM (butorphanol/azaperone/medetomidine) by ZooPharm compounding pharmacy (https://www.zoopharm.com/). Azaperone produces calming effects in commercial pigs and is often used when introducing new pigs to one another, to prevent aggression, and for transportation. Azaperone can produce restlessness (akathisia), which may manifest as pacing and agitation. It is best thought of as a calming agent and is unlikely to be sufficient for sedation in aggressive or frightened animals. Azaperone can alter thermoregulation, and following administration, patients should be protected from extreme temperature fluctuations (heat or cold).

Benzodiazepines (e.g., diazepam, midazolam, zolazepam)

Benzodiazepines are minor tranquilizers that decrease anxiety and produce moderate sedation in minipigs. While the sedative effects of midazolam and diazepam are similar, there are properties of each that might impact the choice of one over the other. Midazolam is water soluble, which supports administration by an extended number of routes: intranasal, SQ, IM, and IV. The bioavailability of intranasal midazolam in pigs was ~65% in one study (Lacoste 2000). Comparatively, diazepam is not water soluble (drug vehicle is propylene glycol) and should be administered by the IV route as any other route might produce unpredictable absorption. Due to the propylene glycol, diazepam should not be mixed with other drugs before administration. Diazepam is bioavailable via rectal administration in people and in other species, so it would likely be effective in a pig too. Zolazepam is only available in combination with tiletamine, sold as Telazol.

Gabapentin

Gabapentin was initially developed for use as an anticonvulsant but is used commonly as a sedative and to provide analgesia, particularly for neuropathic pain. Gabapentin causes sedation due to the activation of GABA receptors (inhibitory neurotransmitters that result in sleepiness). Gabapentin produces analgesia by blocking the alpha-2-delta subunit of voltage-gated calcium channels, which decreases the release of pain-activating neurotransmitters (e.g., Substance P). These particular calcium channels are upregulated in chronic pain states, which might explain why gabapentin appears to provide better analgesia for patients with long-term pain compared with acute pain. Gabapentin is often administered to minipigs in conjunction with other sedatives (e.g., trazodone, acepromazine). With chronic administration, the sedative effects decrease but analgesic effects remain. In humans, gabapentin is excreted unchanged via the kidney but in dogs requires hepatic metabolism. The metabolism and excretion mechanism of gabapentin in pigs is unknown.

Ketamine

Ketamine is a commonly used anesthetic but is unique in a variety of ways; it increases heart rate and blood pressure, provides analgesia, and is effective with IM administration. Ketamine does not provide good muscle relaxation, so the administration of ketamine to minipigs should be in conjunction with other sedatives/muscle relaxers (e.g., midazolam or dexmedetomidine). Ketamine increases both intraocular and intracranial pressure, so it should be used with caution in minipigs with any penetrating eye trauma or CNS disease.

Opioids

Opioids provide sedation and analgesia to minipigs by activating opioid receptors in the brain, spinal cord, and periphery. Pigs have both mu opioid and kappa opioid receptors. The duration and intensity of analgesia are dependent on the particular drug, which opioid receptor is activated, and the dosage used. In general, mu opioid agonists provide more analgesia but cause more side effects (e.g., vomiting, GI stasis, etc.). Interestingly, the side effects associated with mu opioids are more common when they are administered to patients who have minimal pain and less common in patients with significant pain. Butorphanol (kappa), hydromorphone (mu), tramadol (mu and serotonin), and fentanyl (mu) patches are commonly used in minipigs. In mildly painful pigs, butorphanol and tramadol are likely better choices, whereas in pigs with moderate or severe pain, hydromorphone and fentanyl should be chosen. Tramadol is administered orally, which in food-motivated pigs makes treatment easy. Fentanyl patches result in plasma levels that last up to 3 days in minipigs and provide plasma concentrations of fentanyl without an IV catheter or parenteral drug administration.

Propofol

Propofol produces smooth anesthesia in minipigs when administered IV, which limits its use to patients that already have IV access. Propofol can cause significant respiratory depression or apnea. Caution must be used where the ability to intubate the minipig and provide assisted ventilation may be compromised. Propofol can undergo complete extrahepatic metabolism and thus is a good choice for an anesthetic in patients with hepatic dysfunction.

Trazodone

Trazodone is a serotonin (5-HT2) antagonist and reuptake inhibitor, which produces a calming effect and encourages sleep. Trazodone is administered orally and is useful in minipigs when combined with other drugs and administered several hours before presentation. Trazodone has minimal physiologic effects, even at high dosages.

Telazol

Telazol is the proprietary formulation of zolazepam and tiletamine, which pharmacologically is similar to midazolam and ketamine. In pigs, zolazepam has a longer duration of action than tiletamine, which generally results in slow, calm recoveries. Another advantage of Telazol is a small volume per dose and the ability to reconstitute with other anesthetic drugs (e.g., xylazine).

Sedation/Anesthesia Protocols for Minipigs

Inspection of any porcine formulary will identify dozens if not hundreds of drugs and dosages. One goal of this chapter is to provide the minipig practitioner a reasonable number of established sedation protocols. In general, protocols containing a combination of sedatives, anesthetics, and analgesics produce more reliable sedation. In each section below, one or two combinations have been flagged as favorites with an asterisk (*).

ORAL SEDATION

- *Trazodone 10 mg/kg + gabapentin 20 mg/kg +/- acepromazine 0.5 to 1 mg/kg given PO; administered 2 to 3 hours prior to handling
- Diazepam 0.1 to 0.5 mg/kg PO; administered 1 hour prior to handling

INTRANASAL SEDATION

- *Midazolam 0.1 to 0.5 mg/kg, intranasal

INTRAMUSCULAR (IM) SEDATION

- Midazolam 0.1 to 0.5 mg/kg IM
- Midazolam 0.1 to 0.3 mg/kg + butorphanol 0.2 to 0.4 mg/kg + xylazine 1 mg/kg IM
- *Midazolam 0.1 to 0.3 mg/kg + butorphanol 0.2 to 0.4 mg/kg + dexmedetomidine 0.01 to 0.04 mg/kg (10 to 40 mcg/kg) IM
- Acepromazine 0.5 to 1.1 mg/kg + ketamine 15 to 30 mg/kg IM

- Alfaxalone 4 mg/kg + dexmedetomidine 0.02 mg/kg (20 mcg/kg) + butorphanol 0.4 mg/kg IM
- Azaperone 2.2 mg/kg IM
- Azaperone 4 mg/kg + midazolam 0.5 mg/kg +/- atropine 0.04 mg/kg IM
- Azaperone 2 mg/kg + ketamine 15 mg/kg IM
- *Dexmedetomidine 0.01 to 0.04 mg/kg (10 to 40 mcg/kg) + ketamine 5 to 10 mg/kg + midazolam 0.2 mg/kg IM
- Midazolam 1 mg/kg + ketamine 10 mg/kg IM
- Telazol is a mixture of tiletamine and zolazepam sold as a powder that needs to be reconstituted with sterile water
  - TKX= Telazol-ketamine-xylazine
  - Reconstitute powdered Telazol (500 mg) with 2.5 mL (100 mg/mL) ketamine and 2.5 mL (100 mg/mL) xylazine, instead of sterile water; mixture has 50 mg/mL each of tiletamine, zolazepam, ketamine, xylazine
    - TKX (mild to moderate sedation) 0.007 to 0.013 mL/kg IM
    - TKX (profound sedation) 0.03 mL/kg IM
    - NOTE DOSING FOR TKX IS IN MILLILITERS (NOT MG)
- Telazol 0.6 mg/kg + detomidine 0.12 mg/kg + butorphanol 0.3 mg/kg IM
- Telazol 0.6 to 1.0 mg/kg + xylazine 2 to 3 mg/kg + butorphanol 0.3 to 0.4 mg/kg IM
- Xylazine 2 mg/kg + ketamine 5 mg/kg + butorphanol 0.22 mg/kg IM
- Xylazine 1 mg/kg + ketamine 5 to 10 mg/kg + midazolam 0.2 mg/kg IM

ENDOTRACHEAL TUBE INTUBATION

Orotracheal intubation in minipigs is challenging due to the small gape, fleshy neck, presence of a pharyngeal diverticulum, and the presence of a tracheal bronchus. However, minipigs can safely be intubated as long as these considerations are addressed and proper equipment is available. Visualization of the larynx and arytenoids is necessary to assure proper intubation; thus a laryngoscope with a long straight blade and a good light source is required (e.g., Miller blade). For minipigs weighing less than 50 kg, a laryngoscope blade of 180 to 200 mm (7 to 8 inches) should be adequate to facilitate visualization of the larynx, whereas bigger pigs may need blade lengths up to 350 mm (14 inches).

ET tubes can be made of silicone or polyvinyl chloride (PVC) plastic. Silicone tubes are soft and require a stylet for placement, whereas the PVC tubes are rigid and have an arc shape. ET tubes should have a Murphy eye (the hole at the end that can prevent airway obstruction) and be cuffed to allow protection of the airways and allow for positive pressure ventilation. Pigs, in general, have a relatively small sized trachea for their body weight. Most adult minipigs weighing 50 to 100 kg (100 to 220 lbs) require a 6 to 8 mm ID ET tube. Following intubation, the end of the ET tube should lie distal to the larynx and cranial to the tracheal bronchus. The length of the ET tube can be approximated by measuring from the snout to just in front of the shoulder. It is prudent when anesthetizing minipigs to have a variety of diameter and length ET tubes available. Ideally, ET tubes should be sterilized between patients but are often just disinfected.

Desensitization of the larynx is suggested to decrease the risk of laryngospasm and coughing and to make intubation easier. Lidocaine (2% injection) in a syringe with either a catheter or atomizer can be sprayed onto the larynx prior to intubation. Desensitization of the larynx takes time, so after topical administration, the operator should wait 30 to 45 seconds before attempting intubation.

Minipigs can be intubated in ventral or dorsal recumbency, based on the preference of the anesthetist. Once asleep, tape strips or smooth rope can be used to distract the mandible from the maxilla. Pressing a laryngoscope blade to the base of the tongue nearest to the epiglottis allows visualization of the larynx. The epiglottis should not be held down with the laryngoscope blade as that can lead to edema of the epiglottis. Commonly, the epiglottis is entrapped by the soft palate, and the laryngoscope blade or ET tube can be used to release the epiglottis. Two techniques are commonly used to avoid the pharyngeal diverticulum during ET intubation. The first is the use of an arc-shaped ET tube. Following identification of the larynx with a laryngoscope, the ET tube is advanced through the arytenoids with the arc facing down. Once the tube is through the larynx, it is rotated 180 degrees (so the arc faces up), which allows the ET tube to progress into the trachea without entering the diverticulum (Fig. 8.5). Alternatively, a thin, smooth-edged stylet can be placed through the larynx and into the trachea, and an

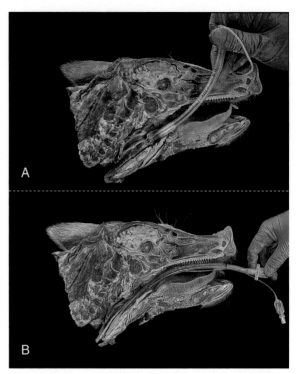

Fig. 8.5 (A) After the endotracheal tube has been advanced through the arytenoids, it is rotated 180 degrees (so the arc faces up), which allows the ET tube to progress into the trachea without entering the diverticulum. Pharyngeal diverticulum identified by green pin. (B) Once the ET tube is within the trachea, it is rotated so the arc faces ventral/down. (Photo credit: Christopher S. Walker.)

ET tube can be threaded over the stylet, avoiding the diverticulum (Fig. 8.6). Proper intubation should be confirmed by hearing air in both lung fields or by identifying carbon dioxide in the exhalation of breath through the ET tube (capnography). The presence of a tracheal bronchus makes it easier to have bronchial intubation in minipigs than in other domestic species. If the ET tube is directed into the tracheal bronchus, then the majority of the lung lobes are not exposed to oxygen and anesthetic gases that can lead to hypoxemia and inadequate anesthetic depth.

Once properly intubated, the ET tube cuff should be inflated to protect the airways from aspiration and to provide a closed circuit that allows for positive pressure ventilation and prevents anesthetic gases from polluting the room. The cuff should be inflated just enough to prevent air from leaking when breaths

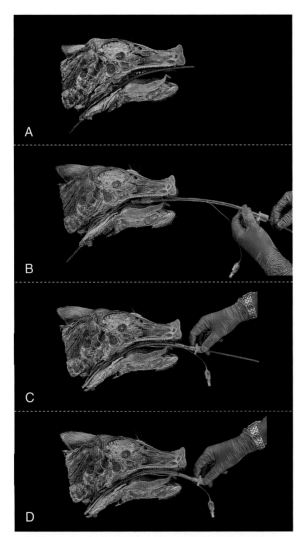

Fig. 8.6 (A) Demonstrates placement of stylet into trachea. (B) Demonstrates guiding endotracheal tube over stylet. (C) Demonstrates advancement of endotracheal tube while withdrawing stylet. (D) Final position of ET tube within the trachea. (Photo credit: Christopher S. Walker.)

are given to an airway pressure of 20 cm H_2O. Overinflation of the ET tube cuff can cause tracheal damage as with other domestic animals.

Minipigs can develop laryngeal edema as a sequela to difficult intubation. The edema can range from mild to life-threatening. It is important to make a conscious decision regarding the number of intubation attempts, and the force used when placing the ET tube. It is better to abort the anesthetic event than create a different and serious issue. Mild cases of edema can be treated with topical phenylephrine drugs (e.g., Neo-Synephrine), whereas laryngeal edema that is affecting breathing should be treated aggressively with IV glucocorticoids, topical phenylephrine, oxygen if needed, and observation to assure adequate ventilation.

INHALANT ANESTHETICS

Inhalant anesthetics such as isoflurane or sevoflurane are useful to induce and then maintain general anesthesia in minipigs but require specialized equipment (anesthesia machine, vaporizer, oxygen supply). Following good sedation, general anesthesia can be produced smoothly with facemask administration of inhalant anesthetics. General anesthesia then can be maintained via the facemask or through an ET tube. Since all inhalants cause respiratory depression, it is important when anesthetizing minipigs with a facemask to have the equipment needed to intubate in the event that ventilation becomes dangerously depressed. An advantage of inhalant anesthesia is the rapid recovery following discontinuation.

Inhalant anesthetics are effective in making patients unconscious but do not produce analgesia. While the patient is anesthetized, they do not feel pain, but the pain pathway can be activated. When the inhalant anesthetic is discontinued, the activated pain pathway will be felt by the patient if other analgesics have not been given [e.g., non-steroidal anti-inflammatory drugs (NSAIDs), opioids].

REVERSAL AGENTS

Following completion of a procedure that required sedation or anesthesia, it might be possible to provide reversal agents to speed the time to recovery. It is important to consider analgesia when reversing drugs such as opioids and alpha-2 agonists as the removal of those drugs from the binding sites will remove the analgesia too. Reversal agents can be administered by two different routes. For example, when administering atipamezole, you can administer 25% of the dose IV and 75% IM.

- Alpha-2 antagonists (reversal of xylazine, dexmedetomidine, detomidine)
  - Atipamezole 0.1 to 0.3 mg/kg IM/IV
  - Yohimbine 0.25 to 0.5 mg/kg IM/IV

- Benzodiazepine antagonist (reversal of midazolam, diazepam)
  - Flumazenil 0.02 mg/kg IM/IV
- Opioid antagonist (reversal of mu opioids, e.g., fentanyl, hydromorphone)
  - Naloxone 0.5 to 2 mg/kg IM/IV

Sedation/Anesthesia Maintenance

A logical progression when sedating or anesthetizing a minipig starts with choosing a location that will facilitate restraint, the procedure, and recovery. Following IM drug administration, the minipig should be observed from afar and left unstimulated until the desired effects are achieved. Stimulation before drugs have taken full effect will often prolong the time to full effect and lead to additional drugs being required. Once sedated, the minipig should be assessed for the level of sedation and have physiologic variables assessed (see below). If the sedation is inadequate, additional drugs should be administered and time given to wait for the full effects.

If the plan is to maintain anesthesia with an inhalant, the minipig can be administered isoflurane with oxygen through a facemask. Anesthesia can be maintained with the facemask or through an ET tube. For longer procedures or for major surgeries, ET tube and IV catheter placement are recommended (see Chapter 7 for IV catheterization details).

Once sedated or anesthetized, the minipig should be placed on a soft or padded surface (e.g., grass, thick blanket). Their eyes should be lubricated, and it is often useful to place their head on a towel to protect the eye facing down and to cover the up-facing eye to minimize light stimulation. Throughout sedation/anesthesia, minipigs should be consistently assessed for anesthetic depth and physiologic stability.

PHYSIOLOGIC VARIABLES TO MEASURE DURING SEDATION OR ANESTHESIA

While anesthetized, minipigs should have physiologic monitoring comparable to other domestic species. The American College of Veterinary Anesthesia and Analgesia recommends basic anesthesia monitoring to include heart rate, respiratory rate, blood pressure, body temperature, and oxygen saturation (SpO_2). Advanced monitoring can also include capnography. The availability of portable, multiparameter monitors makes physiologic monitoring of minipigs more convenient.

Expected Variables in Minipigs While Sedated or Anesthetized

- Heart rate (HR): ~70 to 100 beats/min
- Respiratory rate (RR): ~10 to 20 breaths/min
- Pulse oximetry: SpO_2 >95%
- Capnography: end-tidal CO_2 ($ETCO_2$) 30 to 60 mm Hg
- Blood pressure: MAP (mean arterial pressure) >60 mm Hg
- Body temperature: 37 to 39°C (98.6 to 102.2°F)

Physiologic Complications

- Bradycardia (HR <60) is a common complication associated with anesthesia and sedation but only needs to be treated when negatively affecting cardiac output or causing arrhythmias (e.g., ventricular escape beats). Bradycardia in minipigs can be treated with anticholinergics (atropine/glycopyrrolate).
  - Atropine 0.02 to 0.04 mg/kg SC, IM, IV
  - Glycopyrrolate 0.004 to 0.01 mg/kg SC, IM, IV
- Hypotension (MAP <60 mm Hg) is the most common anesthetic complication. Hypotension can usually be addressed by IV fluid bolus, increasing heart rate with anticholinergics, or use of positive inotropes (e.g., dopamine). Untreated hypotension can contribute to renal dysfunction and myopathies.
- Hypoventilation (CO_2 >60 mm Hg) can be treated by decreasing the depth of anesthesia or by assisting ventilation (in minipigs with ET tubes).
- Hypoxemia (SpO_2 <90%) is life-threatening and should be treated swiftly. Supplemental oxygen by face mask or ET tube is the best choice. If hypoxemia is due to decreased ventilation, then assisting ventilation with supplemental oxygen is recommended. If the minipig is not intubated, then an ET tube should be placed and supplemental oxygen administered with assisted breaths.
- Hypo/hyperthermia can occur in pigs due to environmental factors coupled with the effects of anesthetic drugs. In most patients, the majority of heat loss occurs within the first 15 minutes of

anesthesia, so if hypothermia is a concern, action should be taken as soon as possible after the start of anesthesia. The two biggest causes of heat loss are to the air (radiation) and through cold metal tables (conduction), so the focus should be on covering the patients to prevent radiative losses and making sure the skin does not directly touch metal surfaces (e.g., put a blanket between the metal table and the patient). Since pigs can suffer either complication, it is important to routinely check body temperature and adjust treatment as necessary.

MONITORING ANESTHETIC DEPTH

Depth of anesthesia in minipigs is evaluated similarly to other species, including voluntary movement, muscle tension, palpebral reflex, and changes in physiologic variables. Assessing jaw tone is not a useful indicator of anesthetic depth in minipigs. Corneal reflexes are not useful in assessing the depth of anesthesia in any patient as they reflect brainstem (medulla) function and are not depressed or lost until the patient is dangerously over-anesthetized.

ANALGESIA

As with any other veterinary patient, minipigs should be assessed for and treated for pain. Pre-emptive analgesia (analgesia provided before a painful stimulus) is more effective for the patient, helps prevent central sensitization, and can decrease anesthetic drug requirements. While NSAIDs are effective and routinely used, caution should be used if administering with anesthesia, as hypotension in patients who have been administered NSAIDs can lead to renal compromise.

NSAIDs

- Aspirin 10 to 20 mg/kg PO q6–8h
- Carprofen 2.2 mg/kg SQ q12h or 4.4 mg/kg PO q24h
- Flunixin 1.1 mg/kg IV, IM or SQ q12–24h
- Ibuprofen 10 mg/kg PO q6–8h
- Meloxicam 0.4 mg/kg IM or SQ q24h or 0.1 mg/kg PO q24h

Opioids

- Buprenorphine 0.01 to 0.05 mg/kg IM, SQ or IV q6–12h

- Butorphanol 0.2 to 0.4 mg/kg IV, IM or SQ q2–6h
- Fentanyl transdermal patch, 0.5 to 1 mcg/kg/h for 3 days; ~12 hours to max effect
- Hydromorphone 0.1 to 0.2 mg/kg IV q2h or 0.2 mg/kg IM or SQ q4–6h
- Morphine 0.2 mg/kg IM or SQ q4h
- Tramadol 2 to 4 mg/kg PO q6–24h

RECOVERY FROM SEDATION OR ANESTHESIA

Following discontinuation of the maintenance anesthetic, minipigs should continue to breathe supplemental oxygen (if possible) to compensate for any hypoventilation present until more awake. If the minipig has been intubated, the ET tube should be left in place until the minipig is recovered sufficiently (breathing adequately and able to control its airway). Following extubation, the patient should be monitored for hypoxemia and hypoventilation.

Following recovery from anesthesia, minipigs should be assessed for pain. In addition to the humane implication, allowing patients to remain in pain is associated with increased morbidity and mortality. Pain recognition can be difficult in minipigs since their expression of pain can be quite subtle. Behavioral changes to look for include: decreased appetite, decreased activity level, change in posture (i.e., hunching, kneeling, frequent repositioning when recumbent), change in gait (i.e., stiff-legged, limping, frequent weight shifting), bruxism (teeth grinding), lip-smacking, and vocalizations (Mozzachio 2014). Treatment with analgesics should resolve or attenuate these signs.

DELAYED RECOVERY FROM ANESTHESIA

Most minipigs require moderate to heavy sedation for procedures or to facilitate anesthesia; therefore, it is possible for them to have slow recoveries with a delayed return to function. During the recovery time, pigs should be monitored for physiologic changes and, in particular, temperature as hypothermia can decrease drug metabolism and delay recovery further. In general, pigs should extubate within 30 minutes of discontinuing inhalant anesthesia and should be able to move to sternal recumbency within 45 to 60 minutes. If recovery is delayed, consideration should be given to reversing sedative/anesthetic agents, correcting physiological abnormalities, and investigating if a different problem may be contributing to the slow recovery.

BIBLIOGRAPHY

Baratta JL, Schwenk ES, Viscusi ER. Clinical consequences of inadequate pain relief: barriers to optimal pain management. *Plast Reconstr Surg*. 2014;134(4 Suppl. 2):15S–21S.

Bigby SE, Carter JE, Bauquier S, et al. The use of alfaxalone for premedication, induction and maintenance of anaesthesia in pigs: a pilot study. *Vet Anaesth Analg*. 2017;44(4):905–909.

Claxton-Gill MS, Cornick-Seahorn JL, Gamboa JC, et al. Suspected malignant hyperthermia syndrome in a miniature pot-bellied pig anesthetized with isoflurane. *J Am Vet Med Assoc*. 1993;203(10):1434–1436.

FARAD Food Animal Residue Avoidance Databank. http://www.farad.org/. Accessed May 2021.

Kumar A, Mann HJ, Remmel RP. Pharmacokinetics of tiletamine and zolazepam (Telazol) in anesthetized pigs. *J Vet Pharmacol Ther*. 2006;29(6):587–589.

Lacoste L, Bouquet S, Ingrand P, et al. Intranasal midazolam in piglets: pharmacodynamics (0.2 vs 0.4 mg/kg) and pharmacokinetics (0.4 mg/kg) with bioavailability determination. *Lab Anim*. 2000;34(1):29–35.

Lervik A, Toverud SF, Krontveit R, et al. A comparison of respiratory function in pigs anaesthetised by propofol or alfaxalone in combination with dexmedetomidine and ketamine. *Acta Vet Scand*. 2020;62(1):14.

McInnes EF, McKeag S. A brief review of infrequent spontaneous findings, peculiar anatomical microscopic features, and potential artifacts in Göttingen minipigs. *Toxicol Pathol*. 2016;44(3):338–345.

Mozzachio K, Asseo L. Miniature pigs. In: Carpenter JW, ed. *Exotic Animal Formulary*. Elsevier. 6th ed. In press.

Mozzachio K, Tynes VV. Recognition and treatment of pain in pet pigs. In: Egger CM, Doherty T, Love L, eds. *Pain Management in Veterinary Practice*. Ames, Iowa: John Wiley & Sons, Inc.; 2014:383–389.

Wilkinson AC, Thomas ML III, Morse BC. Evaluation of a transdermal fentanyl system in Yucatan miniature pigs. *Contemp Top Lab Anim Sci*. 2001;40(3):12–16.

Chapter 9

Surgery

Kristie Mozzachio

Neuter

CASTRATION (ORCHIECTOMY)

Castration of male miniature pet pigs is warranted to prevent unwanted pregnancy but undesirable behaviors such as mounting and frequent ejaculation, bad odor, territorial urine marking, and possible aggression must also be considered. Additionally, testicular tumors are common in older males and may be cancerous (Fig. 4.15). Surgery can be performed within the first couple weeks of life as is done in commercial swine but is typically performed around 8 to 12 weeks of age or older in the pet pig (Lawhorn 2013).

Castration is a straightforward surgery in the miniature pig, typically done under general anesthesia (see Chapter 8). Technically speaking, field castration on an unanesthetized, conscious piglet is acceptable and performed as in commercial swine. However, this method is not recommended for minipigs as these animals are beloved pets worthy of the standard of care afforded a dog rather than that afforded livestock. In addition, castration of commercial breed piglets is typically performed within the first 1 or 2 weeks of life, and most miniature pet pigs present at an older age. As weaning should occur around 6 to 8 weeks of age, by the time of adoption or purchase, a piglet will be too old for this method of castration despite his small size.

First and foremost, palpate! Testicles in the porcine descend in the last 30 days of gestation and should be easily palpable within the scrotum from birth. (Note: The Kunekune breed has smaller testicles relative to body size as compared to other pig breeds, but they are still readily identifiable). Ensure two testicles are present within the scrotum and check for hernia prior to incising. Cryptorchidism is common in miniature pigs and if you are uncomfortable performing this surgery, do NOT remove the scrotal testicle while leaving the abdominal testicle behind. Please.

Testicle size in the minipig is quite large relative to body size, and although the incision must be larger to accommodate this, one common castration technique is similar to that used in the canine: prescrotal incision, exteriorization of each testis, ligation of spermatic cords, closure of tunics, fascia, subcutis/skin (Fig. 9.1). Skin sutures are not recommended as the stress of restraint required for removal outweighs benefit. Either open or closed castration can be performed. In field procedures, closed castration might be the better option to avoid exposure of the abdominal cavity. In older males, the increasingly dense fibrous tissue that comprises the vaginal tunic may make open castration easier. Even with open castration, the incised tunic can be pulled back up over the stump of the ligated spermatic cord and sutured closed after removal of the testicle (semi-closed castration). Removal can also be accomplished via separate scrotal incisions made over each testicle. Such incisions may be left open to allow drainage, but the environment and potential for contamination should be considered as well as owner objections to open wounds.

In minipigs, the inguinal ring should be evaluated as inguinal hernia has historically been one of the more common complications. If a finger can easily be inserted through the ring, a suture should be placed to close the gap. In many instances, the stump of the ligated spermatic cord is large enough to fill the ring; if the stump regresses all the way into the abdomen and cannot be palpated after the testicle is removed, closure of the ring should be considered. However, it has been reported that pigs undergoing inguinal ring

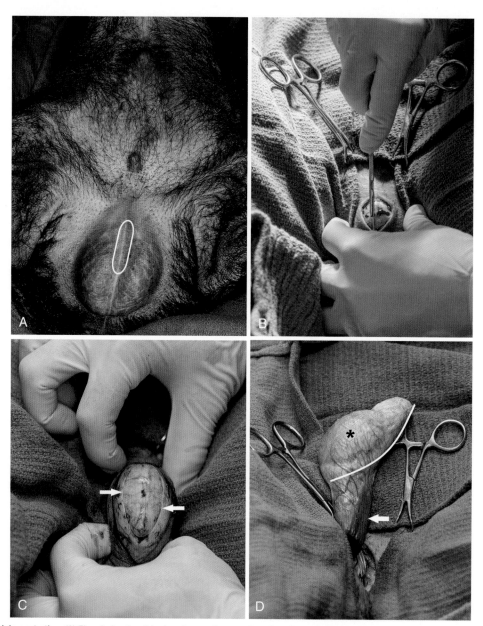

Fig. 9.1 Minipig castration: (A) The pig is placed in dorsal recumbency, clipped, and aseptically prepped. A line block of the intended surgical incision *(circled)* can be performed using a local anesthetic such as lidocaine. Lidocaine can also be injected into each testicle and allowed several minutes to infiltrate the spermatic cord. Multimodal analgesia should also include preoperative (i.e., an opioid such as butorphanol) and postoperative (i.e., NSAID) medications. (B) One testis is maneuvered to midline (to avoid incising over the penis) and an incision made. (C) The testis is squeezed through the incision. The outer fibrous connective tissue layer (external spermatic fascia; *arrows*) can be distinguished from the vaginal tunic that still encloses the testicle (closed technique). (D) The testis has been exteriorized through the midline prescrotal incision, still contained within the vaginal tunic (closed technique); excess adipose and connective tissue have been "stripped" away. The cremaster muscle is clearly visible as a reddish-brown strip *(arrow)*; within the tunic, the outline of the testis *(*)* and epididymis *(curved line)* can be seen.

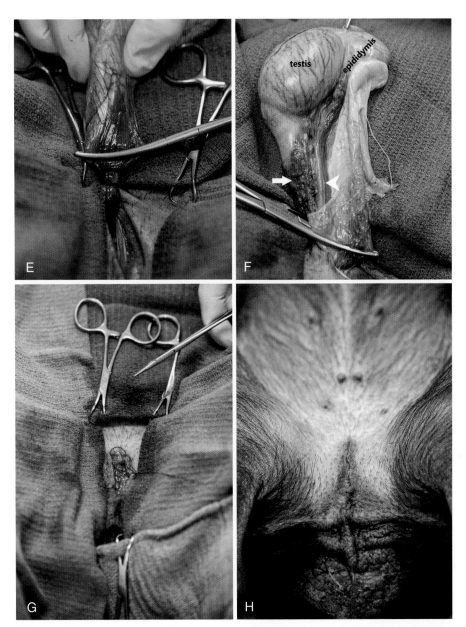

Fig. 9.1, cont'd (E) The spermatic cord has been double ligated as proximal as possible. (F) The second testicle has been exteriorized through the same midline incision, after incising through the external spermatic fascia; the vaginal tunic has been incised and reflected to show the testis, epididymis, pampiniform plexus *(arrow)* and spermatic cord *(arrowhead)*. (G) After spermatic cords have been ligated and both testes removed, the incision is closed. An intradermal (buried) skin closure is recommended due to difficulty of restraint for removal of external skin sutures. **(H)** The incision site post-castration. (B–H, Photo credit: Jennifer L. Davis.)

closure are more likely to experience postoperative complications, so need should be carefully assessed.

Cryptorchid Castration

Cryptorchidism, usually unilateral and more common on the left Wilbers, personal communication), is common in the miniature pig. The cryptorchid testicle is typically found just within the abdomen at the level of the inguinal ring, less commonly in the inguinal canal. Although smaller than the normally descended testicle (Fig. 9.2B), it should be readily identifiable. Paramedian

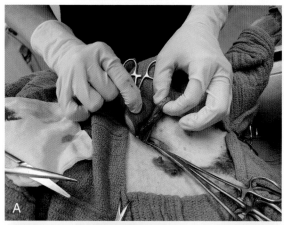

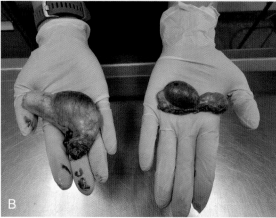

Fig. 9.2 Cryptorchid castration: (A) To remove a cryptorchid testicle, an incision has been made over the inguinal ring and the gubernaculum used to pull the abdominal testicle into the surgical field without entering the abdomen. (B) Size difference between the scrotal testis *(left)* and abdominal testis *(right)*. While significantly smaller, the cryptorchid testicle is easy to identify and is most often located at the abdominal entrance to the inguinal canal.

laparotomy is a standard procedure for removal of a cryptorchid testicle. However, Scollo and colleagues (2016) describe a less-invasive inguinal approach in which traction placed on the gubernaculum through an incision over the inguinal ring pulls the testis to the exterior of the body without breaching the abdominal cavity or enlarging the ring (Fig. 9.2A). Ultrasound examination can be helpful in locating the undescended testicle. A laparoscopic-assisted technique has also been described.

Note: Hyperplastic seminal vesicles may be identified during abdominal surgery to remove a cryptorchid testicle (Fig. 9.3). These can be striking—large, cystic, occupying the entire pelvic region around the bladder—and may appear neoplastic to those unfamiliar with the condition. Hyperplasia is clinically insignificant and will regress following castration.

Inguinal Hernia Repair

The scrotum should be carefully palpated prior to castration so that plans can be made to correct a hernia if present; in commercial swine, inguinal hernias are more common on the left. A hernia can be corrected once the testicle is exteriorized by twisting the spermatic cord, starting at the testicle, to push intestine back into the abdomen. If adhesions are present, an open reduction must be performed. After intestines have been moved back into the abdomen, the inguinal ring must be closed.

SPAY (OVARIOHYSTERECTOMY)

Spay of female miniature pet pigs (Fig. 9.4) is warranted to prevent unwanted pregnancy, but undesirable behaviors such as mounting, inappropriate urination, and nipping—at a frequency of every 21 days—also prompts owners to consider surgery. In addition, uterine pathology is common starting around 3 years of age (Cypher et al. 2017; Ilha et al. 2010; 1–7; Edson M, March 4–8, 2018), especially in nulliparous animals. Tumors are especially prevalent in older females and, while usually benign, can grow large enough (50 to 100 lbs [22 to 45 kg]) to result in death. Removal of both the ovaries and uterus is recommended, as neoplasia of the uterus in aged ovariectomized pigs has been reported. These animals typically present with bleeding from the vulva, and uterine adenocarcinoma is the most commonly identified neoplasm (Fig. 4.6); while metastasis

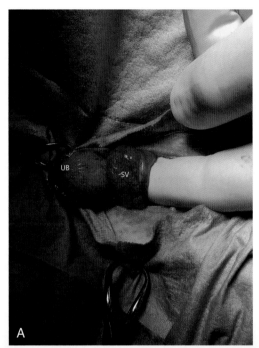

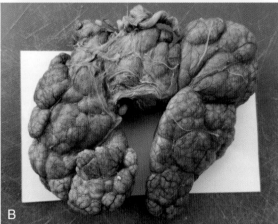

Fig. 9.3 (A) A normal seminal vesicle *(SV)* can be seen at the neck of the urinary bladder *(UB)*. (B) Formalin-fixed hyperplastic seminal vesicles from a cryptorchid 2-year-old pig (on a 3 × 5 in [7.6 × 12.7 cm] index card for size reference). Hyperplasia may be observed during laparotomy to remove a cryptorchid testicle. It can be striking and may resemble neoplasia but is clinically insignificant and will regress following castration. (A, Photo credit: Dr. Matt Edson.)

is rare, a second spay surgery to remove the uterus is indicated.

Miniature pig spay is a more time consuming, more technically difficult surgery than a dog spay due to the abundance of tissue (excessive adipose as well as a dense reproductive tract) and extensive ligation needed, although the overall approach is similar. Some notable details:

- Fat deposition is abundant. In addition to the expected subcutaneous adipose tissue (Fig. 9.4G), there may be a thick layer just beneath the linea, between the linea and the dense peritoneal lining. There may be yet another layer of adipose adhered to the inner peritoneum as well.
- The uterine horns are long and coiled within the caudal abdomen, so the ventral midline abdominal incision is made as for cystotomy. Note: There is often a substantial mid-abdominal scar at the umbilicus. Do not mistake for a spay scar—it's in the wrong location—see Fig. 9.4H.
- A spay hook may or may not be useful as the instrument is not very effective on coiled uterine horns and there is risk of mesenteric rent.
- The long uterine horns may resemble intestine (Fig. 9.5). Uterine horns are turgid, palpate firmly, and have faint longitudinal striations over the surface, while intestines are thin-walled and superficial branching blood vessels are visible.
- There is no suspensory ligament to break down as in the dog. The reproductive tract generally exteriorizes easily in a well-conditioned animal (Fig. 9.4B). Exception: The reproductive tract is quite small in non-cycling piglets under approximately 4 months of age (Fig. 9.6). After a few heat cycles, the tract rapidly enlarges, and surgery may be easier in terms of access and exteriorization. There is no current evidence to indicate that there are any benefits to early spay.
- The ovary is comparatively large, cystic in appearance, and is covered by a large, thin-walled bursa. This is normal. Oviducts are long and coiled. See Fig. 4.2.
- The ovarian pedicle is dense and vascular. A larger suture size than that required for a similarly sized canine is generally needed (Fig. 9.4C). Miller's knots or modified Miller's knots are useful in larger adults due to the abundance of tissue to be crushed.

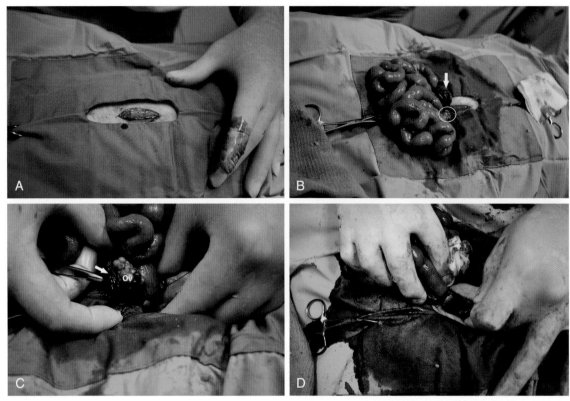

Fig. 9.4 Minipig Spay (5-month-old obese 95 lb pig): (A) A ventral midline abdominal incision is made as for cystotomy to access the caudally-located reproductive tract. Rule of thumb: Identify the "puckered" umbilicus prior to draping [see H below], palpate the pelvic rim, start halfway between these points and cut caudally. Start small—the uterus exteriorizes easily but so do intestines if given the opportunity. The incision can always be extended if needed. (B) The reproductive tract is easily exteriorized in a well-conditioned, cycling pig; both uterine horns, an ovary *(circled)*, and the contralateral oviduct *(arrow)* can be seen in this image (head is to the right and the tract is pulled caudally to access ovaries). (C) A ligature has been placed on the ovarian pedicle proximal to the large, cystic-appearing ovary *(Ov)*; the thin-walled ovarian bursa *(arrow)* has been retracted to allow better visualization for the surgeon. A larger suture size than that required for a similarly sized canine is generally needed; in this case, the surgeon chose to use size 1 polydioxanone to allow ready crushing of tissue. A Miller's knot or modified Miller's knot is useful in larger/older adults OR with smaller suture size due to the thickness of tissue to be crushed. Large suture size in this pig precluded the need for this and allowed a simple encircling ligature to be placed. Note the absence of clamps. We prefer to use clamps only to prevent back bleeding during transection of the tract, but this is simply surgeon preference. (D) After ligating the artery on each side of the uterine body, an encircling ligature has been placed. The double-ligated and transected ovarian pedicles have been released into the abdomen; the surgeon is holding the ovaries (hidden) and uterine horns and is pulling the tract caudally.

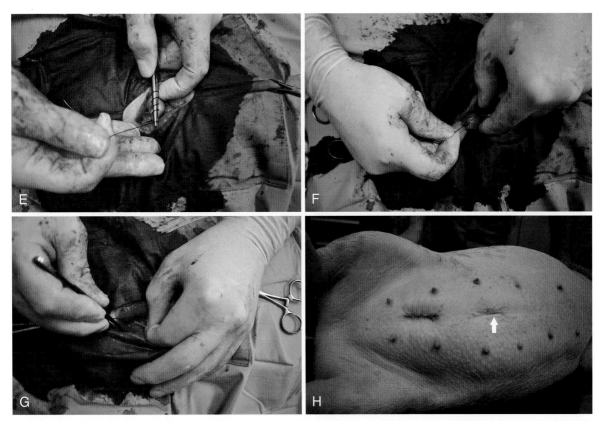

Fig. 9.4, cont'd (E) A continuous line of suture is placed over a clamp on the uterine stump; the ends will then be tightened as the clamp is removed. This is one of several techniques that can be used to oversew the stump and invert mucosa that will lend to adhesion formation if left exposed. This also allows crushing of small oozing vessels that may lead to bleeding from the vulva. (F) Following removal of the clamp, suture ends are tied, and the mucosa of the uterine stump inverted. The stump should be manually replaced beneath the bladder prior to closing the abdomen. (G) Following removal of the reproductive tract, the linea, subcutaneous tissue, and skin are closed as in the canine. The peritoneal lining is thick in the pig and may be closed as a separate layer prior to linea closure or may be included in the linea closure; this reduces intra-abdominal adhesions. The surgeon is holding a glistening pale band of tissue that includes both the peritoneum and linea. Note the deep layer of subcutaneous adipose. (H) Skin sutures are not recommended as the stress of restraint for removal outweighs any benefit. In this image, the incision location relative to the umbilicus *(arrow)* can be appreciated.

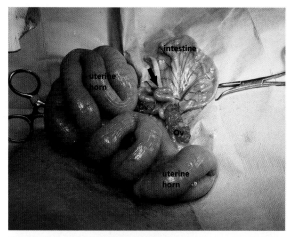

Fig. 9.5 The uterine horns of the pig are extremely long and resemble intestine but are more turgid, palpably firm, and bear faint longitudinal striations. Intestine is more flaccid and exhibits obvious branching blood vessels over the surface. The ovaries *(Ov)* and adjacent long, coiled oviduct are also visible in this image.

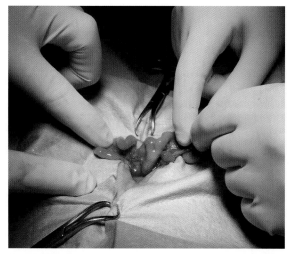

Fig. 9.6 The reproductive tract is quite small in non-cycling piglets under ~4 months of age, sometimes an obstacle in terms of access and exteriorization (in a deep potbelly) but more easily ligated. (Photo credit: Dr. Matt Edson.)

- The broad ligament is dense and highly vascular; it becomes more fibrous with age and vessels become more difficult to visualize. Hint: Position the surgery lamp to provide backlighting of blood vessels to see through the fibrous tissue.

The vascular anatomy includes an arc that allows access "windows" to be made (Fig. 9.7). Broad ligament vessels are large and must be ligated.

- The uterine body is short and the cervix long. Palpate the cervix and ligate between this dense, firm structure and the softer, more pliable uterine body. In smaller pigs, the body can be encircled as in the dog or cat, but in larger animals, this may not be feasible due to tissue thickness (too much to crush). In these animals, the uterine arteries can be ligated on either side and the stump over-sewn using an inverting pattern after removal of the tract. This helps to ligate small vessels that might lead to oozing from the vulva and also inverts the mucosal tissue that lends to adhesion formation if left exposed. The stiff cervix holds its place if exteriorized and should be tucked down under the bladder when spay is complete.
- Closure is similar to the canine. Skin sutures are unnecessary and may be difficult to remove in an awake patient so intradermal skin closure is recommended.

As in other species, analgesics should be used as part of the premedication protocol, intraoperatively (i.e., line block with local anesthetic such as lidocaine along incision and/or application to ovarian pedicle and uterine stump), and postoperatively [injectable non-steroidal anti-inflammatory drug (NSAID) and/or opioid with oral NSAID for 3 to 4 days]. Details on drug options and dosing can be found in Chapter 8.

Postspay complications are uncommon. Pigs are inflexible and cannot chew or paw at the incision. Owners should keep the pig calm and quiet post-surgery and avoid bathing or mud puddles for a week. Owners may be able to monitor the incision for bleeding, swelling, and discharge during a belly rub.

Postoperative vomiting is most common with the use of alpha-2 agonists such as xylazine or dexmedetomidine or with acepromazine; it may also be an issue with inadequate intraoperative pain control as well as motion sickness during transport to the clinic. Maropitant (Cerenia) or ondansetron can be used as needed for control of nausea and vomiting.

Intraoperative bradycardia is a common event and easily treated, if needed, with atropine to effect.

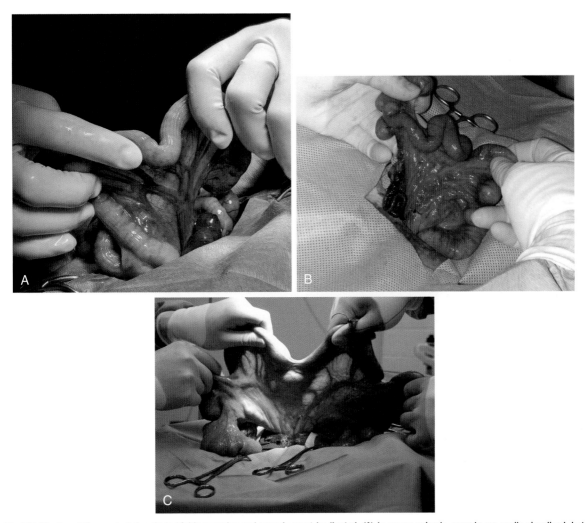

Fig. 9.7 The broad ligament of the pig is highly vascular, and vessels must be ligated. (A) In young animals, vessels are easily visualized, but (B) dense fibrous connective tissue increases with age and reduces visibility. (C) Backlighting can highlight vessels, making access windows more readily identifiable.

Tumor Removal or Pregnancy

Spaying of either a pig in late pregnancy or a pig with a uterine tumor is possible, but care should be taken to place the patient in dorsolateral recumbency to prevent the weight of the uterus from compromising circulation (Fig. 9.8). Aortocaval compression can severely compromise circulation and lead to cardiac arrest, which is a known complication in human obstetrics.

In addition, a prokinetic agent (i.e., metoclopramide) should be considered whenever a large mass (tumor or pregnant uterus) is removed to prevent postoperative ileus.

Note: Many uterine tumors can be readily exteriorized as the common leiomyomas/leiomyosarcomas that develop tend to remain enclosed within a smooth connective tissue covering, thus preventing extensive adhesions to other abdominal organs (Fig. 9.9).

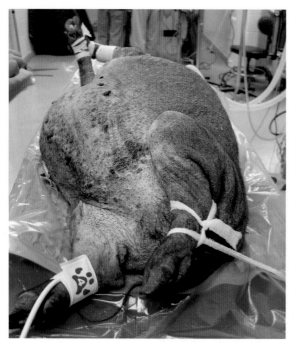

Fig. 9.8 Dorsolateral recumbency is the preferred position for removal of uterine tumors (or for late pregnancy) as aortocaval compression by a heavy uterus can compromise circulation and lead to cardiac arrest.

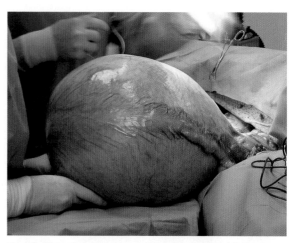

Fig. 9.9 Many uterine tumors can be readily exteriorized, despite potentially large size, as the common leiomyomas/leiomyosarcomas that develop tend to remain enclosed within a smooth connective tissue covering, thus preventing extensive adhesions to other abdominal organs. This 50-lb (23-kg) leiomyoma within the broad ligament was exteriorized onto a Mayo stand during surgical removal through ovariohysterectomy.

Entropion Correction

Entropion is frequently observed in miniature pigs as these animals have abundant periocular fat and a naturally heavy upper lid that cause inward rolling of lashes; the problem is often complicated by obesity. Surgical correction is similar to the canine and commonly employs a Hotz-Celsus technique to remove an elliptical section of skin adjacent to the eyelid margin to roll the cilia away from the cornea. A modification of the Hotz-Celsus procedure that utilizes secondary granulation tissue (i.e., Stades technique) has also been described by Linton and Collins (1993). Some individuals, especially if obese or formerly obese, may also require surgical resection of periocular fat pads to restore vision; details can be found in the listed references. See Fig. 9.10 and also Chapter 10.

Cutaneous Mass Removal (Lumpectomy)

The most common cutaneous neoplasms in the miniature pig (in my experience) are mast cell tumor and melanocytoma (Fig. 9.11), although other differentials exist including cyst, squamous cell carcinoma, cutaneous lymphoma, etc. (see also Chapter 10). Oddly, lipomas are uncommon to rare. Cytologic or histopathologic evaluation must be performed for definitive identification. Many cutaneous tumors, including most mast cell tumors, are benign.

Surgical removal is warranted if the mass is growing in size, ulcerated, interfering with function (i.e., on an eyelid), or becoming traumatized due to location. Removal is similar to that in the canine, although the thickness of the dermis and skin may impede closure depending on location. The skin of the ventrum is relatively thin and skin edges may be apposed post mass removal much like in the dog. However, the skin over the face, shoulders, dorsum, and rump is dense and tightly adhered to the subcutis, with little to no mobility to allow apposition of skin. No worries. These can be allowed to heal by second intention and do not require additional care other than keeping appositions clean (Fig. 9.12). When suturing pig skin, absorbable suture swaged onto a reverse cutting needle is recommended. Pig skin heals remarkably well.

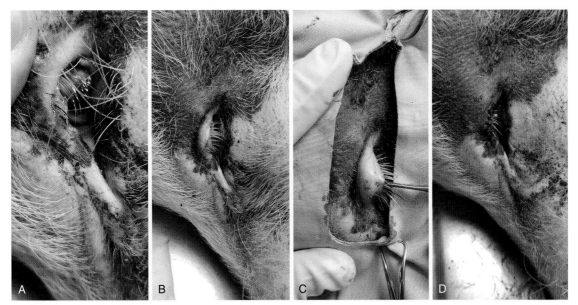

Fig. 9.10 Entropion correction: (A) Entropion is frequently observed in miniature pigs as these animals have abundant periocular fat and a naturally heavy upper lid that cause inward rolling of lashes. Although periocular fat is minimal in this lean, long-snouted pig, the large, recessed upper eyelid allows lashes to contact the corneal surface and subsequent mucoid discharge exacerbates the problem by making the cilia "sticky." Upper eyelids are more commonly affected but lower lid involvement is also possible. (B) Hair has been clipped, ocular discharge cleaned, and the eyelid everted; the entirety of the pale colored skin will be removed in an elliptical section starting adjacent to the eyelid margin (Hotz-Celsus technique). (C) Following clip and surgical prep with a dilute povidone iodine solution, the site is draped, and the surgeon rechecks the amount of lid to be removed. (D) Following removal of an elliptical eyelid section, incised edges have been closed in a simple interrupted pattern using a small size (4-0 or smaller) soft/braided absorbable suture, ensuring that knots and suture tags do not irritate the cornea. We prefer to allow the sutures to dissolve over time rather than anesthetize for removal.

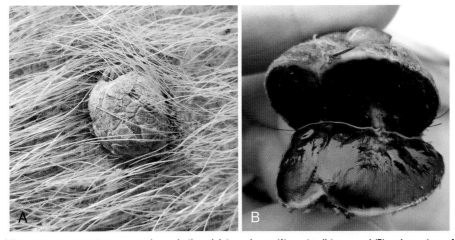

Fig. 9.11 Two of the more common cutaneous neoplasms in the miniature pig are (A) mast cell tumor and (B) melanocytoma. Melanocytoma is black on cut surface and oozes an inky substance, but hemangiosarcoma may appear nearly black as well. Definitive diagnosis cannot generally be made on gross examination alone; cytologic or histopathologic evaluation must be performed.

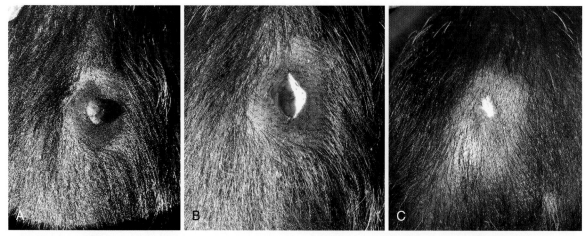

Fig. 9.12 (A) This approximately 3-cm diameter mass, histopathologically identified as a mast cell tumor, is located over the rump—an area with extremely thick skin that is firmly adhered to the underlying subcutis. Removal was deemed necessary as the mass was slowly enlarging, and the pig was traumatizing it by rubbing. (B) The mass has been removed, leaving a deep defect that cannot be closed due to lack of skin mobility, so the site will be allowed to heal by second intention. (C) Healed surgery site several weeks postoperatively. The scar reduced even further over time.

Rectal/Vaginal Prolapse Correction

Rectal (Fig. 9.13) or vaginal (Fig. 9.14) prolapse are both occasionally seen in miniature pigs. Rectal prolapse may occur secondary to straining (i.e., constipation, diarrhea, coughing, cystitis, vaginitis, etc.) or there may simply be a genetic predisposition. Vaginal prolapse is less common and cause is unknown, although inflammation or edema leading to straining (i.e., with vulvovaginitis, zearalenone, estrogenic substances) may predispose. If tissue is viable, the area can be cleaned with cold water and a hygroscopic agent (i.e., sugar, honey) and steady gentle pressure applied to reduce edema and swelling. Following a second rinse, the tissue is manipulated back into a normal position and a purse-string suture placed using non-absorbable suture or umbilical tape. Underlying issues, if identified, must be corrected to prevent recurrence. Anti-inflammatory medication as well as an antibiotic may be indicated.

An alternate method of rectal prolapse correction—especially if tissue is devitalized—is insertion of a rectal ring (commercially available or homemade from PVC) (Fig. 9.15). A rectal ring is an open tube with a central groove, and the largest ring size possible should be used to allow fecal material to pass. The ring is lubricated and inserted into the prolapsed tissue, with the groove next to the anus; viable mucosal tissue should be pulled out from the rectum to the level of the groove and an elastrator band or tight umbilical tape placed around the tissue. The prolapsed tissue should slough off within a week. High-fiber diet (i.e., adding canned pumpkin), a laxative such as mineral oil and/or stool softener should be administered to keep feces soft to allow ready passage through the ring (Edson 2018).

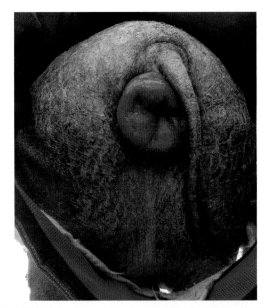

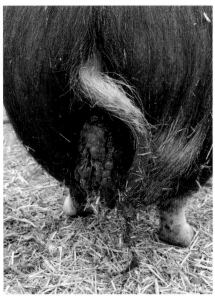

Fig. 9.13 Rectal prolapse may occur secondary to straining (diarrhea, constipation, cough, etc.) but may simply be a genetic predisposition. Reduction followed by placement of a purse string suture is an appropriate treatment in this case as the mucosa is healthy and undamaged. Sugar or honey can facilitate replacement if tissue is edematous. Underlying etiology, if known, should be corrected to prevent recurrence.

Fig. 9.14 Vaginal prolapse is less common than rectal prolapse in miniature pigs, but treatment is similar—clean with cold water, apply a hygroscopic agent such as sugar or honey, rinse, replace, and use a purse-string suture to maintain. In this animal, the vaginal mucosa is abnormal, exhibiting nodular proliferation; hyperplasia secondary to hormonal influence (i.e., estrogenic substances) was considered the likely cause and spay was recommended.

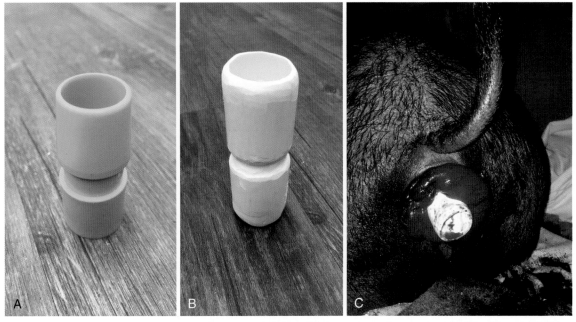

Fig. 9.15 (A) A commercially available rectal ring or (B) one homemade from PVC pipe can be used to correct rectal prolapse (C), especially if tissue is devitalized. (Photo credit: Dr. Matt Edson.)

BIBLIOGRAPHY

Allbaugh RA, Davidson HJ. Surgical correction of periocular fat pads and entropion in a potbellied pig (Sus scrofa). *Vet Ophthalmol.* 2009;12(2):115–118.

Anderson DE, Mulon PY. Anesthesia and surgical procedures in swine. In: Zimmerman JJ, Karriker LA, Ramirez A, et al., eds. *Diseases of Swine.* 11th ed. Hoboken, NJ: John Wiley & Sons, Inc.; 2019:179–181. 11th ed.

Andrea CR, George LW. Surgical correction of periocular fat pad hypertrophy in pot-bellied pigs. *Vet Surg.* 1999;28(5):311–314.

Becker HN. Surgical procedures in miniature pet pigs. In: Reeves DE, ed. *Care and Management of Miniature Pet Pigs.* Santa Barbara, CA: Brillig Hill, Inc.; 1993:67–76.

Cypher E, Videla R, Pierce R, et al. Clinical prevalence and associated intraoperative surgical complications of reproductive tract lesions in pot-bellied pigs undergoing ovariohysterectomy: 298 cases (2006–2016). *Vet Rec.* 2017;181(25):685.

Edson M. When pigs get high—anesthesia and surgery of miniature pigs. Presentation at Western Veterinary Conference; Las Vegas, NV; March 4–8, 2018.

Ilha MR, Newman SJ, van Amstel S, et al. Uterine lesions in 32 female miniature pet pigs. *Vet Pathol.* 2010;47(6):1071–1075.

Lawhorn DB. *Reproduction of potbellied pigs.* Merck Veterinary Manual; Revised June 2013. https://www.merckvetmanual.com/exotic-and-laboratory-animals/potbellied-pigs/reproduction-of-potbellied-pigs. Accessed March 2021.

Linton LL, Collins BK. Entropion repair in a Vietnamese pot-bellied pig. J Small Anim Pract. 1993;2(3):124–127.

Newman SJ, Rohrbach B. Pot-bellied pig neoplasia: a retrospective case series (2004–2011). *J Vet Diagn Invest.* 2012;24(5):1008–1013.

Østevik L, Elmas C, Rubio-Martinez LM. Castration of the Vietnamese pot-bellied boar: 8 cases. *Can Vet J.* 2012;53(9):943–948.

Rosanova N, Singh A, Cribb N. Laparoscopic-assisted cryptorchidectomy in 2 Vietnamese pot-bellied pigs *(Sus scrofa). Can Vet J.* 2015;56:153–156.

Salcedo-Jiménez R, Brounts SH, Mulon PY, Dubois MS. Multicenter retrospective study of complications and risk factors associated with castration in 106 pet pigs. *Can Vet J.* 2020;61(2):173–177.

Scollo A, Martelli P, Borri E, Mazzoni C. Pig surgery: cryptorchidectomy using an inguinal approach. *Vet Rec.* 2016;178(24):609.

Skelton JA, Baird AN, Hawkins JF, Ruple A. Cryptorchidectomy with a paramedian or inguinal approach in domestic pigs: 47 cases (2000–2018). *J Am Vet Med Assoc.* 2021;258(10):1130–1134.

Swindle MM. The reproductive system. In: Swindle MM, Smith AC., eds. *Swine in the Laboratory: Surgery, Anesthesia, Imaging, and Experimental Techniques.* Boca Raton, FL: CRC Press; 2016:191–195.

Tsai PS, Chen CP, Tsai MS. Perioperative vasovagal syncope with focus on obstetric anesthesia. *Taiwan J Obstet Gynecol.* 2006;45(3):208–214.

Wood P, Hall JL, McMillan M, et al. Presence of cystic endometrial hyperplasia and uterine tumours in older pet pigs in the UK. *Vet Record Case Rep.* 2020;8(1). http://dx.doi.org.prox.lib.ncsu.edu/10.1136/vetreccr-2019-000924.

Chapter 10

Illness and Disease

Kristie Mozzachio

This chapter is intended to provide some general guidance and is by no means comprehensive! It is organized to allow quick reference based on disease process or clinical signs and primarily focuses on features unique to, or especially common in, miniature pigs. As always, evaluate as for more familiar companion animal species such as the dog and extrapolate. In most cases, diagnostic testing, differential list, and treatment will be similar even if specific etiology varies.

AGGRESSION

Overview: Human-directed aggression is probably the number one behavioral issue in miniature pet pigs and is especially common in single-pig households. The behavior may begin at an early age but is generally identified as a problem around 2 years of age when the behaviors become an issue for the owner.

Pigs are naturally aggressive to one another and exhibit forceful physical contact from birth (i.e., when establishing a teat order). They continue these behaviors throughout life and will attempt to assert themselves when meeting a new pig; they often exhibit similar assertive behaviors with people and other animals as well. Online resources offer helpful tips for introducing unfamiliar pigs to one another, and this topic will not be covered further. See Chapter 2 for more information.

Signalment	Commonly 2 years of age (and older) but careful observation reveals the behavior in younger pigs; both genders, intact or neutered, are equally affected	Although intact male domestic swine are known to be aggressive to humans, this is uncommon in the miniature pig boar.
History	Single-pig households are a common denominator, with animals in multi-pig environments less commonly affected. By the time an owner recognizes a problem, the behavior is usually advanced with the pig charging, biting, or swiping (lateral movement of the head); the behavior may involve only visitors to the home but may also be directed at family members.	Besides an obvious attempt to bite, an aggressive pig may also chomp at the mouth, rapidly flick the tail or raise it straight out, or raise the mohawk (piloerection of hair on the dorsal neck/shoulders), and swipe the head to the side. However, all behaviors must be interpreted in the proper context. A raised mohawk by itself, for example, may indicate that the pig is relaxed and enjoying being petted; chomping may indicate tooth pain and is also common in intact males.
		The piglet in this video at the following link is showing aggressive behaviors that are being encouraged rather than corrected. While this may be cute in a small pig, the behavior becomes more pronounced and dangerous as the pig matures. https://www.minipiginfo.com/dear-pig-whisperers-blog/aggressive-pig-in-training

Continued

AGGRESSION—cont'd

Physical Exam Findings	Normal exam, although a female in estrus may exhibit behaviors interpreted as aggression
Diagnostics	None needed unless an underlying medical condition is suspected
Treatment	Aggressive behavior can be controlled with training but is best avoided altogether through owner education. Owners that recognize and correct inappropriate behaviors can avoid advanced aggression. These behaviors begin in piglets as they establish pecking order within the litter and represent a form of communication readily understood by conspecifics but often misinterpreted and mishandled by owners. See Chapter 2 for more information. At least one sorting panel should be used for protection when handling an aggressive pig. See Fig. 5.4.
Differentials	Estrus
	Rule out medical issues such as blindness (i.e., fat-blind obese pig) or deafness as well as painful conditions (i.e., tusk growing into the face)
Other	Pigs are social herd animals, and a minimum of two is recommended in any pet household. This is always my first suggestion to new pet pig owners as it is often the easiest way to avoid behavioral issues. Redirecting aggression is especially difficult if the pig accepts the family members but is aggressive towards strangers. It is nearly impossible to train a human visitor to correct a charging, biting pig, and their fearful reactions may further reinforce the behavior. Isolating the animal while "outsiders" visit may be necessary.
	Whenever a pig is removed from its herd (i.e., a visit to the veterinarian), there is a risk that there will be some degree of conspecific aggression upon return. This seems particularly likely when sedation, especially gas anesthesia, is involved, possibly associated with alteration of the pig's odor. Fighting is not as intense as during initial introduction and is typically short-lived, but owners should be forewarned, especially if an animal is recovering from the effects of sedation and/or a surgical procedure.
References	Tynes VV, Hart BL, Bain MJ. Human-directed aggression in miniature pet pigs. *J Am Vet Med Assoc.* 2007;230(3):385–389.
	Tynes VV. Miniature pet pig behavioral medicine. *Vet Clin North Am Exot Anim Pract.* 2021;24(1):63–86.
	https://www.minipiginfo.com/multiple-pig-families.html.

ARTHRITIS (DEGENERATIVE JOINT DISEASE)

See also Lameness

Overview: Arthritis is extremely common in pet pigs, and clinical signs can start as young as 2 years of age. Infectious causes (i.e., erysipelas), as well as metabolic issues (i.e., osteochondrosis/osteochondritis dissecans) or traumatic injury (i.e., humeral condylar fracture), may play a role, but conformation alone is enough to eventually lead to osteoarthritis in nearly all miniature pigs, with small/delicate limbs supporting a large amount of weight in these dwarf animals.

Signalment	8+ years a common signalment, although animals may be affected at a much younger age (2–3 years)

History	Lameness, often unilateral and involving a forelimb but may be shifting to involve multiple limbs; difficulty rising from a lying position or becoming sternal from a lateral position; crawling or frequent kneeling; inability to remain standing for long periods; greater reluctance than usual to move across certain flooring that may be slippery, or reluctance to use a step that has been navigated well in the past; signs become increasingly severe over time and may be exacerbated by cold or wet environmental conditions; end stage—using the bed as a toilet

Fig. 10.1: This pig suffers from moderate osteoarthritis and frequently assumes a "kneeling" posture rather than remain standing; she ambulates stiffly but without a limp.

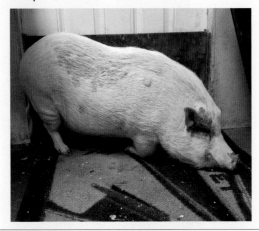

Physical Exam Findings	Limp; stiffness/reduced range of motion, especially of the elbows; hunched posture with the hindlimbs drawn far under the body; frequent "kneeling"; pain or crepitus on palpation; bony enlargement of joints, most commonly the elbow; valgus deformity of the forelimbs; joint swelling possible but less common Full orthopedic exam is generally not feasible in an awake pig

Fig. 10.2: "Classic" hunched posture of a severely arthritic pig, with the hindlimbs tucked beneath the body and the forelimbs held straight, sometimes even lifted off of the ground. Scooting backward is often easier than moving forward in these animals.

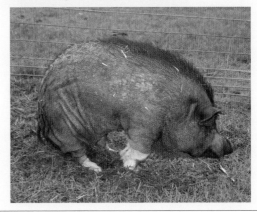

Continued

ARTHRITIS (DEGENERATIVE JOINT DISEASE)—cont'd

Diagnostics   Imaging—radiographs, CT, MRI

Arthrocentesis (joint tap) and cytologic evaluation ± bacterial culture and sensitivity may be helpful, primarily in animals in which an infectious process is suspected. Infectious arthritis is much less common in the minipig than in commercial swine.

Fig. 10.3: Mild bony remodeling (*osteophytosis*) involving the distal forelimb, with valgus deformity distal to the carpus. (*Photo credit: Jennifer L. Davis.*)

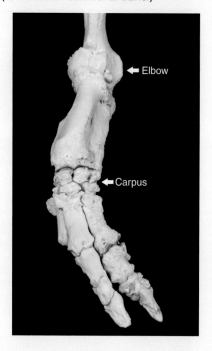

The most commonly affected joints are the elbow, carpus/tarsus, joints of the distal limbs (involving metacarpals/metatarsals and phalanges), and the spine. Bridging spondylosis may be severe and widespread.

Unlike the canine or feline, the hip and stifle joints are typically spared, which might be expected given that pigs carry much of their body weight at the cranial end of the body.

Fig. 10.4: Bridging spondylosis of the spine can range from minimal and multifocal (A, *arrows*) to severe and extensive, nearly fusing the spine (B). See also Fig. 10.48 for radiographic images. (*Photo credit: Jennifer L. Davis.*)

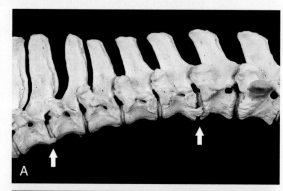

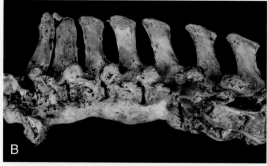

Treatment (Box 10.1)	Multimodal approach including: • Weight management • Pain control: non-steroidal anti-inflammatory drugs (NSAIDs) or steroids; acetaminophen; gabapentin; amantadine; tramadol; low-dose ketamine • Joint injection: intra-articular steroid, hyaluronic acid, platelet-rich plasma (PRP) • Nutritional supplements: glucosamine/methylsulfonylmethane (MSM)/chondroitin, omega-3 fatty acids • Polysulfated glycosaminoglycan (i.e., Adequan) • Alternative therapies: acupuncture, chiropractic, cold laser, massage, Assisi loop, physical therapy • Surgical treatment: arthroscopy to remove injured cartilage or joint mice; arthrodesis (usually reserved for younger animals with congenital or traumatic injury involving a single joint) • Frequent hoof trim • Environmental modification: good traction (stall mat or rubber-backed runner), light exercise, well-cushioned bed, flat/level surfaces (i.e., no ramps, no steep hills in the yard), heated bed	Treatment of osteoarthritis is an art and involves determination of whether changes in ambulation involve active inflammation and pain or are simply mechanical in nature, the result of loss of range of motion ("frozen" joints)—if a joint is immobile, it is no longer painful although gait abnormality persists. The goal is to keep the pig comfortable with the fewest drugs at the lowest dose and frequency, but this requires owner compliance and/or frequent evaluation. In mild cases, I typically start with an oral NSAID plus joint supplements and add additional medications as needed. In severe cases, I start with a tapering course of a steroid before switching to a maintenance NSAID +/− acetaminophen, gabapentin, amantadine, tramadol, acupuncture and cold laser, then begin to taper to an effective treatment once initial pain is controlled. **Weight loss is the single most effective treatment for arthritic pigs that are overweight.**
Differentials	Osteoarthritis, septic or traumatic arthritis, immune-mediated arthritis Osteochondrosis (OCD) Congenital deformity Luxation	Septic arthritis and OCD are common causes of lameness in commercial swine but are far less common in the minipig.
Other	Extrapolate from any species that suffers from arthritis, including humans. Owners are becoming better educated and starting to address the issue earlier with better results (i.e., maintaining appropriate body weight and starting joint supplements earlier in life), but many pigs present with advanced disease, and treatment is palliative to keep the animal comfortable until euthanasia becomes necessary. Osteoarthritis typically only affects mobility, not appetite or demeanor, and owners struggle with the decision to euthanize. Have owner fill out a questionnaire on normal activity levels similar to those designed for dogs or cats—when the pig fails to engage in previously enjoyable activities (such as rooting in the yard or exploring novel areas), it is time to consider euthanasia. As pigs are fastidious animals, euthanasia should be strongly encouraged for any pig that, despite treatment, begins to urinate or defecate in or near the sleeping area.	
References	Epstein ME. Rethinking management of canine osteoarthritis. Oral presentation at: Western Veterinary Conference; February 17–20, 2019; Las Vegas, NV. Mozzachio K, Tynes VV. Recognition and treatment of pain in pet pigs. In: Egger CM, Love L, Doherty T, eds. *Pain Management in Veterinary Practice*. Ames, IA: John Wiley & Sons, Inc.; 2014:383–389. Mozzachio K, Asseo L. Miniature pigs. In: Carpenter JW, ed. *Exotic Animal Formulary*. 6th ed. In press. Papich MG. *Papich Handbook of Veterinary Drugs*. 5th ed. St. Louis, MO: Elsevier, Inc.; 2021.	

BOX 10.1

Treatment of arthritis should be multimodal and includes a number of pain medications, often used in combination, as well as weight management, nutritional supplements, regular hoof care, environmental modifications such as good traction, level surfaces, soft/warm/draft free bed, etc. Alternative therapies including acupuncture, chiropractic, cold laser, massage, Assisi loop, and physical therapy can be added as well. Surgical treatments may be useful but are not commonly offered for the porcine species.

- Pain medications:
  - NSAID
    - Carprofen 2.2 mg/kg PO q12h
    - Grapiprant (Galliprant®) 2 mg/kg PO q24h
    - Meloxicam 0.1–0.2 mg/kg PO q24h
  - Acetaminophen 15 mg/kg PO q8–12h
  - Amantadine 3-5 mg/kg PO q12-24h
  - Gabapentin 5–15 mg/kg PO q12h gradually increased up to 40 mg/kg PO q8–12h if needed
    - Do not discontinue abruptly as rebound pain (pain intensity higher than than original level) may occur
  - Tramadol 2–4 mg/kg PO q6h–24h
- Supplements:
  - Glucosamine 22-44 mg/kg/day PO
  - Polysulfated glycosaminoglycan (Adequan®)
    - Loading dose: 4.4 mg/kg IM once, then 3.3 mg/kg q4d × 7 treatments
    - Maintenance: once per week × 4 wks, then 2 ×/month, then monthly as needed

CONSTIPATION

See also Urolithiasis

Overview: Constipation can be diagnosed and managed as for the dog or cat and is mentioned here only because straining to urinate and straining to defecate appear similar to owners, the former requiring immediate evaluation. Uncomplicated constipation is most commonly related to reduced fluid intake, especially during cold winter weather.

Signalment	Any	
History	Straining to defecate, possibly with grunts or groans; production of small, hard fecal balls	Pregnant sows close to parturition may become constipated as intestinal water absorption increases in response to milk production, changing fecal consistency.
Physical Exam Findings	Physical exam is often unremarkable, except for small, firm fecal balls within the rectum. Dehydration is difficult to identify on PE alone.	Tenesmus may not be observed during the exam as episodes tend to be infrequent. However, a pig straining to urinate will be agitated and repeatedly posturing, often with intense abdominal effort while straining.

Diagnostics

Imaging (i.e., radiographs) to evaluate for obstruction or foreign body; if uncomplicated constipation, imaging will be unremarkable, although a large amount of feces is expected to be present in any pig.

Complete blood count (CBC), serum chemistry may confirm dehydration but results otherwise unremarkable.

Fig. 10.5: Normal abdominal radiographs in an adult pig—right lateral (A), ventrodorsal (B), and left lateral (C) views.

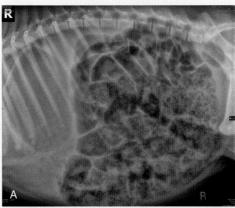

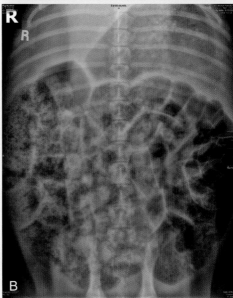

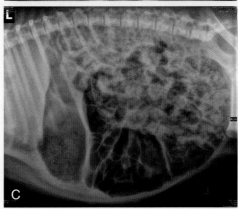

Continued

CONSTIPATION—cont'd

Treatment	Fluid therapy to correct dehydration; enema; adjust diet to increase fiber and fluid intake (i.e., add canned pumpkin or psyllium to the diet and flavor room temperature water with juice to encourage intake); regular exercise Stool softeners may be useful for more severe cases.	A ride in the car frequently stimulates defecation in pet pigs that are unaccustomed to transport. Environmental modification may be needed to prevent yearly recurrence during cold weather. Outdoor pets, especially, are less active in the cold and drink less, particularly if water is cold or frozen. Livestock water heaters can at least keep water from freezing, and owners can offer room temperature water during the day or add water to feed to encourage intake. Increasing dietary fiber can also be helpful. Multiple meals or snacks fed at a distance from the sleeping area can encourage brief exercise and more frequent potty breaks. For breeding females, increase dietary fiber in late pregnancy and ensure adequate fluid intake.
Differentials	Urinary tract obstruction, especially in males Neoplasia, foreign body, or stricture causing mechanical obstruction Motility disorder	
Other	The majority of constipation cases are medically managed through rehydration and increased fluid and fiber intake. If an animal is also anorexic or vomiting or fails to respond to treatment, further work-up is needed as more severe underlying issues may be present.	
References	Bassett JR, Mann EA, Constantinescu GM, McClure RC. Subtotal colectomy and ileocolonic anastomosis in a Vietnamese pot-bellied pig with idiopathic megacolon. *J Am Vet Med Assoc.* 1999;215(11):1640–1643. Farmer C, Maes D, Peltoniemi O. Mammary system. In: Zimmeran JJ, Karriker LA, Ramirez A, et al., eds. *Diseases of Swine.* 11th ed. Hoboken, NJ: John Wiley & Sons, Inc.; 2019:328–329.	

DENTAL DISEASE

See also Chapter 7; Epistaxis; Tusk Abscessation

Overview: As with other pets, miniature pigs suffer from dental disease, and severity increases with age. Prophylactic care similar to that recommended for dogs and cats should be considered and promoted; however, clinics willing and able to provide this level of care to pet pigs are limited. At a minimum, a thorough oral exam under anesthesia may be warranted every few years for pigs over the age of 6–8 years, with extraction of grossly diseased teeth. Quick evaluation of the oral cavity on a "flipped" pig (see Chapter 5) may allow determination of disease level and risk versus benefit of additional diagnostics and treatment, including the necessary sedation. Dental disease can be severe enough in some animals to warrant euthanasia if treatment is not pursued.

Signalment	Middle-aged to older animals, with disease severity increasing with age (8+ years), although gingivitis and periodontitis have been reported as early as 6 months of age, becoming serious by 16 months

History

Foul odor emanating from the mouth; eating more slowly; refusing crunchy/hard food items; abnormal behaviors such as chewing on one side of the mouth, head shake or tilt while eating, lip-smacking, teeth grinding; excessive salivation; tooth loss; facial swelling ± drainage; epistaxis

Fig. 10.6: This swelling along the jawline (*arrow*) palpated as soft, fluctuant, and fine needle aspirate confirmed an abscess. While an uncomplicated superficial abscess is one differential, oral exam ± skull radiographs should be performed to rule out underlying dental disease. (*Photo credit: Leanne Jones.*)

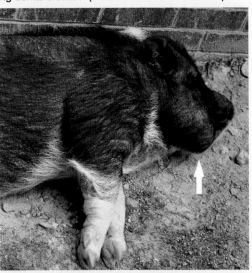

Physical Exam Findings

Brown to black tooth discoloration or excessive tartar accumulation; loose, fractured, or missing teeth; deep gingival pocketing with entrapped feed material and hair; "wave mouth" (sharp points on premolars and molars due to malocclusion); gingival proliferation ± associated palpable bony lysis

Kunekune breed: Facial swelling, especially near the ear base/angle of the jaw, and possibly discharging feed material

Fig. 10.7: The trimmed surface of tusks in the male, especially upper tusks, may turn black, but discoloration alone is not indicative of a diseased tooth.

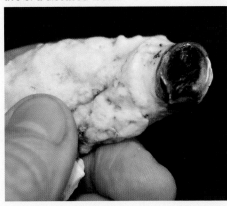

Fig. 10.8: Although a pig may open the mouth widely to accept a treat and allow a glimpse (pictured), complete examination of the oral cavity must be done under anesthesia, especially given the narrow "gape" that limits access.

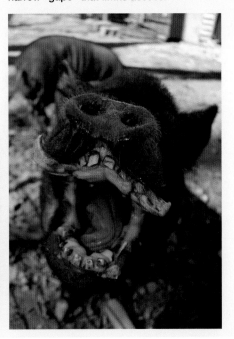

Continued

DENTAL DISEASE—cont'd

Fig. 10.9: The lower incisors frequently break along visible horizontal demarcations (pictured) or simply may wear excessively—nearly ALL pigs will eventually exhibit this; pulp exposure is extremely common and readily noted on physical exam. The issue may be clinically benign but warrants treatment if discomfort is observed.

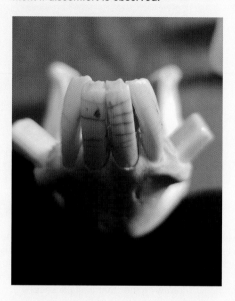

Fig. 10.10: Broken/worn lower incisors in an 11-month-old pig.

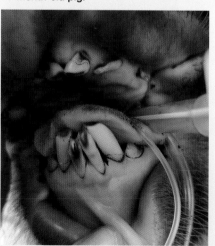

Fig. 10.11: Tartar covering canine and premolars in a 4-year-old pig.

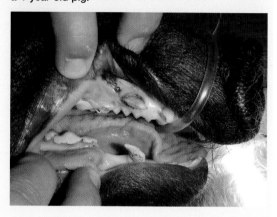

Fig. 10.12: Periodontal pocketing (*arrowhead*) and generalized, smooth, bulbous gingival proliferation in a 13-year-old pig. Note also malocclusion of lower canine/tusk causing damage to maxillary gum tissue (*arrow*).

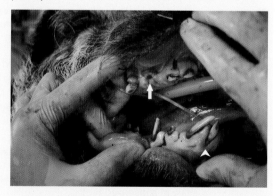

Diagnostics   Radiographs, possibly CT

Endoscopy can allow better visualization of caudal oral cavity

Biopsy suspicious lesions

Fig. 10.13: Radiographs of an 18-year-old castrated male pig with left mandibular tusk abscess as well as nasal squamous cell carcinoma, the latter seen as a soft tissue swelling over the rostral snout (*arrow*) in the lateral view (A); the infected right mandibular tusk had been extracted 5 years prior, and bony remodeling of the mandible (*arrow*) is evident in the ventrodorsal view (B). (*Photo credit: Leanne Jones.*)

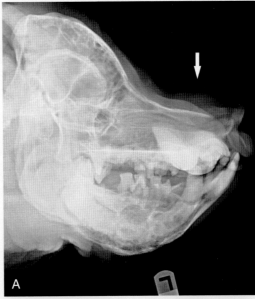

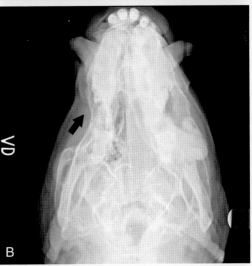

Continued

DENTAL DISEASE—cont'd

Treatment	Scale and polish; extract diseased teeth; lightly file points on premolars and molars if indicated to improve bite or reduce traumatic damage	A combination of small animal and equine dental instruments may be helpful as access is severely limited due to narrow gape; caudal molars may be inaccessible.
	Trim tusks if contributing to malocclusion	
	Drain abscess(es)	
	Antibiotics and analgesic medications if warranted	
Differentials	Oral neoplasia—squamous cell carcinoma is common in aged miniature pigs and is often indistinguishable from severe dental disease in which osteomyelitis and/or gingival hyperplasia is present	Miniature pigs are dwarf animals and frequently suffer from facial deformities such as a shortened maxilla and resultant malocclusion. Misalignment can lead to "wave mouth" with sharp points on teeth that traumatize soft tissues and lead to ulceration, feed impaction, infection, etc. The short-snouted Kunekune breed, in particular, has been reported to suffer from an inheritable malocclusion in which a deformed mandible leads to abnormal positioning of caudal molars. An "opening just lateral to the last visible molar at the junction of the body and ramus of the mandible" (Archer) allows feed to become impacted, with enlargement of both soft tissue and bony pockets over time, and eventually leading to the formation of fistulous tracts. The deformity is bilateral even though the clinical presentation may be initially unilateral. Treatment is difficult, and although a cure has not been reported, management is possible.
	Abscessation of the canine (tusk) in the male seems to be related to open-rooted confirmation rather than secondary to periodontal disease, although extensive osteomyelitis in advanced infection will affect adjacent teeth.	
Other	As with any species, pet pigs should be intubated for dental procedures, and this may limit service offerings given intubation difficulties. Refer to Chapter 8 for more details on intubation in the pig.	
References	Archer RM, Weston JF, Herdan CL, Owen MC. Facial swelling and discharging lesions associated with abnormalities of the mandible in Kunekune pigs. *N Z Vet J.* 2012;60(5):305–309. Baumgardner R, Ziegler J, Shannon D, et al. Mandibular feed impaction resulting in fistulous tract development in a Kunekune sow [*Sus scrofa domesticus*]. *J Exot.* 2020;35:80–81. Eubanks DL. Dental anatomy, radiography, and extraction of mandibular premolar teeth in Yucatan minipigs. *J Vet Dent.* 2013;30(2):96–98. Smith MA, Rao S, Rawlinson JE. Dental pathology of the domestic pig [Sus Scrofa Domesticus]. *J Vet Dent.* 2021 Feb 19:898756421989097. doi:10.1177/0898756421989097. Wang S, Liu Y, Fang D, Shi S. The miniature pig: useful large animal model for dental and orofacial research. *Oral Dis.* 2007;13(6):530–537.

DIARRHEA

Overview: Pet pigs occasionally present with diarrhea and should be treated as for any species. Care is generally supportive, and etiology is often undetermined. Numerous infectious diseases cause diarrhea in the commercial industry and are associated with significant morbidity and/or mortality, but these rarely cause issues in the miniature pig population.

Signalment	Any, but young piglets more commonly affected	
History	Soft to liquid feces ± increased frequency of defecation ± straining; possible loss of appetite; lethargy	
	Possible history of newly introduced animal(s) into the herd that may be clinically normal or similarly affected	
Physical Exam Findings	Affected pigs range from clinically normal except for loose stool to lethargic, depressed, and hyporexic; fever may be present.	
Diagnostics	CBC, serum chemistry including electrolytes	Identification of a specific etiologic agent might be useful in a herd health situation (i.e., rescue/sanctuary) as this may allow for better control in the future (i.e., through vaccination). A variety of antemortem tests are offered through the Iowa State University Veterinary Diagnostic Laboratory. Diarrheal disease in swine is often diagnosed on post-mortem evaluation.
	Fecal flotation ± direct smear	
	Fecal testing for infectious agents possible but not generally indicated	
Treatment	Primarily supportive: bland diet such as chicken and rice, eggs, oatmeal, yogurt	Diarrhea is often self-limiting, as in other species. However, more aggressive treatment is indicated if the animal is clinically depressed and inappetent, there is blood in the feces, or there are comorbidities that might contribute to rapid decline (neonate, emaciation, concurrent disease).
	Fluid therapy (SQ, IV, or oral such as water flavored with juice or Pedialyte/Gatorade)	
	GI protectants: kaolin-pectin, bismuth subsalicylate (Pepto Bismol), sucralfate, famotidine, omeprazole	
	Maropitant (Cerenia)	
	Antibiotics may be warranted in some instances but use judiciously	
	If a causative agent is identified in a larger "open" herd with a regular influx of new animals, vaccination may be prudent. However, it is not recommended to vaccinate without identification of a specific agent.	
Differentials	Infectious (viral, bacterial, parasitic less common)	The underlying etiology of minipig diarrhea is frequently undetermined. GI parasites are often a "go-to" for diagnosis and treatment but uncommonly cause issues in pet pigs.
	Moldy feed or plant material	
	Dietary indiscretion	
	Systemic disease such as organ dysfunction, endocrinopathy, etc.	
Other	Metronidazole is a commonly used medication in canine diarrhea cases; however, this drug is illegal for use in food animals in the US.	
References	https://vetmed.iastate.edu/vdpam/FSVD/swine/index-diseases/diarrheal-diseases https://vetmed.iastate.edu/vdpam/research/disease-topics/bacterial-susceptibility-profiles	

DIPPITY PIG (ACUTE DERMATITIS; ERYTHEMA MULTIFORME)

Overview: "Dippity Pig" is the common name given this unusual condition based on clinical signs—a "dipping" movement in which the pig repeatedly flattens or arches the back and either sits down or lowers the body toward the ground, often appearing weak or painful in the hind end, and sometimes vocalizing in distress/pain. Within approximately 12 hours, extremely painful, serosanguinous lesions may develop along the dorsum. The condition is precipitated by a stressful event and resolves spontaneously within about 2–4 days. Etiology is unknown.

Signalment	More frequently affects younger pigs, <3 years of age, although any age pig may be affected
History	Acute onset
	Precipitated by a stressful event such as a fight with another pig, transport, introduction of a new human or pet to the household, thunderstorm, any sudden deviation from normal routine

Physical Exam Findings

Repeated flattening or arching of the back, with simultaneous sitting or lowering of the body to the ground; in between these "dipping" episodes, the pig can ambulate normally

Distress vocalizations

Weeping serosanguinous lesions, typically along the dorsum and often exhibiting a unique, horizontally-oriented "grill mark" appearance; ± Fever

Severe pain along the dorsum, especially over the lumbar area (even in the absence of visible skin lesions)

Appetite typically unaffected

Video of affected pigs can be found at the following links:
https://www.youtube.com/watch?v=e568j5P494M
http://www.youtube.com/watch?v=_4QDDn169ho

Fig. 10.14: Horizontally-oriented "grill mark" lesions along the dorsum, primarily over the lumbar region (*arrowheads*). These late-stage Dippity Pig lesions are crusted over and no longer painful in this animal.

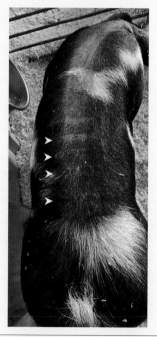

Diagnostics	None needed as clinical signs are distinctive and sufficient for diagnosis

Treatment	Analgesic (i.e., NSAID)	As appetite is typically normal, oral medications are preferred over injectable drugs to reduce handling stress for administration.
	Antipyretic if warranted	
	Topical ointments such as lanolin cream or lidocaine gel	
	Reduce stress by providing a dimly lit, temperature-controlled, quiet environment	
	Keep patient out of the sun	
Differentials	Traumatic injury	
	Intervertebral disk disease (IVDD)	
	Sunburn	
Other	Dippity Pig has been termed erythema multiforme, and although clinical disease (acute, self-limiting) is most similar to that observed in humans, gross lesions are dissimilar to both human and canine disease. Acute dermatitis in the Göttingen minipig most closely resembles Dippity Pig. I personally liken the condition to shingles. Skin biopsy can confirm diagnosis and may enhance understanding of the disease.	
References	https://www.minipiginfo.com/dippity-pig-syndrome.html Grand N. Diseases of minipigs. In: McAnulty PA, Dayan AD, Ganderup N, Hastings K, eds. *The Minipig in Biomedical Research*. Boca Raton, FL: CRC Press; 2012:60. Yager JA. Erythema multiforme, Stevens-Johnson syndrome and toxic epidermal necrolysis: comparative review. *Vet Dermatol*. 2014;25(5):406-e64.	

ENTROPION

See also Chapter 9

Overview: Entropion is commonly identified in miniature pet pigs and may be conformational (primary) or may be secondary to rolling of the lids with excessive weight gain in the face. Despite lashes contacting the corneal surface, many pigs remain subclinical, and the condition is identified during routine examination. Squinting and epiphora may be noted, and behavioral changes associated with reduced vision may be reported by the owner.

Signalment	Any, young pig if genetic; prevalent in obese (or formerly obese) animals	
History	Squinting; ocular discharge; irritable, aggressive, or "jumpy" behavior due to reduced vision and/or pain	
Physical Exam Findings	Eyelids roll such that lashes rotate toward, or contact, the corneal surface; upper lids are more commonly affected, but lower lids may be involved as well; mucoid discharge; epiphora; ulceration uncommon; cornea may exhibit opacity or brown pigmentation from chronic insult in obese animals	Pigs have abundant periocular fat and a naturally heavy upper lid, and evaluation must determine whether this presents a problem to the individual.

Continued

ENTROPION—cont'd

Note: Pigs appear to have much lower corneal sensation as compared to other species, and expected clinical signs of entropion may be absent, despite corneal microabrasions.

Fig. 10.15: With upper lid entropion, lashes clumped with mucoid discharge may be "tucked under" (situated along the conjunctival surface of) the lower lid.

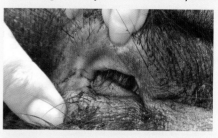

Fig. 10.16: Primary entropion of the lower lid.

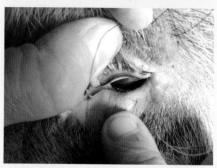

Diagnostics	Fluorescein stain to evaluate for corneal ulceration; slit lamp may be needed to detect subtle changes
Treatment	Surgical correction [i.e., Hotz-Celsus most common technique in which an elliptical section of eyelid is removed; Stades forced granulation method; combination technique (Linton)] In young animals that may outgrow the condition, surgical tacking may be performed to temporarily evert the eyelid margins. Weight loss in obese animals

In obese animals—or formerly obese animals that still maintain a heavy brow—surgical removal of periocular fat pads may be necessary ± entropion correction to restore vision.

Fig. 10.17: Heavy upper lid causing inward rolling of lashes (A); surgical correction performed using Hotz-Celsus technique (B).

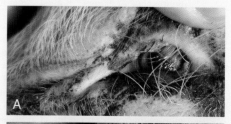

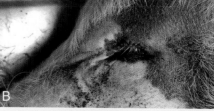

Differentials	Obesity—weight loss is preferred prior to surgery as the condition may correct on its own
	Spastic entropion caused by ocular irritation (including foreign body, ectopic cilia, etc.)
References	Allbaugh RA, Davidson HJ. Surgical correction of periocular fat pads and entropion in a potbellied pig [Sus scrofa]. *Vet Ophthalmol*. 2009;12(2):115–118.
	Andrea CR, George LW. Surgical correction of periocular fat pad hypertrophy in pot-bellied pigs. *Vet Surg*. 1999;28(5):311–314.
	Ehall H. Ocular examination and background observations. In: McAnulty PA, Dayan AD, Ganderup N, Hastings K, eds. The Minipig in Biomedical Research. Boca Raton, FL: CRC Press; 2012:293-303.
	Linton LL, Collins BK. Entropion repair in a Vietnamese pot-bellied pig. *J Small Exotic Anim Med*. 1993;2(3):124–127.

EPISTAXIS

See also Neoplasia—Squamous Cell Carcinoma

Overview: Epistaxis is occasionally observed in miniature pet pigs, and diagnosis and treatment are similar to the canine, although underlying etiology seems to be less varied in the pig. Neoplasia is by far the most common cause of nasal bleeding and is often highly aggressive; however, other differentials exist, and biopsy may be needed for definitive diagnosis.

Signalment	Typically middle-aged to older animals (8+ years)
History	Intermittent bleeding from the nares; sneezing; snoring or raspy breathing; rubbing the face; focal snout swelling

Physical Exam Findings	Physical exam may be normal, especially if there is no active bleeding
	Reduced airflow from the nares, often unilateral
	Swelling over the dorsal snout
	Sedated oral exam may be necessary to evaluate for contributing dental disease or oral neoplasia.

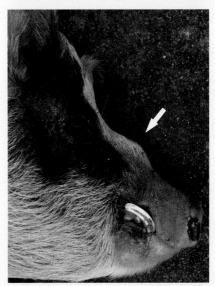

Fig. 10.18: Domed swelling over the dorsal snout (*arrow*). This rapidly growing mass was diagnosed as nasal squamous cell carcinoma (SCC), and extensive osteolysis of underlying bone was present at necropsy.

Continued

EPISTAXIS—cont'd

Diagnostics   Imaging of the head (radiographs, CT, MRI)

Rhinoscopy

Biopsy

CBC to evaluate for anemia and thrombocytopenia, especially with severe bleeding; coagulation profile

Thoracic radiographs may be indicated to evaluate for pulmonary metastasis, but most nasal tumors, while locally invasive, do not metastasize.

Although pigs spend a significant amount of time rooting, nasal foreign body is (unexpectedly) uncommon.

Fig. 10.19: Right lateral radiograph (A) shows a slightly raised, mixed opacity mass on the dorsal snout *(arrow)*; DV view (B) highlights a hazy region of soft tissue opacity in the rostral nasal cavity (*circled*). This mass was diagnosed as nasal SCC through biopsy of a polypoid mass removed from the nasal passage.

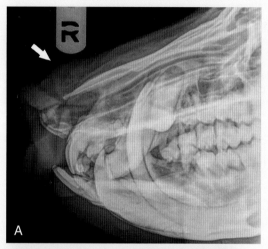

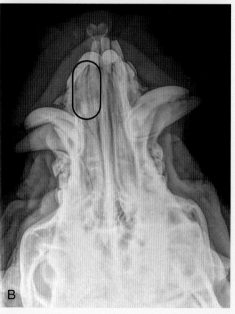

Treatment	Depends on underlying etiology	Avoid drugs such as NSAIDs that may predispose to hemorrhage
	Yunnan Baiyao (Chinese medicine formula) ± acupuncture can provide symptomatic treatment and reduce bleeding	
	Masses can be surgically debulked, but cancerous lesions tend to be highly aggressive, with rapid (re)growth; histopathology should always be performed as pigs also develop inflammatory masses that appear cancerous grossly but are readily cured with excision ± antibiotic treatment.	
	Antifungal or antibiotic treatment as indicated based on cytologic or histopathologic evaluation; secondary bacterial infection is common, and antibiotics may help temporarily alleviate clinical signs	
	Radiation treatment for cancerous lesions	
Differentials	Neoplasia, most commonly nasal squamous cell carcinoma	
	Inflammatory nodules comprised of exuberant granulation tissue admixed with inflammatory cells ± bacterial colonies	
	Fungal or bacterial rhinitis	
	Foreign body	
	Dental disease	
	Trauma	
Other	Coagulopathy, vasculitis, or another systemic disease (i.e., African swine fever) can potentially cause epistaxis but are rare in minipigs; additional clinical signs would be expected.	
References	Newman SJ, Rohrbach B. Pot-bellied pig neoplasia: a retrospective case series (2004–2011). *J Vet Diagn Invest.* 2012;24(5):1008–1013.	

ERYSIPELAS (SEPTICEMIA)

Overview: Erysipelas, caused by the gram-positive rod *Erysipelothrix rhusiopathiae,* appears to be one of the more common infectious diseases seen in pet pigs. The organism is ubiquitous and often carried asymptomatically, transmitted through feces or oral/respiratory secretions; it also affects multiple species and persists in the soil, so infection does not necessarily require pig-to-pig contact.

Early treatment typically yields a rapid response, and a preventative vaccine is available. Note: This diagnosis is suppositional as erysipelas cannot be clinically differentiated from other causes of septicemia. Other bacterial septicemias should be on the differential list, but confirmatory testing is not generally performed, especially with rapid response to treatment.

This disease has zoonotic potential. It causes erysipeloid, a localized skin lesion primarily seen in workers handling meat, fish, poultry, or lobster, as well as leather workers and veterinarians. Endocarditis is a rare manifestation in humans.

Continued

ERYSIPELAS (SEPTICEMIA)—cont'd

Signalment	Any

History	Acute onset of lethargy and anorexia is the most common presenting complaint; stiffness or lameness involving multiple limbs may be observed as the disease can affect joints; acute death is possible without prior clinical signs; abortions can occur	Erysipelas causes acute or subacute septicemia as well as chronic proliferative lesions, including synovitis and endocarditis. Chronic infection can follow acute, subacute, or subclinical infection, and arthritis can be seen as soon as 3 weeks post-infection. The role of this organism in chronic arthritis in pet pigs is unknown.
Physical Exam Findings	High fever often >105°F (40.6°C); depression; stiff gait, if the pig can be made to rise at all; dusky appearance to snout or pinnae; firm, raised, rhomboid "diamond-shaped" skin lesions are nearly pathognomonic but uncommon	**Fig. 10.20:** Acute erysipelas lesions consist of raised, erythematous, diamond-shaped, firm areas on the skin. (*Photo credit: https://www.minipiginfo.com/.*) Raised skin lesions on a darkly pigmented pig may not be easily visible but will be readily palpable. Following clinical resolution, these areas may slough.

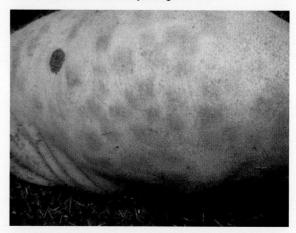

Fig. 10.21: Resolving diamond-shaped erysipelas lesion that will eventually slough before healing completely. (*Photo credit: https://www.minipiginfo.com/.*)

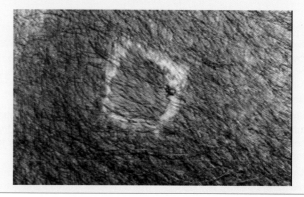

Diagnostics	History and clinical signs are adequate to begin empirical treatment. If no response, bloodwork (CBC, serum chemistry) can be performed to further assess the clinical condition and direct additional treatment. Polymerase chain reaction (PCR) assay on blood can confirm a diagnosis of acute disease.	The organism cannot generally be cultivated from the blood a few days post-infection but can persist in joints. Culture is not recommended due to difficulties in obtaining samples as well as rapid response to treatment. Serology tests cannot ensure a diagnosis as many animals are healthy carriers but may be useful to determine vaccination response in a herd as antibody titers should increase post-vaccination.
Treatment	Beta-lactam antibiotic to combat infection; NSAID to treat fever—expect rapid response Organism is usually sensitive to penicillin—the treatment of choice—as well as cephalosporins, lincosamides, macrolides, quinolones, and tetracyclines If non-responsive to initial treatment, hospitalization with supportive care such as IV fluids and an antibiotic switch may be warranted; treat as for septicemia in any patient Institute vaccination protocol in affected households, especially with multiple pigs; immunity is reported to last 6–12 months, so vaccination boosters may be needed semiannually; both oral and injectable vaccines are available	An injectable antibiotic dose followed by oral medication as soon as the pig is eating is preferred to multiple injections (especially if the owner is expected to continue treatment). Affected pigs rapidly respond to the reduction of fever with an NSAID and begin eating, so an oral beta-lactam antibiotic such as amoxicillin can be administered to complete the treatment course. An oral NSAID or acetaminophen may also be needed for the first several days to reduce fever.
Differentials	Other bacterial septicemia (i.e., *Salmonella choleraesuis, Streptococcus suis, Actinobacillus* spp., etc.) or viral disease (i.e., porcine circovirus or classical swine fever in countries outside of the United States)	
Other	Pigs are the primary reservoir for *Erysipelothrix rhusiopathiae,* and acutely infected animals shed copiously in feces, urine, saliva, and nasal secretions. This should be taken into consideration in multi-pig households and biosecurity measures implemented to prevent spread between pigs and humans (isolate sick pigs, wear separate clothing and shoes to handle the sick animal, and wash hands after handling).	
References	Forde T. Swine erysipelas. In: *Merck Veterinary Manual*. https://www.merckvetmanual.com/generalized-conditions/erysipelothrix-rhusiopathiae-infection/swine-erysipelas. Revised May 2020. Accessed February 2021. Opriessnig T, Coutinho TA. Erysipelas. In: Zimmeran JJ, Karriker LA, Ramirez A, et al., eds. *Diseases of Swine.* 11th ed. Hoboken, NJ: John Wiley & Sons, Inc.; 2019:835–843. Opriessnig T, Forde T, Shimoji Y. Erysipelothrix spp.: past, present, and future directions in vaccine research. *Front Vet Sci.* 2020;7:174. doi:10.3389/fvets.2020.00174.	

Continued

GASTROINTESTINAL TRACT OBSTRUCTION

See also Neoplasia—Intestinal; Vomiting

Overview: Obstruction within the gastrointestinal tract is relatively common in minipigs and may be caused by a foreign body, traumatic stricture, focal abscessation, as well as neoplasia in aged animals. Presentation, diagnostic testing, and treatment are similar to the dog.

Signalment	Any	
History	Intermittent or finicky appetite to anorexia; lethargy; vomiting, ranging from occasional to intractable; intermittent diarrhea or constipation; reduced fecal output; weight loss if chronic	Owners should be questioned on the pet's living arrangements (i.e., Are blankets used for bedding? Does the pig tend to rip carpets when rooting?). While pigs do not tend to purposely ingest foreign material, blanket or carpet pieces can be accidentally ingested as pigs not only root but use the mouth to manipulate nesting materials. Owners should also be questioned on diet as some unwittingly feed hazardous items such as corn cobs or pitted fruits (avocados, peaches).
Physical Exam Findings	Patient QAR (quiet, alert, responsive) to depressed; lip-smacking, teeth grinding, excessive salivation, and/or pressing the snout to the floor may be indicative of nausea; pain on abdominal palpation; abdominal distension Vitals may be normal, or heart and/or respiration rates may be elevated due to pain and/or nausea	While dehydration can be severe, this is best detected through clinical pathology evaluation rather than from a physical exam.
Diagnostics	CBC, serum chemistry—values may be unremarkable, or abnormalities associated with dehydration may be noted; imaging (radiographs, ultrasound); barium contrast study; endoscopy Refer to Fig. 10.5 for normal abdominal radiographs. Note: The torus pyloricus is a sessile protuberance in the pyloric region, along the lesser curvature of the stomach—do not confuse for a mass (i.e., during endoscopy or gastrotomy).	**Fig. 10.22:** Right lateral radiograph from a pig with a mid-jejunal, mineralized mass *(circled)*; bowel orad to the obstruction is mildly dilated. As the mass only partially occluded the intestinal lumen, clinical signs of anorexia and reduced fecal output were more chronic (2 weeks duration). 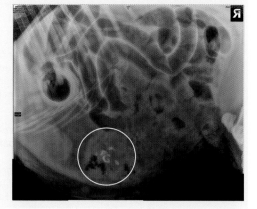

Fig. 10.23: Barium study in a pig presenting for acute vomiting; a piece of fabric torn from bedding—clearly outlined with contrast material—was removed surgically. (*Credit: Harley Swan.*)

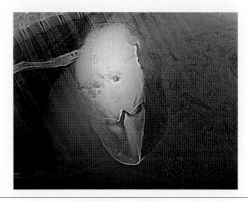

Treatment	Surgery (i.e., gastrotomy/enterotomy to remove foreign body, intestinal resection and anastomosis for stricture or mass)—post-operative care may include: fluid therapy, prokinetic agents (i.e., metoclopramide), maropitant (Cerenia) or ondansetron for nausea, ± antibiotics; analgesia (opioids, gabapentin ± NSAID if eating well and not dehydrated—use judiciously due to potential GI side effects); acupuncture may help with GI motility and pain control

Differentials	Foreign body Stricture (non-neoplastic) Intussusception Volvulus Abscess/Granuloma Neoplasia	Pigs readily deposit dense fibrous connective tissue, and traumatic injury to the bowel (i.e., abrasive or penetrating foreign material) can cause a stricture ± mass of connective tissue that mimics neoplasia. As intestinal neoplasia can be accompanied by a similar (scirrhous) reaction, histopathology may be necessary to distinguish.

Other	Pigs readily scar and form abdominal adhesions post-celiotomy; there is a risk of stricture at anastomosis site(s) as well. Intraperitoneal (IP) administration of sodium carboxymethylcellulose prior to manipulation of the intestine and immediately before closure of the abdominal wall can help to reduce adhesion formation (Ludwig). Other options to reduce the risk of adhesions include the use of atraumatic surgical technique, moistening of tissues, lavage, closing the dense peritoneum separately from the body wall, and giving anti-inflammatory drugs post-operatively.

References	Ehrle A, Gillespie A, Rubio-Martinez LM. Management of a linear foreign body gastrointestinal obstruction in a miniature pig. *Vet Rec Case Rep*. 2019. doi:10.1136/vetreccr-2018-000791. Ludwig EK, Byron CR. Evaluation of the reasons for and outcomes of gastrointestinal tract surgery in pet pigs: 11 cases (2004–2015). *J Am Vet Med Assoc*. 2017;251(6):714–721. Reed SK, Middleton JR, Ringen D, Nagy D. Use of cecal bypass via side-to-side ileocolic anastomosis without ileal transection for treatment of ileocecal intussusception in a Vietnamese pot-bellied pig [*Sus scrofa*]. *J Am Vet Med Assoc*. 2012;241(2):237–240. Sipos W, Schmoll F, Stumpf I. Minipigs and potbellied pigs as pets in the veterinary practice–a retrospective study. *J Vet Med A Physiol Pathol Clin Med*. 2007;54(9):504–511.

LAMENESS

See also Arthritis; Dippity Pig; Erysipelas; Paresis/Paralysis

Overview: Minipigs frequently present with complaints of lameness/limping that often involve one limb (i.e., traumatic) but may involve multiple limbs (i.e., infectious, degenerative joint disease [DJD]). Evaluate as for a dog, including physical exam and radiographs at a minimum. Treatment is also similar to that used in other species, so go ahead and extrapolate!

Signalment	Any age or gender can be affected. Young, rambunctious piglets (1 year of age or less), as well as older, arthritic animals (8–10+ years), may be overrepresented. Obesity may be a factor.	
History	Variable. A young pig may present with acute onset lameness of a single limb, more commonly the forelimb. An older animal may have a history of being chronically stiff or limping, with either acute exacerbation or slowly worsening clinical signs. Cold or wet weather may exacerbate the problem in chronic cases.	Known trauma may result in soft tissue injury or fracture as with any animal.
Physical Exam Findings	Observe the awake patient ambulating as much as possible (i.e., along the length of a carpet runner or gym/stall mat to provide traction). With a calm pig during a belly rub (see Chapter 5), a thorough evaluation of each limb may be done to assess soft tissues and joints for pain, swelling, heat, crepitus, range of motion. Standing exam is more limited but possible in a tractable patient. A complete orthopedic examination is not typically feasible. If the pig is not amenable to an evaluation while awake, the necessary sedation can impede evaluation. Systematically examine every part of the affected limb(s) as well as normal limbs for comparison. Uneven hoof wear may be noted in chronic cases—either overgrown claws on weight-bearing toes of the affected limb or short squared toes worn nearly to the quick from scraping the ground while trying to ambulate with a "stiff" limb.	In young pigs with acute forelimb lameness, the elbow joint is the most likely to be traumatically injured (see Other below). The elbow is often the most severely affected joint in chronic DJD (see Arthritis).
Diagnostics	Imaging including radiographs, CT, MRI; arthrocentesis (joint tap), especially if infectious etiology is suspected; testing for tick-borne disease has not been established for pigs; routine blood work (CBC, serum chemistry) if systemic infection or metabolic disease suspected	In older pigs, arthritis is typically most severe in the elbow, carpus, tarsus and distal phalanges, as well as the entire spine. Unlike the canine, shoulders, hips, and stifle are much less affected if not spared altogether. As in other species, the severity of radiographic signs does not necessarily correlate with clinical condition.

Fig. 10.24: Deformities of the shoulder joint are one of the more common developmental/congenital defects and can be unilateral or bilateral (see Other below). This pig started showing nearly imperceptible signs of lameness at 8 months of age and became increasingly worse, likely due to the inability to compensate at a heavier weight as she grew. Affected limb (A) versus contralateral limb (B).

Fig. 10.25: Fractures in two acutely non-weight-bearing lame pigs (*arrows*). One was due to severe osteopenia of undetermined etiology (diagnosed at necropsy) (A) and the other due to traumatic damage from inter-pig aggression (B). (*B, Photo credit: Ross Mill Farm.*)

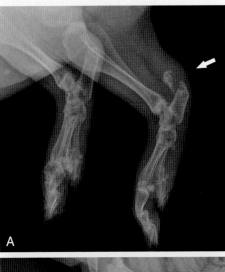

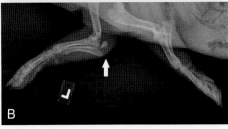

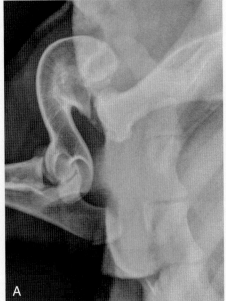

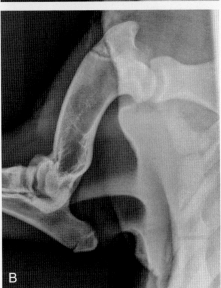

Continued

LAMENESS—cont'd

Treatment	Pain medications including NSAID; acetaminophen; gabapentin; amantadine; tramadol, fentanyl patch, or other opioids; low-dose ketamine injection

Joint-penetrating systemic antibiotic if suspected bacterial etiology; appropriate antibiotic if a tick-borne illness is suspected or soft tissue infection is identified; joint lavage

Fracture of the distal humeral condyle is best repaired with surgery; healing will eventually occur regardless, but early arthritis will be a sequela. There is a high risk that the contralateral condyle will also fracture as the pig starts bearing more weight on the unaffected limb.

Fracture in other locations may also be best treated with surgery, although conservative management consisting of rest and pain medications is an option. External fixation with casts or splints will only be effective if the joints above and below can be stabilized, difficult in the pig except for the most distal limb (below carpus or tarsus).

Chronic osteoarthritis treatment is more complicated, and a variety of drugs, supplements, and complementary treatments are available (see Arthritis).

Amputation (i.e., severe fracture, neoplasia) is not recommended in the pig (see Other below).

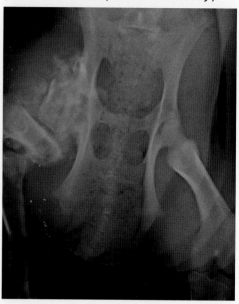

Fig. 10.26: The femur of this pig has been destroyed, apparently due to a traumatic gunshot injury. However, this rescue animal presented for evaluation of only a mild limp and continued to ambulate well despite the extent of the injury. (*Photo credit: Blind Spot Animal Sanctuary.*)

Differentials	Arthritis Congenital deformity, esp. shoulder Fracture, esp. distal humeral condyle Hoof overgrowth or injury Infection, incl. tick-borne disease Luxation Neoplasia Nutritional, incl. obesity Sprain/soft tissue injury

Mycoplasma is considered a top differential for arthritis in commercial swine; however, this organism has not been overwhelmingly identified in survey necropsy cases and is not considered a major contributor to miniature pig arthritis. Other causative agents such as *Streptococcus suis* are also uncommon. *Erysipelothrix rhusiopathiae*, on the other hand, is a ubiquitous organism that affects multiple species and might be considered a more likely differential for infectious arthritis in pet pigs.

If there is a history of tick exposure, tick-borne illness should be on the differential list, especially with shifting leg lameness or multiple affected limbs. Other systemic infections (see Erysipelas) should be on the differential list as well.

Hoof injuries may be identified but are less common causes of lameness.

If the pig is completely non-weight-bearing, acute fracture or luxation are top differentials.

Other	Fracture of the distal humeral condyle is one of the most common fractures in young/immature pigs due to late or incomplete ossification centers susceptible to injury, even without excessive force. Pain can readily be localized to the elbow, but fracture can be surprisingly difficult to identify on survey radiographs due to limited flexibility of the pig forelimb for positioning. CT or MRI may be best for diagnosis, especially if surgical fixation is pursued. The medial condyle is more commonly affected.
	Congenital malformations of the shoulder joint are also common and are easily identified on radiographs. Unless the animal is very young, it is generally not possible to determine whether an individual was born with the defect or suffered a chronic, healed, traumatic injury as both can be similar in appearance. Most of these pigs are medically managed with pain medications throughout life and frequently suffer severe limb deformities at an early age (valgus deviations, limb contracture, extreme loss of range of motion).
	Amputation: Pigs can and have survived limb amputation, although they more easily acclimate to loss of a hind limb as much of their weight is carried in the front half of the body. However, these animals are quite limited in ambulation ability as they reach their mature weight at 3–5 years of age and will suffer joint laxity and arthritis in the contralateral limb as a result. Owners and veterinarians should carefully consider the ramifications of amputation in a pet pig before opting for this treatment, particularly if the pig hasn't yet attained adult size. This is one instance in which extrapolation from canine and feline patients does not correlate well.
References	Dubois MS. Surgical arthrodesis for treatment of chronic shoulder joint luxation in a Vietnamese potbellied pig. *J Am Vet Med Assoc.* 2020;257(7):750–754.
	Høy-Petersen J, Smith JS, Merkatoris PT, et al. Case Report: trochlear wedge sulcoplasty, tibial tuberosity transposition, and lateral imbrication for correction of a traumatic patellar luxation in a miniature companion pig: a case report and visual description. *Front Vet Sci.* January 13, 2021;7:567886. doi:10.3389/fvets.2020.567886. PMID: 33521073.
	Payne JT, Braun WF, Anderson DE, Tomlinson JL. Articular fractures of the distal portion of the humerus in Vietnamese pot-bellied pigs: six cases (1988–1992). *J Am Vet Med Assoc.* 1995;206(1):59–62.
	Rölfing JHD, Swindle MM. Musculoskeletal system and orthopedic procedures. In: Swindle MM, Smith AC, eds. *Swine in the Laboratory: Surgery, Anesthesia, Imaging, and Experimental Techniques.* 3rd ed. Boca Raton, FL: CRC Press; 2016:325–329.
	Rubio-Martínez LM, Rioja E, Shakespeare AS. Surgical stabilization of shoulder luxation in a pot-bellied pig. *J Am Vet Med Assoc.* 2013;242(6):807–811.
	Samii VF, Hornof WJ. Incomplete ossification of the humeral condyle in Vietnamese pot-bellied pigs. *Vet Radiol Ultrasound.* 2000;41(2):147–153.

MASS/SWELLING, FACIAL

See also Dental Disease; Epistaxis; Neoplasia—Squamous Cell Carcinoma; Tusk Abscessation

Overview: Swelling/mass on the head/face/snout is addressed as in any other species, and differentials include uncomplicated cutaneous abscess, dental issues, traumatic injury, neoplasia, etc. In addition to physical examination, evaluation of the oral cavity under anesthesia, fine needle aspirate (FNA) or biopsy, and/or imaging may be required, and treatment determined based on findings.

Minipigs can develop tumor-like masses comprised of exuberant granulation tissue (akin to equine proud flesh), often admixed with bacterial colonies and sometimes lacking significant inflammation (so FNA may be unrewarding and histopathology needed); these inflammatory masses can appear anywhere on the body, but the face is a common site. Treatment may require surgical debulking in addition to antibiotic therapy.

The Kunekune breed exhibits an inheritable malocclusion in which deformity of the mandible and associated malpositioning of teeth leads to traumatic injury of soft tissues, feed impaction, extensive infection and fistula formation, especially near the ear base/angle of the jaw.

Continued

MASS/SWELLING, FACIAL—cont'd

Signalment	Usually adult animals; middle-aged to older males (8+ years) more commonly affected by swelling associated with tusk abscessation; Kunekune breed especially prone
History	Facial swelling; scratching at the face; foul odor or discharge; epistaxis; altered eating/chewing patterns if dental in nature

Fig. 10.27: This pig presented with a large, multi-lobulated, firm mass compressing one side of the snout (A); biopsy revealed this to be an inflammatory mass with intralesional cocci—without bony involvement based on skull radiographs—and surgical debulking plus antibiotic treatment was curative (B). (*B, Photo credit: Ross Mill Farm.*)

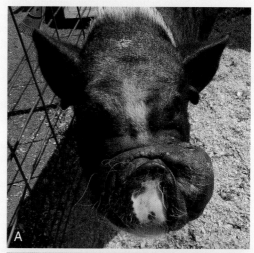

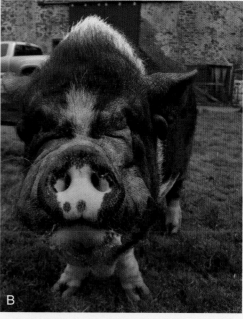

| **Physical Exam Findings** | PE is often unremarkable except for swelling/ mass (see also Figs. 10.6 and 10.18); possible epistaxis or mucoid nasal discharge; decreased air flow from naris, usually unilateral

Kunekune breed: Facial swelling, especially near the ear base/angle of the jaw, and possibly discharging feed material | **Fig. 10.28:** This hard swelling over the forehead (A) was diagnosed at necropsy as an osteoma. On sagittal section of the skull (B), the extent of bony proliferation can be appreciated relative to the brain case *(star)*. |

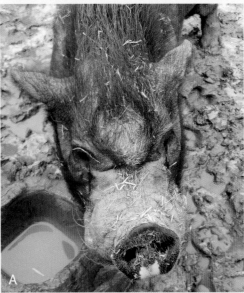

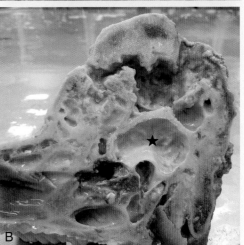

Continued

MASS/SWELLING, FACIAL—cont'd

Diagnostics	FNA or biopsy ± culture and sensitivity; radiographs; advanced imaging such as CT or MRI	See also Figs. 10.13, 10.19 and 10.65
Treatment	Depends on underlying etiology Antibiotics and pain medications as needed Drain and flush abscess Dental cleaning with removal of diseased teeth Surgical debulking, especially of inflammatory lesions; neoplasia often highly aggressive and debulking not recommended in these cases	
Differentials	Cutaneous abscess Tusk (or other tooth) abscess Inflammatory mass (bacterial, fungal, foreign body granuloma) Neoplasia, squamous cell carcinoma is the most common Trauma	*Actinomyces suis/denticolens* is a filamentous organism that contaminates wounds and leads to tumor-like proliferations. Facial masses are similar to lumpy jaw in cattle, but the condition in minipigs is typically confined to the skin, without bony involvement. This organism is anaerobic and difficult to culture.
References	Archer RM, Weston JF, Herdan CL, Owen MC. Facial swelling and discharging lesions associated with abnormalities of the mandible in kunekune pigs. *N Z Vet J.* 2012;60(5):305–309. Baumgardner R, Ziegler J, Shannon D, et al. Mandibular feed impaction resulting in fistulous tract development in a kunekune sow [*Sus scrofa domesticus*]. *J Exot.* 2020;35:80–81. Scott DW. Porcine. In: *Color Atlas of Farm Animal Dermatology.* 2nd ed. Hoboken, NJ: John Wiley & Sons, Inc.; 2018:235–292. Smith G. Actinomycosis in cattle, swine, and other animals. In: *Merck Veterinary Manual.* https://www.msdvetmanual.com/generalized-conditions/actinomycosis/actinomycosis-in-cattle,-swine,-and-other-animals. Revised July 2020. Accessed March 2021.	

NEOPLASIA—CUTANEOUS MAST CELL TUMOR

See also Chapter 9 and Fig. 9.12

Overview: Neoplasia is a broad term, and miniature pigs can suffer from any number of neoplastic diseases—only the most common are highlighted here. Evaluation and diagnostic testing are similar to that used in any species (physical exam, clinical pathology evaluations, imaging, tissue sampling, etc.), and treatments can be extrapolated as well.

Mast cell tumor (MCT) is one of the most common cutaneous neoplasms in the minipig and can be solitary or multifocal. The majority are benign, but rare cases of disseminated disease have been confirmed.

Signalment	Usually adult animals affected (not necessarily aged)
History	Slowly growing skin mass(es) anywhere on the body

Physical Exam Findings	PE generally unremarkable except for cutaneous mass(es)—single to multiple, discrete, domed to sessile, firm, sometimes ulcerated (most commonly from self-trauma, but sometimes associated with neoplastic mast cell degranulation)	**Fig. 10.29:** Two mast cell tumors (*arrows*) on the forelimb of a miniature pet pig. Gross appearance is not specific for MCT. 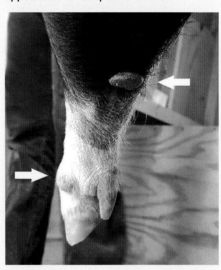
Diagnostics	Fine needle aspirate (FNA) or biopsy	
Treatment	Watch and wait—no treatment may be necessary Surgical removal, especially if traumatized or interfering with function (i.e., near the eye)	
Differentials	Melanocytoma, squamous cell carcinoma, or other tumor Cyst Hematoma Abscess Granuloma	
Other	Treatment options used for canine mast cell tumors, such as prednisone, CCNU (lomustine), toceranib phosphate (Palladia), or tigilanol tiglate injection (Stelfonta), may prove useful in miniature pig patients as well, especially with disseminated disease or non-resectable tumors (i.e., on the distal limb where closure may be problematic). Always keep in mind that use is extra-label in food animals, and some drugs may be prohibited. There is no grading scheme for cutaneous mast cell tumors in the miniature pig.	
References	Newman SJ, Rohrbach B. Pot-bellied pig neoplasia: a retrospective case series (2004–2011). *J Vet Diagn Invest.* 2012;24(5):1008–1013. Rasche BL, Mozzachio K, Linder KE. Cutaneous mast cell tumors in miniature pigs: a retrospective study. Draft manuscript submitted to JVDI. Williams F, Annetti K, Nagy D. Cutaneous mast cell tumour and renal tubular adenocarcinoma in a Vietnamese potbellied pig. *Vet Rec Case Rep.* 2018;6:e000533. doi:10.1136/vetreccr-2017-000533.	

NEOPLASIA—HEPATIC

Overview: Neoplasia is a broad term, and miniature pigs can suffer from any number of neoplastic diseases—only the most common are highlighted here. Evaluation and diagnostic testing are similar to that used in any species (physical exam, clinical pathology evaluations, imaging, tissue sampling, etc.), and treatments can be extrapolated as well.

Hepatic neoplasia is common in aged miniature pigs, but clinical signs may be subtle, are non-specific, and often don't appear until late in the disease course.

Signalment	Older pigs, starting around 10 years of age, often 16–18+ years

History	Intermittent or finicky appetite to anorexia; lethargy; distended abdomen; weight loss	With many cancers, a pig will demonstrate a finicky appetite—refusing pig food and eating only certain foods items offered, switching food preferences every few days. Owners sometimes fail to recognize that a finicky appetite is abnormal.

Physical Exam Findings

Patient QAR (quiet, alert, responsive) to depressed; abdominal distension; palpable mass in cranial abdomen; engorgement of subcutaneous abdominal veins

Icterus is underwhelming if present at all, with only a pale yellow discoloration of mucous membranes

Fig. 10.30: Grossly apparent yellow discoloration (icterus) is uncommon in the minipig.

Fig. 10.31: Distension of subcutaneous abdominal veins is an indication of abdominal pathology, including hepatic neoplasia, but is non-specific. See also Fig. 7.23.

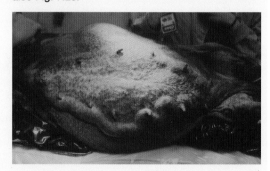

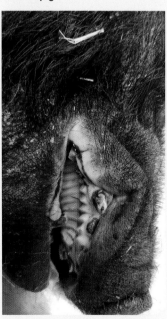

Diagnostics	Clinical pathology evaluation (CBC, serum chemistry, urinalysis); imaging (radiographs, ultrasound); ± biopsy; ± thoracic radiographs (pulmonary metastasis has been reported but is rare)	**Fig. 10.32:** Two large neoplastic liver masses (*stars*) are present in addition to numerous metastatic nodules throughout all lobes; a large cholelith is also identified *(arrow)*.

Normocytic, normochromic (non-regenerative) anemia may be present; liver enzymes may be elevated but are often within reference ranges

On ultrasound, disseminated hyperechoic nodules may be seen as intrahepatic metastasis is common; distension of the bile duct may also be present as concurrent cholelithiasis is frequent. Areas of necrosis or abscessation within large tumors may be present, and draining lymph nodes may be enlarged.

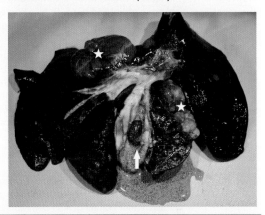

Treatment	Supportive care Euthanasia	As clinical signs are usually not observed until late in the disease course, euthanasia is often recommended over supportive care. Many aged pigs also have concurrent illness such as arthritis, tusk abscess or severe dental disease, other neoplasms, etc., that contribute to clinical decline.
Differentials	Hepatocellular carcinoma; biliary (cholangio) carcinoma Metastatic neoplasia Hepatic abscess(es) Granulomatous disease	

References	Haddad JL, Habecker PL. Hepatocellular carcinomas in Vietnamese pot-bellied pigs [Sus scrofa]. *J Vet Diagn Invest.* 2012;24(6):1047–1051. Morrow JL. Hepatocellular carcinoma and suspected splenic hemangiosarcoma in a potbellied pig. *Can Vet J.* 2002;43(6):466–468. Newman SJ, Rohrbach B. Pot-bellied pig neoplasia: a retrospective case series (2004–2011). *J Vet Diagn Invest.* 2012;24(5):1008–1013.

NEOPLASIA—INTESTINAL

See also Gastrointestinal Tract Obstruction; Vomiting

Overview: Neoplasia is a broad term, and miniature pigs can suffer from any number of neoplastic diseases—only the most common are highlighted here. Evaluation and diagnostic testing are similar to that used in any species (physical exam, clinical pathology evaluations, imaging, tissue sampling, etc.), and treatments can be extrapolated as well.

Intestinal neoplasia is relatively common in miniature pet pigs, affecting both small and large bowel. Surgery may be curative but depends on a location amenable to resection (i.e., duodenum or jejunum); the anatomy of the spiral colon does not allow for resection with neoplastic disease. However, with some non-neoplastic strictures, bypass through anastomosis may be considered as described for the treatment of ileocecal intussusception (Reed). Older animals frequently have concurrent disease, including multiple unrelated neoplasms or evidence of distant metastasis, so this should be taken into consideration in terms of treatment options and prognosis.

Signalment	Aged pigs, 10–12+ years	
History	Intermittent or finicky appetite to anorexia; lethargy; weight loss; reduced fecal output; intermittent vomiting, less commonly diarrhea or constipation	With many cancers, a pig will demonstrate a finicky appetite—refusing pig food and eating only certain foods items offered, switching food preferences every few days. Owners sometimes fail to recognize that a finicky appetite is abnormal.
Physical Exam Findings	Patient QAR (quiet, alert, responsive) to depressed, although PE may be within normal limits; increased gut sounds; palpable abdominal mass	
Diagnostics	CBC, serum chemistry—values may be unremarkable, or abnormalities associated with dehydration may be noted; imaging (radiographs, ultrasound); barium contrast study Refer to Fig. 10.5 for normal abdominal radiographs.	**Fig. 10.33:** Marked gas distension of bowel (A) in a 10-year-old pig presenting with anorexia, intermittent vomiting, and reduced fecal output of 2 weeks duration. At necropsy, a thickened, strictured area was identified at the ileocolic junction (B) and histopathology confirmed mucinous adenocarcinoma. (*Photo credit Dr. Janice Raab.*)

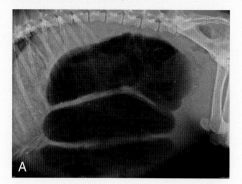

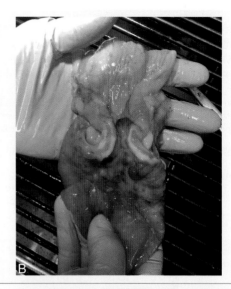

Treatment	Surgery (i.e., resection and anastomosis)—post-operative care may include fluid therapy, prokinetic agents (i.e., metoclopramide), maropitant (Cerenia) or ondansetron for nausea, ± antibiotics; analgesia including opioids, gabapentin ± NSAID if eating well and not dehydrated—use judiciously due to potential GI side effects; acupuncture may help with GI motility and pain control	Many affected pigs are elderly (15+ years) and have substantial concurrent disease (arthritis, severe dental disease, tusk abscess, other neoplastic diseases, etc.), which must be taken into consideration in terms of treatment and prognosis.
	Euthanasia	Evaluate the entire gastrointestinal tract as neoplastic masses may be multiple (metastasis versus de novo formation); prognosis is worse with multiple masses, even if resectable, as more are likely to develop.
Differentials	(Adeno)carcinoma Sarcoma Lymphoma Stricture (non-neoplastic) Abscess/Granuloma Foreign body	Pigs readily deposit dense fibrous connective tissue, and traumatic injury to the bowel (i.e., abrasive or penetrating foreign material) can cause a stricture ± mass of connective tissue that mimics neoplasia. As intestinal neoplasia can be accompanied by a similar (scirrhous) reaction, histopathology may be necessary to distinguish.
Other	Before offering treatment options to elderly animals, consider that concurrent disease is likely, and euthanasia may be in the best interest of the pig. My 22-year-old pig—with clinical signs restricted to anorexia and related to a resectable jejunal sarcoma—also had osteoarthritis, multiple intervertebral disc protrusions, hepatocellular carcinoma, mandibular squamous cell carcinoma, hepatic necrosis of unknown etiology, and pulmonary and myocardial fibrosis. He was clinically normal, only a little stiff-gaited, until he became anorexic. I find that substantial comorbidities are extremely common in very old pigs based on hundreds of post-mortem examinations.	
References	Corapi WV, Rodrigues A, Lawhorn DB. Mucinous adenocarcinoma and T-cell lymphoma in the small intestine of 2 Vietnamese potbellied pigs [Sus scrofa]. *Vet Pathol.* 2011;48(5):1004–1007. McCoy AM, Hackett ES, Callan RJ, Powers BE. Alimentary-associated carcinomas in five Vietnamese potbellied pigs. *J Am Vet Med Assoc.* 2009;235(11):1336–1341. Newman SJ, Rohrbach B. Pot-bellied pig neoplasia: a retrospective case series (2004–2011). *J Vet Diagn Invest.* 2012;24(5):1008–1013. Reed SK, Middleton JR, Ringen D, Nagy D. Use of cecal bypass via side-to-side ileocolic anastomosis without ileal transection for treatment of ileocecal intussusception in a Vietnamese pot-bellied pig [Sus scrofa]. *J Am Vet Med Assoc.* 2012;241(2):237–240.	

NEOPLASIA—LYMPHOMA

See also Paresis/Paralysis

Overview: Neoplasia is a broad term, and miniature pigs can suffer from any number of neoplastic diseases—only the most common are highlighted here. Evaluation and diagnostic testing are similar to that used in any species (physical exam, clinical pathology evaluations, imaging, tissue sampling, etc.), and treatments can be extrapolated as well.

Lymphoma is not as prevalent in miniature pet pigs as in other companion animal species. Spinal lymphoma, presenting as paraparesis, may be the most common. Involvement of internal organs may be seen, but clinical signs are non-specific. Peripheral lymph node involvement is uncommon to rare.

Signalment	Middle-aged to older animals (8+ years)	
History	Anorexia; lethargy; weight loss; weakness or limp progressing to paraparesis or tetraparesis if spinal	With many cancers, a pig will demonstrate a finicky appetite—refusing pig food and eating only certain foods items offered, switching food preferences every few days. Owners sometimes fail to recognize that a finicky appetite is abnormal.
Physical Exam Findings	Para-/tetraparesis to paralysis if spinal involvement; depression; rarely, palpable lymph node enlargement	Peripheral lymph nodes are generally not palpable in minipigs, so those readily identified are either reactive or neoplastic. Internal organ involvement is usually multicentric, affecting parenchymal tissue yet unlikely to form a discretely palpable mass.
Diagnostics	CBC, serum chemistry—often unremarkable although hypercalcemia may be present; imaging—ultrasound to scan for nodules/masses or enlargement/distortion of abdominal organs (i.e., lymph nodes, liver, kidney); CT or MRI for spinal involvement as radiographs are typically non-diagnostic	Fig. 10.34: MRI from a tetraparetic pig with spinal lymphoma. (A) A mass along the vertebral column infiltrates into adjacent epaxial muscles; (B) Severe compression of the cervical spinal cord as well as a mass ventral to the cerebellum and brain stem. (*Photo credit: Dr. Lauren Powers/Carolina Veterinary Specialists.*)

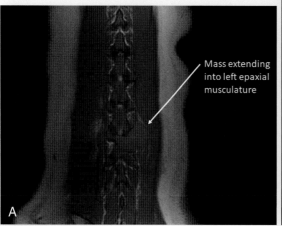

Mass extending into left epaxial musculature

A

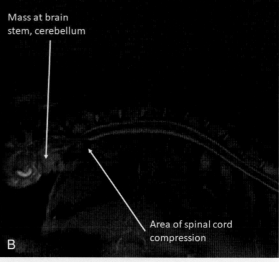

Mass at brain stem, cerebellum

Area of spinal cord compression

B

Treatment

Lymphoma is often identified in the late stages of the disease. It is unknown whether treatment modalities used in other species might be effective in pigs.

Anecdotally, prednisone has been effective for short-term palliation.

Fig. 10.35: Lymphoma involving only peripheral and internal lymph nodes—an unusual presentation. Nodes along the ventral neck region were massively enlarged and readily palpable; a single node (*circled*) is surrounded by adjacent, enlarged, sometimes abscessed nodes.

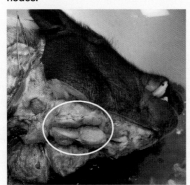

Fig. 10.36: Renal lymphoma (also affecting the liver, lungs, and internal lymph nodes—splenic involvement is uncommon to rare). Note: Abscesses or granulomas are grossly similar in appearance; fine needle aspirate or touch impression can differentiate from neoplasia.

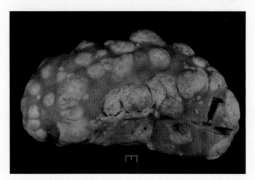

Differentials

Spinal form: IVDD (intervertebral disc disease); fibrocartilaginous embolism (FCE); traumatic injury including fracture; infectious including meningitis or osteomyelitis

Other abdominal neoplasia; bacterial infection causing multifocal abscesses or granulomas

Other

Lymphoma has been reported as a common neoplasm in domestic swine, often presenting in young animals less than 1 year of age; viruses and hereditary components have been identified as contributing factors (Robinson). Thus far, this form has not been reported in the miniature pet pig population.

Continued

NEOPLASIA—LYMPHOMA—cont'd

References	Corapi WV, Rodrigues A, Lawhorn DB. Mucinous adenocarcinoma and T-cell lymphoma in the small intestine of 2 Vietnamese potbellied pigs [*Sus scrofa*]. *Vet Pathol*. 2011;48(5):1004–1007.
	Robinson NA, Loynachan AT. Cardiovascular and hematopoietic systems. In: Zimmeran JJ, Karriker LA, Ramirez A, et al., eds. *Diseases of Swine*. 11th ed. Hoboken, NJ: John Wiley & Sons, Inc.; 2019:232.
	Skavlen PA, Stills Jr HF, Caldwell CW, Middleton CC. Malignant lymphoma in a Sinclair miniature pig. *Am J Vet Res*. 1986;47(2):389–393.

NEOPLASIA—SQUAMOUS CELL CARCINOMA

Cutaneous; Nasal; Oral

See also Dental Disease; Epistaxis; Mass/Swelling, Facial; Skin (Dermatologic) Issues

Overview: Neoplasia is a broad term, and miniature pigs can suffer from any number of neoplastic diseases—only the most common are highlighted here. Evaluation and diagnostic testing are similar to that used in any species (physical exam, clinical pathology evaluations, imaging, tissue sampling, etc.), and treatments can be extrapolated as well.

Squamous cell carcinoma (SCC) is a common neoplasia in aged pet pigs (8–10+ years), and the skin, nasal cavity, and oral cavity are the primary locations. Cutaneous SCC is seen in lightly pigmented animals and is frequently multifocal, with encrusted to ulcerated lesions over the body; sun exposure is likely a contributing factor. Nasal SCC typically presents as a rapidly enlarging swelling over the snout and/or epistaxis. Oral SCC is often subclinical and identified as part of a routine oral exam or during dental prophylaxis. Severe dental disease may complicate the issue, especially as gingival hyperplasia and neoplasia might not be readily differentiated on gross evaluation.

Signalment	Aged pigs, usually 8–10+ years; lightly-colored (white/pink) pigs more commonly affected by cutaneous form	
History	Abnormal eating/chewing behavior, dysphagia, bad odor from the mouth, excessive salivation with oral form; intermittent epistaxis or swelling of the snout with nasal form; presence of increasing numbers of ulcerated skin nodules in cutaneous form	With nasal or oral forms, animals may exhibit an intermittently finicky appetite associated with painful oral lesions or episodes of epistaxis.

Physical Exam Findings	<u>Cutaneous:</u> Multiple ulcerated skin lesions; evidence of solar dermatitis (crusting over sun-exposed areas, especially the dorsal pinnae and skin over the lateral flanks). See Fig. 10.58C and D. <u>Nasal:</u> Swelling over dorsal snout ± epistaxis ± reduced air flow from naris, usually unilateral. See Fig. 10.18. <u>Oral form:</u> Sedated oral exam is necessary, especially as tumors are commonly found in the caudal oral cavity; findings include firm, smooth nodules that resemble gingival hyperplasia to plaque-like mucosal thickening to soft, friable, multinodular masses; tumors are often associated with bony lysis identified through palpable sharp fragments or probing—many tumors are much larger and more invasive than that visibly apparent; associated teeth may be loose or missing.

Fig. 10.37: (A) Oral SCC manifesting as a "crater" with impacted feed material and palpable osteolysis (sharp-edged bone fragments). Despite the focal appearance, the tumor was extensive, crossing to the opposite arcade beneath the hard palate mucosa. All premolars and molars were missing at the time of necropsy, and the tumor was an incidental finding. (B) Oral SCC comprised of an irregularly nodular, soft, friable proliferation that extends along the lower arcade and into the root of the tongue. This pig presented with difficult/painful chewing.

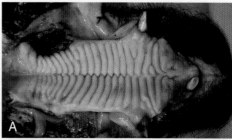

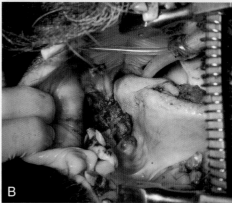

Fig. 10.38: Solar dermatitis +/ SCC over the dorsal pinna—the presence of neoplasia cannot be determined on gross exam alone.

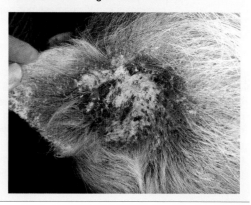

Continued

NEOPLASIA—SQUAMOUS CELL CARCINOMA—cont'd

Diagnostics	Fine needle aspirate (FNA) or biopsy; radiographs or other imaging for nasal and oral forms (CT/MRI may be needed to determine the extent of bony destruction); thoracic radiographs to evaluate for metastasis	Nasal and oral SCC rarely metastasize except to local lymph nodes, although pulmonary metastasis has been reported. Both are rapidly-growing, locally aggressive tumors. Pigs with cutaneous SCC often continue to develop increasing numbers of small tumors, but this is likely de novo formation rather than metastasis.
Treatment	Anti-inflammatory and pain medications (NSAID, opioid, gabapentin, etc.); antibiotic for secondary bacterial infection; Yunnan Baiyao for bleeding masses Electrochemotherapy for cutaneous SCC has been described (Weissman), and other treatment modalities might be extrapolated as well; reduce sun exposure (apply sunscreen, provide shade, limit outdoor activity at peak exposure times, provide protective clothing) Surgical debulking for nasal/oral forms is not recommended for palliative treatment as rapid regrowth is common. However, surgery plus radiation or chemotherapy may be effective.	Nasal and oral SCC are aggressive tumors that rapidly progress and may warrant euthanasia very near the time of diagnosis (weeks to a few months).
Differentials	Cutaneous: solar dermatitis, mast cell tumor, pyoderma Nasal: fungal or bacterial rhinitis; foreign body; granuloma Oral: gingival hyperplasia associated with dental disease; periodontitis; epulis, odontoma, or other benign dental tumors	
References	Kleinschmidt S, Puff C, Baumgärtner W. Metastasizing oral squamous cell carcinoma in an aged pig. *Vet Pathol*. 2006;43(4):569–573. Newman SJ, Rohrbach B. Pot-bellied pig neoplasia: a retrospective case series (2004–2011). *J Vet Diagn Invest*. 2012;24(5):1008–1013. Swenson J, Carpenter JW, Ragsdale J, et al. Oral squamous cell carcinoma in a Vietnamese pot-bellied pig (Sus scrofa). *J Vet Diagn Invest*. 2009;21(6):905–909. Weissman M, Donnelly LL, Branson K, et al. Electrochemotherapy for a cutaneous squamous cell carcinoma in a Vietnamese pot-bellied pig [*Sus scrofa*]. *J Exot Pet Med*. 2020;34;34:37–43.	

NEOPLASIA—UTERINE

Overview: Neoplasia is a broad term, and miniature pigs can suffer from any number of neoplastic diseases—only the most common are highlighted here. Evaluation and diagnostic testing are similar to that used in any species (physical exam, clinical pathology evaluations, imaging, tissue sampling, etc.), and treatments can be extrapolated as well.

Uterine tumors are extremely common in miniature pigs, especially in nulliparous animals, so early ovariohysterectomy (OHE; spay) is recommended for all pets. Smooth muscle tumors are most commonly identified but, while benign, can grow to extreme sizes that may lead to death. Surgical excision through ovariohysterectomy is often curative.

Signalment	Intact, typically nulliparous, middle-aged to older females (6–8+ years)	
History	Abdominal enlargement; general discomfort (i.e., frequent repositioning when lying down); intermittent, abnormal (bloody or purulent) vaginal discharge; anorexia and lethargy in end-stage disease	Weight loss in advanced disease is common, but many owners fail to recognize this in the presence of a large belly.
Physical Exam Findings	Abdominal distension, often asymmetrical, possibly painful on palpation; palpable abdominal mass; if the animal can be observed in a recumbent position, the presence of a mass may be easier to discern; distension of subcutaneous abdominal veins (see Figs. 4.5A, 7.23 and 10.31); thin body condition despite enlarged abdomen	**Fig. 10.39:** Abdominal distension due to uterine neoplasia; OHE was curative in this pig. See also Fig. 4.5B.
Diagnostics	Imaging such as radiographs or ultrasound	
Treatment	OHE (spay)	**Fig. 10.40:** Dorsolateral recumbency is the preferred position for the removal of uterine tumors to prevent aortocaval compression (see also Chapter 9 and Fig. 9.8). This leiomyoma extended into the broad ligament along one uterine horn (*star*) and was easily exteriorized; the spiral colon can be seen at the cranial aspect of the surgical incision *(arrow)*.

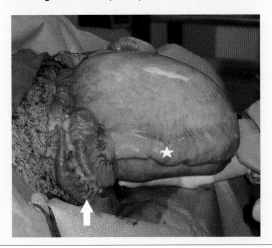

Continued

NEOPLASIA—UTERINE—cont'd

Differentials	Leiomyoma/Leiomyosarcoma Adenocarcinoma Other abdominal masses (i.e., ovarian) Pregnancy
Other	Benign smooth muscle tumors are by far the most common in the uterus of the miniature pig, but adenoma, endometrial adenocarcinoma, and choriocarcinoma-like tumor have also been reported. Even with malignancies, surgery may be curative or might offer relatively long-term palliation; metastasis, however, has been reported. Uterine tumors may be identified incidentally during spay surgery. Expect some sort of reproductive pathology when spaying a pig over 5–6 years old, with the likelihood increasing with age. See Fig. 4.4.
References	Cypher E, Videla R, Pierce R, et al. Clinical prevalence and associated intraoperative surgical complications of reproductive tract lesions in pot-bellied pigs undergoing ovariohysterectomy: 298 cases (2006–2016). *Vet Rec*. 2017;181(25):685. Golbar H, Izawa T, Kuwamura M, et al. Uterine adenocarcinoma with prominent desmoplasia in a geriatric miniature pig. *J Vet Med Sci*. 2010;72(2):253–256. Harmon BG, Munday JS, Crane MM. Diffuse cystic endometrial hyperplasia and metastatic endometrial adenocarcinoma in a Vietnamese pot-bellied pig [*Sus scrofa*]. *J Vet Diagn Invest*. 2004;16(6):587–589. Hirata A, Miyazaki A, Sakai H, et al. Choriocarcinoma-like tumor in a potbellied pig [*Sus scrofa*]. *J Vet Diagn Invest*. 2014;26(1):163–166. Ilha MR, Newman SJ, van Amstel S, et al. Uterine lesions in 32 female miniature pet pigs. *Vet Pathol*. 2010;47(6):1071–1075. Mozzachio K, Linder K, Dixon D. Uterine smooth muscle tumors in potbellied pigs [Sus scrofa] resemble human fibroids: a potential animal model. *Toxicol Pathol*. 2004;32(4):402–407. Wood P, Hall JL, McMillan M, et al. Presence of cystic endometrial hyperplasia and uterine tumours in older pet pigs in the UK. *Vet Rec Case Rep*. 2020. doi:10.1136/vetreccr-2019-000924.

OBESITY

See also Chapter 3

Overview: Obesity has historically been a common problem in the miniature pet pig population. Contributing factors include: pigs are "easy keepers" that readily gain weight; pigs lead sedentary lifestyles; miniature pigs do not voluntarily limit feed intake based on energy requirements; pigs are purposely fed to an overweight body condition based on misconceptions held by owners.

Signalment	Any, although active, growing piglets are less commonly affected
History	Owners may be completely unaware of the level of obesity of their pet, including failing to recognize when the animal has become "fat blind." Owners may notice decreased activity, loud/labored breathing or snoring, lameness, or aggressive behaviors but are unaware of the underlying cause.

Physical Exam Findings

Rotund face with deep folds on the forehead and jowls; periocular fat partially to completely obscuring the eyes; ears pushed laterally into a horizontal position; belly near to or dragging the ground; tailhead buried in dimpled skin folds; inability to ambulate well; impaired vision (bumps into walls or furniture, swings the head or snaps when approached); possibly hearing impaired

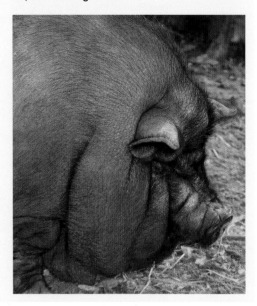

Fig. 10.41: This obese pig exhibits a bulging forehead, fat folds over the cheeks/jowls, a sagging neck, and the ears have been pushed into an abnormal horizontal position by surrounding fat; see also Fig. 3.12C.

Continued

OBESITY—cont'd

Fig. 10.42: The darker pig (A) is slightly over-weight. This is not as obvious as more extreme obesity, but when compared to the ideal body condition of the white pig (B), the rump is clearly more rounded, and the belly sags between the hind legs.

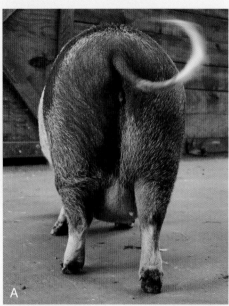

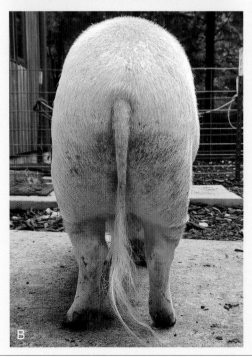

Fig. 10.43: When each pig from Fig. 10.42 is viewed from the side, the difference in body condition is even more subtle. The slightly over-weight dark gray pig (A) is "blockier," with heavier jowls, a less distinct neck, and rounded rump and shoulders, but the difference might be hard to see without a comparison (B). A pig should be viewed from all angles to determine body condition score (BCS), and I personally recommend that owners take monthly pictures from the front, side, and back—at pig level—to monitor weight gain/loss.

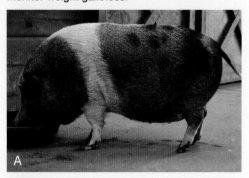

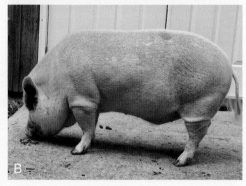

Diagnostics	No specific tests recommended—there is rarely (ever?) an underlying medical condition leading to obesity
Treatment	Diet and controlled exercise
Differentials	NA
Other	General guidelines for maintenance feeding of commercial miniature pig feeds: • Young piglet: ½ cup per 15–25 lb (7–11 kg) body weight/day • Adult: 1 cup per 50–80 lb (23–36 kg) body weight/day However, feed restriction of an obese animal may require reduction to as little as ¼ maintenance rations with certain snacks added to provide satiety (see Chapter 3). Ross Mill Farm, located near Philadelphia, PA, USA, is one location that provides a fee-based weight reduction program ("piggy fat camp") and has a very successful history of returning obese animals to a healthy body condition.
References	Armstrong S. *How to diet the obese potbellied pig*. Swine Medical Database website. https://swinemedicaldatabase.org/how-to-diet-the-obese-potbellied-pig-by-susan-armstrong/. Accessed February 2021. Bollen PJA, Madsen LW, Meyer O, Ritskes-Hoitinga J. Growth differences of male and female Göttingen minipigs during ad libitum feeding: a pilot study. *Lab Anim*. 2005;39(1):80–93. Minipig body condition score is based on the 5-point scale used in commercial swine, with 3 or slightly under considered ideal. Both written and pictorial descriptions of minipig body condition scores can be found at the following link: https://www.minipiginfo.com/mini-pig-body-scoring.html. Dieting an obese pet pig. Ross Mill farm website. https://rossmillfarm.com/2019/06/dieting-an-obese-pet-pig/. Published June 2019. Accessed February 2021.

PARASITES, EXTERNAL

Mange; Pediculosis (lice)

See also Chapter 7; Pruritis

Overview: The most common external parasites in minipigs are mange mites and lice; ticks are occasionally problematic, and although fleas may bite pigs, they are not the source of infestation, and treatment is best addressed for other animals in the household.

Sarcoptic mange, *Sarcoptes scabiei* var. *suis*, can be acute or chronic. The acute presentation is more common and similar to that seen in the dog; patients present with intense pruritis, excoriations, erythema, alopecia, crusting. Chronic carriers are subclinical and may exhibit non-pruritic, patchy hyperkeratosis; these animals can serve as a reservoir for infection of naïve pigs.

Swine lice, *Hematopinus suis*, are species-specific and blood-sucking; severe infestation can lead to clinically relevant anemia (weakness, lethargy, pallor).

Continued

PARASITES, EXTERNAL—cont'd

Signalment	Any, but mange more common in younger animals
History	History of contact with other pigs (close contact needed for transmission between animals) or history of a recent stressor (illness, transport, introduction of new person/pet, recent neuter) as stress may allow subclinical Sarcoptes infestation to manifest
	History of weakness, lethargy, general ill-thrift may be noted with louse infestation as well as severe mange

Physical Exam Findings

<u>Acute mange:</u> Uncontrollable pruritis, excoriations, erythema, alopecia, papules, crusting (see also Fig. 7.5)

<u>Chronic mange:</u> Few, thick, scaly, non-pruritic plaques

<u>Lice:</u> Swine lice are visible to the naked eye, and long, gray-brown, flat-bodied adults can be seen moving over the body of the pig, nits can be seen attached to the lower part of hair shafts (see Fig. 7.4); ± pruritis; ± clinical signs associated with blood-loss anemia such as lethargy, weakness, pallor, elevated heart rate

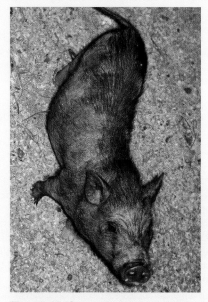

Fig. 10.44: A mildly affected mangy piglet with diffuse erythema and loss of hair along the flanks from excessive scratching.

Fig. 10.45: Severe mange in a piglet. (*Photo credit: Dr. Matt Edson.*)

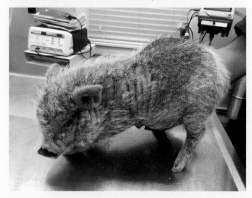

Diagnostics	Skin scrape for mange—mites are numerous with the chronic form, but the acute form involves a hypersensitivity reaction, so mites may be few and difficult to recover. Visual exam alone can confirm lice.	The inside of the pinna is often high yield for Sarcoptes mites. If mange is suspected, treat even if skin scrape is negative.
Treatment	Avermectin (ivermectin, doramectin) Topical treatment (i.e., permethrin) for lice Environment, including bedding, as well as other pigs/pets in the household, should be treated.	See Table 7.2 for a list of medications and dosages Severely debilitated animals, especially young piglets, may require supportive care and/or additional treatment (i.e., for secondary bacterial infection).
Differentials	Bacterial or fungal dermatitis, including exudative dermatitis (greasy pig disease); parakeratosis; photosensitization; cutaneous lymphoma; allergic disease (less common and not fully elucidated in pet pigs)	Mange should rapidly respond to treatment. If there is no response, further diagnostics (i.e., biopsy; culture) are indicated.
Other	While lice are species-specific, Sarcoptic mange has zoonotic potential.	
References	Arends JJ, Skogerboe TL, Ritzhaupt LK. Persistent efficacy of doramectin and ivermectin against experimental infestations of *Sarcoptes scabiei* var. *suis* in swine. *Vet Parasitol.* 1999;82(1):71–79. Brewer MT, Greve JH. External parasites. In: Zimmeran JJ, Karriker LA, Ramirez A, et al, eds. *Diseases of Swine.* 11th ed. Hoboken, NJ: John Wiley & Sons, Inc.; 2019:1005–1014. Grahofer A, Bannoehr J, Nathues H, Roosje P. Sarcoptes infestation in two miniature pigs with zoonotic transmission—a case report. *BMC Vet Res.* 2018;14(1):91. doi:10.1186/s12917-018-1420-5.	

PARASITES, INTERNAL (GASTROINTESTINAL)

See also Chapter 7

Overview: Parasites of the gastrointestinal tract are less of a problem in miniature pigs than in other species and are frequently an incidental finding not associated with clinical signs. Deworming should be based on fecal flotation performed as part of a routine evaluation; a minimum of yearly testing is recommended. Most individual pet households are closed herds (no contact with outside pigs), and these animals may not require regular treatment, especially as overuse of dewormers contributes to parasite resistance. In open herds such as a pig sanctuary/rescue or breeding operation, routine fecal flotation should be used to guide medication choice and frequency, and biosecurity measures should also be evaluated and refined as needed (i.e., isolation and testing of newly arriving pigs, frequent poop scooping, pasture rotation).

Signalment	Young piglets and otherwise sick animals are most affected

Continued

PARASITES, INTERNAL (GASTROINTESTINAL)—cont'd

History	Often an incidental finding on routine fecal float Young piglets may be poor doers, not growing as well as expected

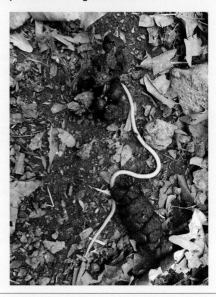

Fig. 10.46: Owners may report large white worms in the feces though this is more common post-deworming treatment.

Physical Exam Findings	PE usually unremarkable; possibly slight ascites (i.e., seen during OHE or open castration); ill-thrift/poor growth, generalized piloerection
Diagnostics	Fecal flotation, possibly sedimentation

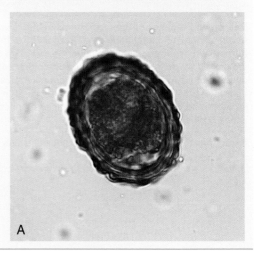

A

Fig. 10.47: Fecal flotation can be performed as in the dog, and ova have a similar appearance, with ascarid and strongyle-type ova most common. Ascarid ovum (A); Strongyle-type ovum (B).

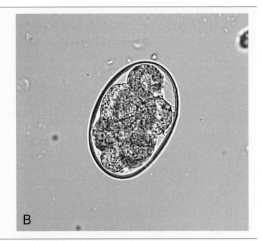

B

Treatment	Avermectin (i.e., ivermectin, doramectin); fenbendazole; pyrantel	See Table 7.2 for a list of medications and dosages.
		Most pigs will readily ingest flavored liquid dewormers considered palatable to humans or horses.
Differentials	NA	
Other	In my experience, internal parasites are very often an incidental finding. In hundreds of miniature pig necropsies, GI parasites were identified only a handful of times and always in animals debilitated for another reason. If a miniature pig presents with clinical signs of illness (diarrhea, abdominal distension, lethargy, inappetence), look for another underlying cause or comorbidity even if parasites are present. Amoebae may be occasionally identified on fecal evaluation, but most are not pathogenic.	
	Note: I have personally found that the Kunekune breed tends to carry a higher parasite load (but still subclinical), and these pets may require more frequent fecal sampling and deworming.	
References	Ballweber LR. Overview of gastrointestinal parasites of pigs. *Merck Veterinary Manual*. https://www.merckvetmanual.com/digestive-system/gastrointestinal-parasites-of-pigs/overview-of-gastrointestinal-parasites-of-pigs. Revised May 2015. Accessed April 2021.	
	Brewer MT, Greve JH. Internal parasites. In: Zimmeran JJ, Karriker LA, Ramirez A, et al., eds. *Diseases of Swine*. 11th ed. Hoboken, NJ: John Wiley & Sons, Inc.; 2019:1028–1040.	
	Tynes VV. Preventive health care for pet potbellied pigs. *Vet Clin North Am Exot Anim Pract*. 1999; 2(2):495–510.	

PARESIS/PARALYSIS

See also Dippity Pig; Neoplasia—Lymphoma; Rabies

Overview: Minipigs commonly present as "down in the back end." Sometimes the pig simply squeals and collapses, while other times, the pig acutely loses hindlimb function after a minor slip or sudden turn. Occasionally, the problem is more insidious, with the pig appearing weak, ataxic, or lame over days to weeks before losing hindlimb function.

Signalment	Usually adult animals, not necessarily aged

Continued

PARESIS/PARALYSIS—cont'd

History	Acute to subacute loss of hindleg movement. In acute cases, loss of function may occur after the pig steps in a hole, slips on leaves, or fights with another pig, but some simply collapse, usually following intense vocalization (pain). Affected animals typically assume a dog-sitting position. With a more insidious onset, owners may report the pig to be wobbly, weak, or intermittently dragging the toes for days to weeks before becoming unable to use the legs.	Dippity Pig can have a similar presentation, but the animal is able to repeatedly rise and walk, then seems to temporarily lose function of the hindlimbs before getting up and walking again.
Physical Exam Findings	Complete (paralysis) or partial (paresis) loss of hindlimb function; tetraparesis is possible depending on lesion location but is uncommon to rare; fever is possible with infectious etiology, and tachypnea is common if painful.	Pain on spinal palpation may be difficult to elicit unless a fracture is present; reflexes are also difficult to assess in a pig. Affected pigs often remain continent and maintain anal tone, although chronic urinary tract issues are a problem in animals affected longterm.
Diagnostics	Imaging: MRI or CT preferred; radiographs may be helpful but are often non-diagnostic; myelography may be useful; cerebrospinal fluid analysis (CSF tap)	**Fig. 10.48:** (A and B) Aged minipigs frequently exhibit bridging spondylosis (*arrowheads*) that is typically incidental despite severity. 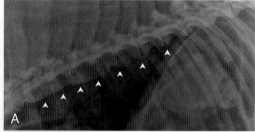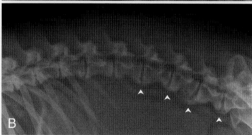
Treatment	<u>Trauma/IVDD/FCE:</u> Conservative including anti-inflammatory medications (i.e., steroid or NSAID), gabapentin, methocarbamol; acupuncture, cold laser, herbal supplements, physical therapy, hyperbaric oxygen, or other alternative treatment <u>Spinal neoplasia (see Fig. 10.34):</u> Euthanasia recommended, although prednisone may provide temporary palliation; often multifocal and rapid to return if surgical debulking performed; more common in middle-aged to older animals (8+ years); lymphoma most common	Repair of traumatic fracture or surgical decompression of the spinal cord (i.e., with disc rupture) is possible, but post-operative care must be carefully considered, especially in larger/heavier animals.

Differentials	Intervertebral disc disease (IVDD) Fibrocartilaginous embolism (FCE) Spinal neoplasia (i.e., lymphoma) Traumatic injury including fracture or luxation Infection including meningitis or osteomyelitis Congenital malformation
Other	Hindlimb paresis/paralysis can be seen in rabid pigs. While this is extremely rare in North America, it should be considered as a differential.
References	Castel A, Doré V, Fazio C. Spinal stabilisation using a polyvinilidine (Lubra) plate in a pot-bellied pig. *Vet Rec Case Rep*. 2020. doi:10.1136/vetreccr-2019-000990. Castel A, Doré V, Vigeral M, Hecht S. Magnetic resonance imaging findings in 13 neurologic pot-bellied pigs. *Front Vet Sci*. 2020. doi:10.3389/vets.2020.00021. Darby S, Gomez DE, Hobbs K, et al. Presumptive fibrocartilaginous embolic myelopathy in a pot-bellied pig. *Can Vet J*. 2021;62(2):167–172. Lapointe JM, Summers BA. Intervertebral disk disease with spinal cord penetration in a Yucatan pig. *Vet Pathol*. 2012;49(6):1054–1056.

PROLAPSE, RECTAL (OR VAGINAL)

See also Chapter 9

Overview: Rectal or, less commonly, vaginal prolapse are occasionally observed in miniature pet pigs and may occur secondary to straining (i.e., constipation, diarrhea, coughing, cystitis, vaginitis, etc.), or there may simply be a genetic predisposition.

Signalment	Any
History	Straining, sometimes with temporary and repeated protrusion of mucosa prior to prolapse; coughing, diarrhea, constipation; recent parturition
Physical Exam Findings	Protrusion of mucosa from anus or vagina

Fig. 10.49: (A) Rectal prolapse; (B) Vaginal prolapse of polypoid mucosa.

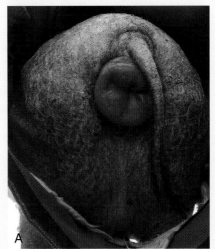

A

Continued

PROLAPSE, RECTAL (OR VAGINAL)—cont'd

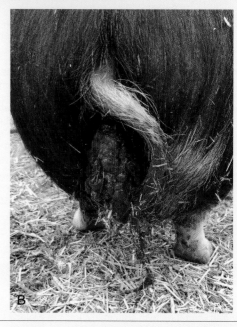

Diagnostics	None required except as needed to diagnose the underlying cause (i.e., fecal flotation if parasitism suspected)

Though gastrointestinal parasitism can lead to rectal prolapse, this is uncommon to rare in miniature pet pigs. Dehydration with ensuing constipation is much more common.

Treatment	Reduce prolapse (with the aid of a hygroscopic agent such as sugar or honey as well as cold water to reduce edema and swelling), then place a purse-string suture to maintain proper position
	Correct rectal prolapse through the placement of a rectal ring, especially if tissue is devitalized (see Chapter 9 for details)
	Surgical treatment for severely traumatized tissue (rectal amputation) or repeat prolapse following initial correction (rectopexy)
	Anti-inflammatory medication (i.e., NSAID)
	Fluid therapy to correct underlying dehydration
	Enema to relieve primary or secondary constipation
	Antibiotic (typically reserved for suspected underlying infection)
	Correct underlying issues if warranted. For rectal prolapse: deworm, increase dietary fiber, give stool softeners and/or laxatives, encourage fluid intake by flavoring water with juice or adding water to pelleted feed. For vaginal prolapse: identify and remove exogenous estrogens, treat any underlying infection, spay.

Differentials	NA
References	Ames NK. Rectal prolapse repair. In: *Noordsy's Food Animal Surgery*. 5th ed. Ames, IA: John Wiley & Sons, Inc.; 2014:139–143.
	Anderson DE, Mulon PY. Anesthesia and surgical procedures in swine. In: Zimmerman JJ, Karriker LA, Ramirez A, et al, eds. *Diseases of Swine*. 11th ed. Hoboken, NJ: John Wiley & Sons, Inc.; 2019: 179–181.
	Becker HN. Surgical procedures in miniature pet pigs. In: Reeves DE, ed. *Care and Management of Miniature Pet Pigs*. Santa Barbara, CA: Brillig Hill, Inc.; 1993:67–76.
	Njoku NU, Kelechi TJ, Rock OU, Orajaka, CF. A case of complete rectal prolapse in an in-gilt. *Case Rep Vet Med*. 2014. http://dx.doi.org.prox.lib.ncsu.edu/10.1155/2014/812340.

PRURITIS

See also Parasites, External; Skin (Dermatologic) Issues

Overview: Pigs have naturally dry skin and like to occasionally scratch themselves on items in the environment. However, pruritic skin conditions leading to excessive scratching above the normally low levels should be investigated. Sarcoptic mange is a top differential in extremely pruritic animals (especially if skin lesions are prominent), but louse infestation, pyoderma, or shedding are also possible.

Signalment	Any	
History	Excessively itchy pig, often with excoriation due to self-trauma; recent introduction of new pig(s); history of a recent stressor (illness, transport, introduction of new person/ pet, recent neuter)	Introduction of a new pig(s) can be a stressor or a source of contagious disease.
		Sarcoptes infestation can be subclinical until the pig becomes stressed.
Physical Exam Findings	Erythema, alopecia, scaling, small papules, excoriations, multifocal crusting or hyperkeratotic plaques; obvious pruritis—scratching on furniture or leaning into/kicking at handler during palpation/petting; easily epilated hair if shedding; adult lice and nits are visible to the naked eye when present	**Fig. 10.50:** Shedding may cause mild pruritis but not to the point of self-trauma. Time of year, as well as easy epilation of hair (pictured), may point to this. 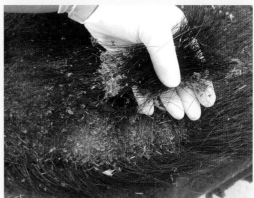

Continued

PRURITIS—cont'd

Diagnostics   Skin scrape for mange—the acute, intensely pruritic form involves a hypersensitivity reaction, so mites may be few and difficult to recover

Visual exam alone can confirm lice

Cytology for bacterial or fungal agents

Culture, biopsy—usually reserved for conditions that are unresponsive to initial treatment

Fig. 10.51: Hyperkeratosis, fissuring, crusting, and severe pruritis led to suspicion of mange and warranted empirical treatment despite negative skin scrape. However, as there was no response to ivermectin, a biopsy was performed and identified severe eosinophilic dermatitis (etiology unknown) and secondary pyoderma. Treatment included prednisone to control itch and amoxicillin to treat pyoderma. Investigation into the underlying cause was then pursued though allergies are uncommon in pigs, and there is no historical data on likely etiology in the species (i.e., food vs. environmental).

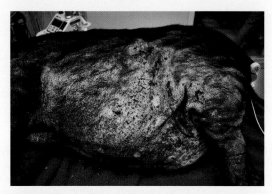

Fig. 10.52: Intact pustules on the medial leg of a pruritic pig with bacterial pyoderma. (*Credit Refuge GroinGroin.*)

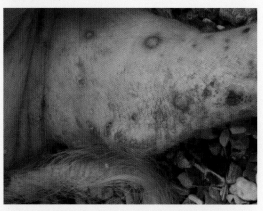

Treatment   Depends on etiology: Avermectin (mites, lice), antibiotic (pyoderma), topical shampoo/ointment/wipes, steroid to control itch

Clinical signs may warrant empirical treatment for mites even if none are identified on skin scrape. Bacterial infection can be a primary issue or secondary to mite infestation, so systemic antibiotics may be helpful in addition to an antiparasitic. Amoxicillin is a good choice for treatment of likely organisms (i.e., *Staphylococcus* spp.).

Differentials	*Sarcoptes scabiei* var. *suis* (mange mite)
	Hematopinus suis (louse)
	Bacterial pyoderma
	Shedding
	Allergies manifesting as pruritis are uncommon in the pig but possible.
	Fleas do not infest pigs but will bite if present in the environment. Raised papules may be noted (especially along the ventrum), but the pig is not overly pruritic.

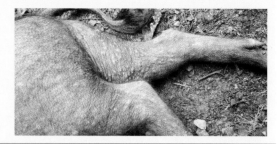

Fig. 10.53: Insect bites (fleas, ants, flies, ticks, etc.) may present with obvious papules (pictured), especially along the ventrum where the point of contact is greatest and skin relatively thin, but—though often dramatic in appearance—these are uncommonly pruritic.

References   Brewer MT, Greve JH. External parasites. In: Zimmeran JJ, Karriker LA, Ramirez A, et al., eds. *Diseases of Swine*. 11th ed. Hoboken, NJ: John Wiley & Sons, Inc.; 2019:1005–1014.
Scott DW. *Porcine. Color Atlas of Farm Animal Dermatology*. 2nd ed. Hoboken, NJ: John Wiley & Sons, Inc.; 2018:235–292.

RABIES

See also Paresis/Paralysis

Overview: Rabies has only been rarely reported in pigs in North America and is sporadically reported in other countries. However, due to the fatality rate and potential for human exposure, it should be on the differential list for any neurologic pig patient, especially those with hindlimb paresis/paralysis.

Signalment	Any	
History	Outdoor environment especially (but not exclusively), with potential or known interaction with wildlife; lack of prior rabies vaccination; hindlimb paralysis; abnormal behavior including aggression, restlessness or hyperactivity, head rubbing, vocalizations, intense itching	The incubation period for rabies is variable and has been most commonly given as 2–3 weeks in swine, although an incubation period of nearly 5 months has been reported in 1 case (DuVernoy).
Physical Exam Findings	Hindlimb paresis/paralysis; fever; depression; ptyalism; aggression; pruritis	In swine, rabies more commonly manifests as the "dumb" form (posterior paresis).
Diagnostics	Submission of the brain to an appropriate laboratory for rabies testing	Fluorescent antibody testing for rabies virus on fresh brain or immunohistochemistry on formalin-fixed tissue can confirm a rabies diagnosis, but the former is preferred.

Continued

RABIES—cont'd

Treatment	Euthanasia, if clinical Quarantine and post-exposure vaccination, if non-clinical with possible exposure, and by permission of the appropriate authorities	There is no approved rabies vaccine for pigs, and there are no swine-specific guidelines following suspected (or known) exposure in vaccinated animals. Anecdotally, some US states have allowed post-exposure vaccination with on-site quarantine and surveillance for a specified period of time. Without prior vaccination in the face of likely exposure to a rabid animal, euthanasia may be requested—if not required—by authorities. There is one report of apparently successful post-exposure treatment in a group of unvaccinated farm pigs in Thailand using equine rabies immune globulin together with vaccination (Mitmoonpitak). If such treatment is possible close to the time of exposure, it may be another option in unvaccinated pets in countries where such treatment may be allowable.
Differentials	Hindlimb paresis/paralysis: IVDD (intervertebral disc disease), fibrocartilaginous embolism (FCE), spinal neoplasia (i.e., lymphoma), trauma, infection Neurologic signs: other viral encephalitides (i.e., pseudorabies, eastern equine encephalitis (EEE), teschovirus A, etc.) or other CNS infection (i.e., bacterial, such as *Streptococcus suis,* or fungal)	
Other	Microscopically observed Negri body inclusions—nearly pathognomonic for rabies virus infection—are not typically present in porcine cases.	
References	de Macedo Pessoa CR, Cristiny Rodrigues Silva ML, de Barros Gomes AA, et al. Paralytic rabies in Swine. *Braz J Microbiol.* 2011;42(1):298–302. DuVernoy TS, Mitchell KC, Myers RA, et al. The first laboratory-confirmed rabid pig in Maryland, 2003. *Zoonoses Public Health.* 2008;55(8–10):431–435. Madson DM, Arruda PHE, Arruda BL. Nervous and locomotor system. In: Zimmeran JJ, Karriker LA, Ramirez A, et al., eds. *Diseases of Swine.* 11th ed. Hoboken, NJ: John Wiley & Sons, Inc.; 2019: 339–372. Mitmoonpitak C, Limusanno S, Khawplod P, et al. Post-exposure rabies treatment in pigs. *Vaccine.* 2002;20(16):2019–2021. Siepker CL, Dalton MF, McHale BJ, et al. Neuropathology and diagnostic features of rabies in a litter of piglets, with a brief review of the literature. *J Vet Diagn Invest.* 2020;32(1):166–168.	

RESPIRATORY ISSUES

Cough; Dyspnea; Pneumonia

Overview: Minipigs occasionally present with respiratory issues, including coughing and dyspnea, with bacterial pneumonia the most common underlying cause. However, respiratory disease in the pet population is much less common than in commercial swine. Diagnosis and treatment should be performed as for the dog.

Signalment	Any, although more common in younger animals
History	Cough, labored breathing (rapid, shallow, open mouth); lethargy; anorexia sometimes reported and may be intermittent

Physical Exam Findings	Depression; cough, dyspnea, tachypnea (RR often >60–70/min); tachycardia; pyrexia; decreased spO$_2$; visible cyanosis of the snout or mucous membranes **Pigs are nasal breathers, and open-mouth breathing should be immediately evaluated.**

Fig. 10.54: (A) Cyanosis of the snout/lips (due to severe laryngospasm (which is rare!) on anesthetic induction for routine castration, not underlying pulmonary disease). (B) Return to normal color following application of topical lidocaine and endotracheal tube placement.

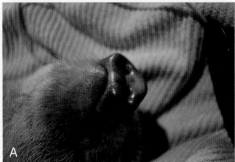

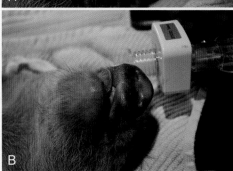

Diagnostics	Imaging (radiographs, thoracic ultrasound, CT) CBC, serum chemistry, arterial blood gas Evaluation of larynx under sedation (for obstructive foreign body or edema) Transtracheal wash, bronchoalveolar lavage, or thoracocentesis with cytologic evaluation ± culture	Although antemortem testing such as culture or PCR on nasal swabs is available, these tests are more commonly used in larger commercial herds as the etiologic agent is not of great concern in pet pigs unless symptomatic treatment is failing.

Continued

RESPIRATORY ISSUES—cont'd

If multiple animals in a large rescue or breeding herd are affected, necropsy should be performed on animals that die spontaneously or are euthanized and should include culture and sensitivity on lung tissue at a minimum. Bacterial agents are most likely to cause clinical disease, but underlying or coexisting viral disease should be investigated as well. Parasitic disease leading to respiratory distress is rare in pets.

Fig. 10.55: Thoracic radiograph from a pig presenting with anorexia, dyspnea, and tachypnea, with intermittent cough and occasional expulsion of thick mucus from the mouth. Mycoplasma pneumonia was suspected based on necropsy findings in other herd members that died. Note gas-distended stomach from aerophagia. (*Photo credit: Quakertown Veterinary Clinic.*)

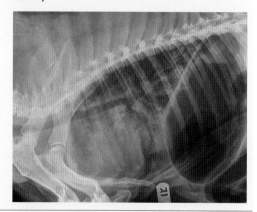

Treatment	
	Supplemental oxygen
	Broad-spectrum antibiotic(s); anti-inflammatories including steroids or NSAIDs; bronchodilators (i.e. terbutaline); expectorant (i.e. guaifenesin)
	Fluids (IV, SQ, rectal, oral) to rehydrate and loosen respiratory secretions
	Coupage
	Humidifier (to provide moist air)
	Nebulization (for targeted drug delivery)
	Acupuncture
	Aromatherapy (topical application) (i.e., in combination with coupage) or nebulization with an essential oil like eucalyptus or menthol
	Controlled, light exercise

Cough suppressants or antihistamines are generally contraindicated as these can suppress mucokinesis and the removal of airway exudates.

Differentials	Bacterial Fungal Viral Pulmonary abscess Neoplasia (rare) Parasitic (rare) Laryngeal, tracheal, bronchial foreign body	Differentials are less varied in the pet pig than in the dog, as most respiratory signs are due to primary pulmonary disease. However, keep other differentials (i.e., cardiovascular disease) in mind too. Although numerous bacterial causes of pneumonia exist for commercial swine, there is no one agent that is prevalent in the miniature pet pig population.
Other	Nasal discharge is not typically observed with primary pulmonary disease. For more information on differentials for nasal discharge, see Neoplasia—SCC and Epistaxis. Upper airway disease, such as rhinitis with associated mucoid or mucopurulent discharge, would be evaluated and treated as for the canine and is not discussed further.	
References	Evans DE, Kawabata A, Wilson LD, et al. Entomophthoromycosis and mucormycosis as causes of pneumonia in Vietnamese potbellied pigs. *J Vet Diagn Invest*. 2018;30(1):161–164. Heller M, Busch R, Koehne A, et al. Unusual severe fungal pneumonia in Vietnamese potbelly pigs: two cases. *Vet Rec Case Report*. 2020;8:e001095. doi:10.1136/vetreccr-2020-001095. Kim JI, Lee YA, Lee JW, et al. Use of ^{18}F-fluorodeoxyglucose positron emission tomography-computed tomography in a miniature pig [*Sus scrofa domestica*] with pneumonia. *Comp Med*. 2012;62(3):203–208. Valussi M, Antonelli M, Donelli D, Firenzuoli F. Appropriate use of essential oils and their components in the management of upper respiratory tract symptoms in patients with COVID-19. *J Herb Med*. 2021;28:100451. doi:10.1016/j.hermed.2021.	

SALT TOXICITY (WATER DEPRIVATION; SODIUM ION TOXICOSIS; HYPERNATREMIA)

Seizures

Overview: Salt toxicity may occasionally be seen in pet pigs as the porcine is the most sensitive species to this condition and may occur with reduced water intake or excessive salt intake. Clinical signs include seizures, blindness, recumbency, paddling, etc., and gradual rehydration is the primary treatment.

Signalment	Any, but young animals are more susceptible	
History	Limited access to water (i.e., pig dumps its only water source, especially on a hot day, and is without water for several hours; freezing limits its access to water in winter); history of feeding high salt foods like potato chips or dog/cat food, especially to very young pigs; owner may observe disorientation, blindness, wobbly/drunk gait (ataxia), recumbency, seizures.	If the owner has attempted rehydration by allowing the pig to drink excessively (i.e., after discovering loss of water source), clinical signs may be exacerbated, and blood sodium levels may be lower than expected. Initially, the pig may be very thirsty, anorexic, or constipated, then progress to a "down" animal that may be ataxic or recumbent ± paddling and seizing; this progression may take several days.
Physical Exam Findings	Recumbent, paddling animal; opisthotonos (arching of the neck with snout pointed up); seizures; head tremors or head pressing; blindness; deafness; absence of menace response and/or pupillary light reflex	

Continued

SALT TOXICITY (WATER DEPRIVATION; SODIUM ION TOXICOSIS; HYPERNATREMIA)—cont'd

Diagnostics	Serum chemistry (including electrolytes)—sodium level above 160 mEq/L is diagnostic

Treatment	Gradual rehydration, IV preferred, but SQ, oral, and/or rectal can also be effective; a slightly hypertonic (sodium-rich) solution[a] is recommended, but normal saline or LRS can be used as well (5% dextrose solutions should be avoided as there is too much free water available which will lower sodium levels too quickly)	Rapid hydration can lead to cerebral edema and exacerbate clinical signs or lead to death. Rehydration should be performed over 48–72 hours, and serum electrolytes should be monitored daily, if possible.
	Mannitol or glycerin, dexamethasone, dimethyl sulfoxide (DMSO), thiamine may help with cerebral edema	"Tailor a sodium-containing fluid that contains sodium equal to 95%–100% of the patient's serum sodium concentration. If history and clinical signs lead you to believe that hypernatremia is present and you are unable to measure serum sodium, start with a fluid containing around 170 mEq sodium per liter." (Angelos)
	Diazepam as needed to control seizures	

Differentials	With history and elevated sodium levels, salt toxicity is a top differential.
	If not clear-cut, any differential for seizures should be considered, including hypoglycemia, toxin, hepatic encephalopathy, head trauma, bacterial or fungal infection, neoplasia, idiopathic, etc. with diagnosis and treatment as for the dog.

Other	Hospitalization is required for appropriate treatment, which may last several days. Prognosis is reportedly poor in animals exhibiting severe clinical signs. However, most clinical cases have been identified in commercial swine in which aggressive treatment was not pursued. Literature reports in potbellied pig patients suggest that recovery is possible with appropriate treatment.

References	Angelos SM, Van Metre DC. Treatment of sodium balance disorders. Water intoxication and salt toxicity. *Vet Clin North Am Food Anim Pract.* 1999;15(3):587–607.
	Banks P, Roussel Jr AJ, Mealey RH. High-sodium crystalloid solution for treatment of hypernatremia in a Vietnamese pot-bellied pig. *J Am Vet Med Assoc.* 1996;209(7):1268–1270.
	Ensley SM, Radke SL. Noninfectious disease. In: Zimmeran JJ, Karriker LA, Ramirez A, et al., eds. *Diseases of Swine.* 11th ed. Hoboken, NJ: John Wiley & Sons, Inc.; 2019:1082–1083.
	Holbrook TC, Barton MH. Neurologic dysfunction associated with hypernatremia and dietary indiscretion in Vietnamese pot bellied pigs. *Cornell Vet.* 1994;84(1):67–76.

[a]A high-sodium crystalloid solution containing approximately 175 mEq/L of sodium and 150 mEq/L of chloride can be made by adding 25 mL of 8.2% $NaHCO_3$ (bicarbonate) solution (25 mEq of Na^+) to 1000 mL of 0.9% NaCl (154 mEq of Na^+ and Cl^-) (Banks).

SKIN (DERMATOLOGIC) ISSUES

See also Dippity Pig; Erysipelas; Neoplasia—Cutaneous Mast Cell Tumor; Neoplasia—Squamous Cell Carcinoma; Parasites, External; Pruritis

Overview: Pet pigs commonly suffer from dermatologic issues, including sunburn, cutaneous abscesses, dermatophytosis, pyoderma, neoplasia, and benign but concerning-to-owners dry flaky skin and plate-like ichthyosis. This is, of course, an extremely broad category and will not be covered in depth as diagnostic testing and treatment follow those employed for the dog.

Signalment	Any, but especially common in aging pets	
History	Light-colored animal with a history of sun exposure (though dark-skinned animals can also suffer from thermal injury)	As with any skin disease, take note of duration, pruritis, seasonality, areas of the body affected, etc., to help narrow differentials.
	Skin that is increasingly dry/flaky, especially in cold winter weather, in low humidity environments, in animals with chronic sun damage, sometimes in animals with nutritional imbalances	
	Slow-growing nodules, single or multiple; a more sudden appearance may be indicative of abscessation	
Physical Exam Findings	See Figs. 10.56 through 10.59	Many dermatologic issues in the minipig are restricted to the skin rather than representing a cutaneous manifestation of systemic disease (so endocrinopathies or food allergies are less likely than in the dog). Any differentials for the canine should still be considered for a pig, though the likelihood of a given disease differs between the species.

Continued

SKIN (DERMATOLOGIC) ISSUES—cont'd

Fig. 10.56: (A) Yeast dermatitis is frequently seen in intertriginous areas of the face and presents as a moist to waxy, reddish-brown accumulation. Secretions build up in the periocular region and can form thick crusts that irritate underlying skin on removal. In severe cases, secretions can adhere lashes/eyelids to one another and impair vision. Regular cleaning with a soft cloth or pet wipe is recommended. (B) Waxy, dark brown aural secretions are ubiquitous and although numerous yeast may be identified on cytologic evaluation, this is an expected finding; frequent budding, however, may indicate active infection. Treatment is necessary only with clinical signs (i.e., head shaking or rubbing, head tilt, scratching at the ears), and clinical disease associated with ear infection is uncommon. (C) Reddish-brown flakes or pinpoint crusts are common in the axilla and groin and are often referred to as "pig rust" by owners; dermatophytosis or yeast (i.e., *Candida* spp.) are likely etiologies. The condition is non-pruritic and is of concern to owners but does not cause issues for the animal. Bathing removes the "rust" temporarily, but discoloration rapidly returns. Systemic (i.e., terbinafine) or topical antifungal may be effective for treatment. (D) Ichthyosis in an aged pig. While aesthetically displeasing, this condition does not appear to bother the animal. Owners can bathe with an appropriate shampoo or apply oil to moisten and loosen flakes which will temporarily improve the appearance, but plate-like scales rapidly return. It should be noted that the thick scales provide protection from the sun and removing them may allow the animal to become sunburned.

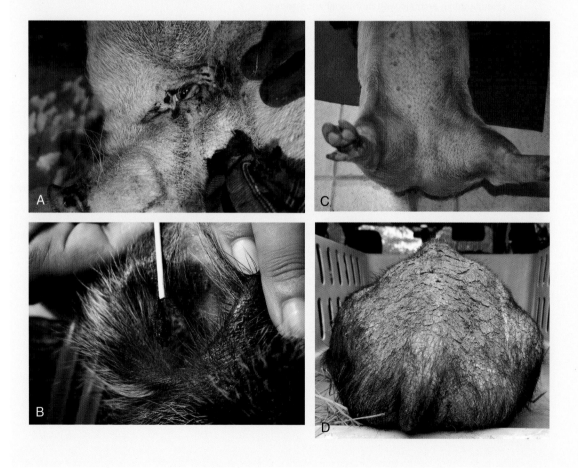

Fig. 10.57: (A, B) Skin scrape yielded numerous *Sarcoptes* spp. mange mites in this pruritic pig with patchy, brownishyellow crusting and hyperkeratosis, primarily on the distal limbs and rump. Treatment with injectable doramectin yielded rapid resolution. (C) Focal swelling of the jaw due to abscessation. (D) Tumor-like mass associated with infection by filamentous bacteria (diagnosis made through biopsy). These masses remain confined to the skin and do not invade underlying bone so may be amenable to surgical removal which can be curative. Inset: Cut surface of one such facial mass. (E) Multifocal, discrete, round, ulcerated skin lesions associated with (presumed) mild bacterial pyoderma. This was successfully treated with an oral antibiotic (amoxicillin BID x 7 days) and no further diagnostic testing was necessary. The lateral flanks, shoulders, and face tend to be affected and microtrauma (i.e., from coarse straw bedding, interpig fighting, or scratching on rough surfaces such as tree bark) may predispose. (F) Cutaneous aspergillosis in a pig with severe dyspnea –ultimately fatal. Inset: Close-up view of lesion. (*Photo credit (C): Leanne Jones; (F) Refuge GroinGroin.*)

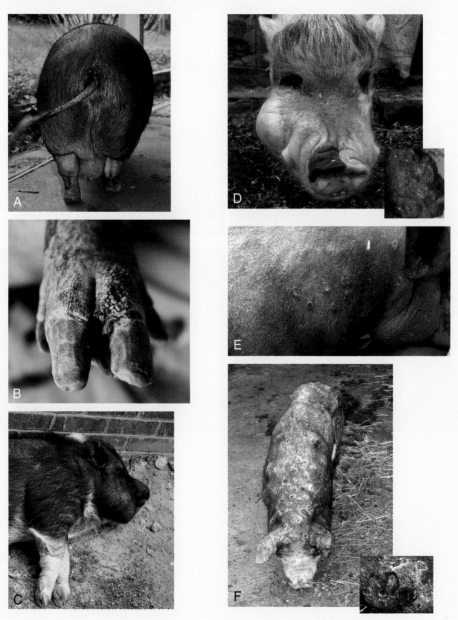

Continued

SKIN (DERMATOLOGIC) ISSUES—cont'd

Fig. 10.58: (A) Numerous, relatively uniform, domed nodules covered the ventrum and medial legs in this pig. Insect bites (likely ants) were suspected based on history but contact dermatitis was also a differential. These were not pruritic, and the pig seemed unbothered; lesions resolved without treatment within a few days. (B) Unusual cutaneous manifestation of lymphoma. This pig ultimately succumbed to systemic neoplastic disease involving multiple internal organs; lymph nodes were not involved. (C) This crusting over the dorsal pinna, affecting only the lightly-pigmented skin, is due to sun damage. Regular application of sunscreen is recommended as well as reduced exposure (i.e., provide shade, bring indoors), especially during peak times (i.e., late afternoon). (D) This pig suffers from extensive scaling and crusting over the lightly-pigmented, sun-exposed areas of the body (flanks, face, and ears, with the ventrum and medial legs unaffected). The multifocal ulcerated lesions were diagnosed as cutaneous squamous cell carcinoma on biopsy and are presumed secondary to chronic solar damage.

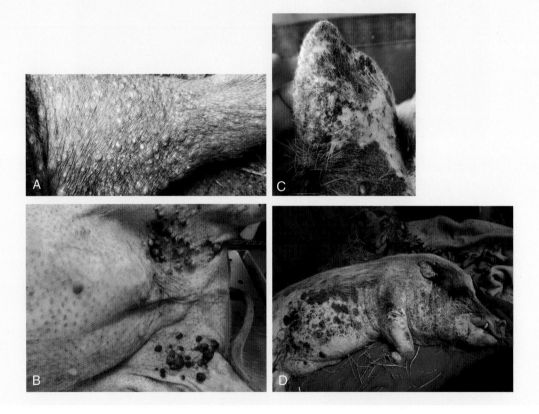

Fig. 10.59: This pig was initially treated for suspected sarcoptic mange due to clinical signs of pruritis and extensive crusting and hyperkeratosis, despite negative skin scrape—a very reasonable protocol with expected rapid resolution. When treatment failed, biopsy was taken (results: widespread moderate eosinophilic, histiocytic and lymphoplasma-cytic dermatitis with epidermal hyperplasia and follicular atrophy) ultimately followed by extensive work-up including bacterial and fungal cultures, blood work, repeated skin biopsies, liver biopsy (to rule out secondary photosensitiza-tion), and multiple dermatology referrals. Treatments included prednisone to control itch, antibiotics for secondary bac-terial infection, antifungals, antiparasitics, medicated baths, dilute topical bleach spray, zinc, fatty acid and Vitamin E supplements, and more. Currently, the pig has suffered from this condition for nearly 10 years and is managed with medication to control itch and regular bathing to remove crusts. The skin becomes painful if crusts build up and are traumatized or manually removed; however, bathing and/or applying baby oil allows the crusts to soften and be readily wiped off with a soft cloth, revealing intact, only slightly erythematous underlying skin. Etiology was never determined.

Moral of this story: Follow a logical, systematic approach as for any companion animal species and provide symptomatic treatment in the meantime. In most cases, the underlying etiology can be identified and specific treatment provided to control or correct the issue.

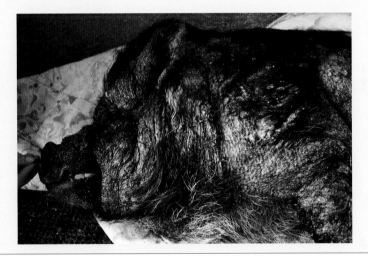

Continued

SKIN (DERMATOLOGIC) ISSUES—cont'd

Diagnostics   Biopsy is a staple for most skin issues

Fine needle aspirate, skin scrape, culture if warranted

+/− CBC, serum chemistry

Additional testing may be needed to evaluate for suspected endocrinopathy; however, reference ranges for the porcine may not be available.

Fig. 10.60: Pigs usually produce thick, pasty pus (A) - use a large–bore needle, 18 g or bigger, to aspirate - but may occasionally produce inspissated secretions (B) that are too solid to yield a diagnosis on fine needle aspirate.

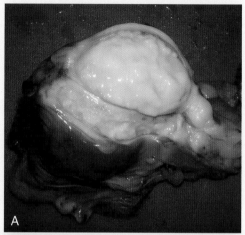

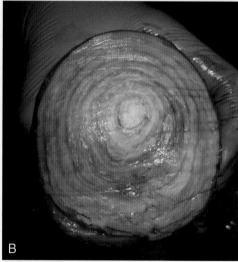

Treatment   Depends on diagnosis

Dry, flaky skin is typical of pet pigs and worsens with age, further complicated by chronic sun damage and age-related, permanent hair loss (i.e., over the rump). Numerous nutritional supplements (top dressing feed with oil or giving other fatty acid supplements) and topical treatments (moisturizers such as Humilac spray) have been tried—some anecdotally have a good response, others do not, and there is no consistency in reported effects. If it works in dogs or humans or some other species, give it a try!

Differentials	Normal pig skin	Lipomas are, oddly, uncommon in the pet pig.
	Photodermatitis (sunburn)	
	Photosensitivity	
	Dippity Pig	
	Insect bite hypersensitivity	
	Nodule/Mass: abscess, granuloma, mast cell tumor, melanocytoma, squamous cell carcinoma, lymphoma, etc.	
Other	There are numerous skin conditions reported in commercial swine (greasy pig disease, vesicular diseases, pityriasis rosea, swine pox, porcine dermatopathy and nephropathy syndrome, etc.), and while these should be included on the differential list, they are uncommon to rare in the pet population.	
References	https://www.minipiginfo.com/common-mini-pig-skin-concerns.html Bollen PJA, Madsen LW, Mortensen JT, et al. Investigation of the involvement of candida albicans in hyperkeratosis of the Gottingen Minipig. *Scand J Lab Anim* 1998;25:150–153. Frank LA, McCormick KA, Donnell RL, Kania SA. Dorsal black skin necrosis in a Vietnamese pot-bellied pig. *Vet Dermatol.* 2015;26(1):64–67, e23. doi:10.1111/vde.12181. Goulding JM, Todkill D, Carr RA, Charles-Holmes R. Pustules, plaques and pot-bellied pigs: difficulties in diagnosing tinea faciei. *Clin Exp Dermatol.* 2010;35(3):e10–e11. doi:10.1111/j.1365-2230.2008.03200.x. Jackson PGG, Cockcroft PD. Diseases of the skin and the pet pig. In: *Handbook of Pig Medicine.* Philadelphia, PA: Elsevier Limited; 2007:112–127;212–219. Scott DW. *Porcine. Color Atlas of Farm Animal Dermatology.* 2nd ed. Hoboken, NJ: John Wiley & Sons, Inc.; 2018:235–292. Scott DW, Miller Jr WH. Non-neoplastic skin diseases in potbellied pigs: report of 13 cases. *Jpn J Vet Dermatol.* 2015;21(4):223–228.	

TRAUMA—DOG ATTACK

Overview: Pet pigs occasionally present for traumatic injury, with dog attacks by far the most common. In many instances, the pig is attacked by dogs within their own household. Owners should be cautioned that pigs and dogs do not make good companions and should never be left together unsupervised. Outdoor pets should be protected from roaming predators by appropriate fencing (tall and secured at ground level to prevent digging underneath ± electrified wire).

Signalment	Any	
History	Pig and dog(s) interact within the household; loose dog/ stray gets into outdoor pig enclosure	Inter-pig aggression is common as minipigs often fight on initial introduction. However, injury is typically minor and may not warrant medical care; it is rarely (if ever) severe enough to be life-threatening.

Continued

TRAUMA—DOG ATTACK—cont'd

Physical Exam Findings

Traumatic injury inflicted by a dog most commonly involves the ears, limbs, and hind end (as the pig attempts to run away) as well as puncture wounds and deep scratches on the dorsal neck region; puncture wounds in the axilla and groin are also common.

Pig skin is thick/tough and tends to separate from underlying subcutaneous tissue when force is applied (i.e., dog grips the hindleg as the pig is moving away), so a focal laceration might be expected to have extensive undermining.

Patient is typically depressed and painful; anorexia may or may not be present.

Fig. 10.61: (A) Damage to the pinna is common in dog attacks. In this case, amputation was necessary. (B) Healing amputation site of the same pig 1 week later. (C) Gouging from claws—multiple, superficial, uniformly parallel wounds—is commonly seen on the dorsal neck region; this pig was cornered in his house facing the attacking dog, so claw marks are present over the snout.

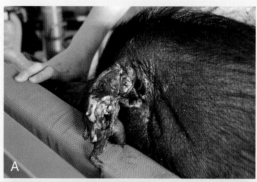

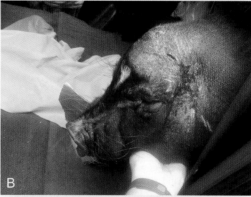

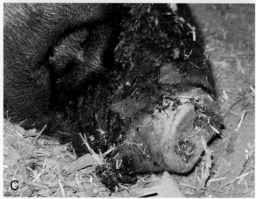

Fig. 10.62: (A) This small laceration on the lateral hindlimb was associated with extensive separation of skin from subcutaneous tissue (B); as a result, drain placement was necessary. Fig. 10.63 shows the progression of wound healing on this limb. (C) This pig sloughed damaged skin at the site of a small puncture wound and developed necrosis of underlying adipose 24 days after initial presentation. (D) The dead tissue was simply removed during a belly rub to reveal a healing bed of granulation tissue; no sedation or further debridement was necessary. (E) The same area 3 weeks later.

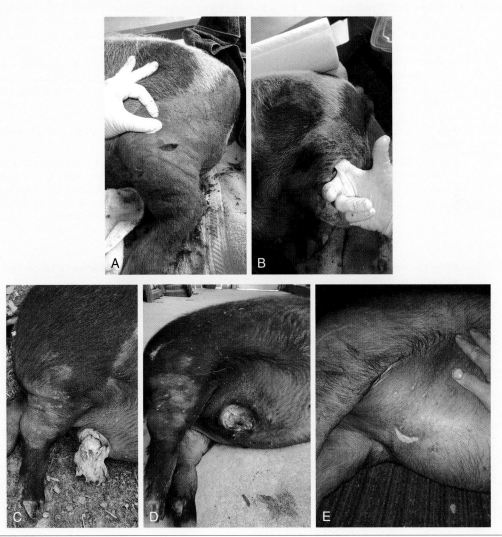

Continued

TRAUMA—DOG ATTACK—cont'd

Diagnostics	Radiographs if fracture or penetration of body cavity suspected	
Treatment	Standard wound care as for any animal—clip, clean and debride wounds, place drain(s) if needed; antibiotics; analgesics (NSAID, opioid); supportive care for severe injury (i.e., warming, fluid therapy) ± rabies vaccination Sugar + betadine or honey application can speed wound healing. Remedy the home environment to prevent future attacks.	If a pig is severely injured, stabilization may be difficult (even if soft tissue injury is not life-threatening) as treatment of shock is problematic due to limited IV access, especially if the pinnae have been damaged. See Chapter 7 for IV catheterization details. For discharged patients, I often have owners flush the wound with warm water and Epsom salt solution, made fresh every time according to label instructions. This helps to draw out fluids and dry oozing tissues and allows the owner to participate in their pet's care in a benign manner. Owners otherwise tend to devise their own treatment plan (i.e., using hydrogen peroxide or antibiotic ointment), which may impede the healing process. After initial treatment, wounds may "declare themselves" within ~2–3 weeks and require additional debriding (see Fig. 10.63). Owners should be forewarned as the wounds look nasty and smell like "rotten flesh," although there tends to be only necrosis without infection if antibiotic treatment has been instituted.
Differentials	NA	
Other	Other traumatic injury is seen on occasion (inter-pig fighting, hit by car, caught on a fence, etc.) and should be evaluated and treated as for any companion animal species.	

Fig. 10.63: This pig was attacked by dogs and suffered extensive injury to the hindleg (see Fig. 10.62 A, B) that required drain placement. (A) About 10 days after initial treatment, the wound exhibits tatters of darkened, firm, necrotic tissue, but there is no infection and the pig is clinically normal except for a slight limp. (B) Following removal of dead tissue, it becomes apparent that the wound is healing well and exhibits a clean bed of granulation tissue. (C) One week later, the wound is increasingly contracted, but the pig is buckling on the limb when ambulating, so sugar + betadine paste was applied and the leg wrapped. (D) After wrap removal the following day, the wound is further contracted, and ambulation is nearly normal.

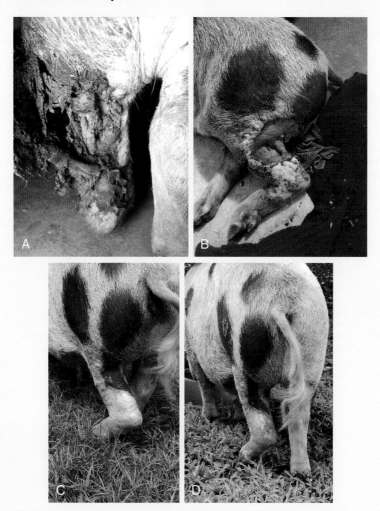

Continued

TRAUMA—DOG ATTACK—cont'd

References	https://www.minipiginfo.com/dangers-of-mini-pigs-and-dogs.html#.
	Di Stadio A, Gambacorta V, Cristi MC, et al. The use of povidone-iodine and sugar solution in surgical wound dehiscence in the head and neck following radio-chemotherapy. *Int Wound J.* 2019;16(4):909–915.
	Knutson RA, Merbitz LA, Creekmore MA, Snipes HG. Use of sugar and povidone-iodine to enhance wound healing: five year's experience. *South Med J.* 1981;74(11):1329–1335.
	Tynes VV. Miniature pet pig behavioral medicine. *Vet Clin North Am Exot Anim Pract.* 2021;24(1):63–86.

TUSK ABSCESSATION

See also Chapter 7

Overview: Abscessation of the tusk(s), most commonly the lower or mandibular tusk, is a common problem in the male minipig. This typically presents as an abscess along the chin or cheek that recurs following medical management (i.e., draining and antibiotics). Oral examination may be unremarkable (especially with early disease), and the pig may exhibit few to no clinical signs, even with the extensive infection and bony lysis seen in advanced disease.

Signalment	Older male (8+ years)	Females occasionally exhibit canine tooth root abscessation, which may be identified during a routine dental evaluation. However, as the tusk root in the female closes at maturity, treatment would involve extraction similar to that performed in the dog.
History	Draining tract or focal swelling along the jaw/chin/cheek; foul odor emanating from the mouth	
Physical Exam Findings	Abscess or draining tract along the mandible, palpable bony distortion (see Fig. 7.15); multiple loose premolars or molars along the lower arcades; erosion of oral mucosa under the tongue, with exposure of underlying bone	Mandibular tusk root abscess is frequently bilateral. Abscess of the upper tusk is possible but much less common. **Fig. 10.64:** The jaw is misshapen in this pig and bears a deep draining tract. The obvious "swelling" (*curved line*) is not an abscess but, rather, bony remodeling of the mandible due to chronic tusk infection. 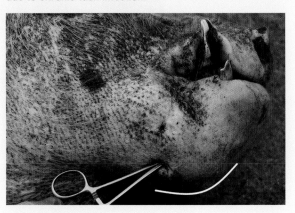

Diagnostics	Radiographs; CT or MRI helpful if extraction planned Culture typically yields a mixed bacterial population and is generally reserved for an infection that does not respond to initial treatment. Biopsy may be indicated as neoplasms can arise within proliferative tissue (i.e., gingiva).	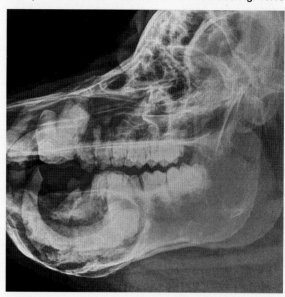 **Fig. 10.65:** Skull radiograph showing advanced tusk infection. (*Photo credit: Dr. Shannon Swink. See also Fig. 10.13.*)
Treatment	Extraction; pulse antibiotic therapy (see Other below)	More advanced dental procedures such as pulpectomy may be possible, although there are no literature reports of attempted treatment in pigs by such measures. However, tusk removal via alveolotomy and an internal collapsing technique has been described in a babirusa (Steenkamp). Other techniques utilized for elephant or walrus tusks may be suitable for minipigs, but again, there are no literature reports on this possibility.
Differentials	Cutaneous abscess Neoplasia	Squamous cell carcinoma of the oral cavity is common in miniature pigs, and chronic infection may predispose to development. Bony tumors are also possible but rare.
Other	Tusk abscess in the male minipig is extremely difficult to manage. Ideal treatment would include extraction of the diseased tooth and treatment of associated osteomyelitis. However, the tusk is semicircular, sometimes spiraling at the caudal end, and extends along the ramus of the mandible to about the level of the first or second molars (see Fig. 7.17). The root remains open throughout life and blurs indistinctly into the surrounding bone until osteomyelitis becomes severe enough to obliterate all attachment. Even then, extraction of this large tooth is technically difficult. Note: The diseased tooth often provides stability to the jaw, and collapse is common with extraction; despite this, pigs heal remarkably well once the diseased tooth and bone have been removed and the residual infection treated. Although extraction is ideal and the only definitive treatment, this may not be possible given technical or financial limitations, advanced patient age, or comorbidities. In this instance, pulse (intermittent) antibiotic therapy may provide some relief in terms of keeping the infection under control, reducing foul-smelling drainage, and preventing large abscesses from forming. As infection typically involves multiple organisms, the antibiotic choice should be based on flora expected in the oral cavity, and occasional rotation of different drugs may help prevent resistance. Although the pig may not appear overtly painful, pain management should be considered. Euthanasia may be best for animals with advanced disease, but it is often difficult to convince owners to consider this option as the pet exhibits few clinical signs, eats well, and does not appear sick.	

Continued

TUSK ABSCESSATION—cont'd

References	Fecchio R, Gioso MA, Bannon K. Exotic animals oral and dental diseases. In: Lobprise HB, Dodd JR, eds. *Wiggs's Veterinary Dentistry: Principles and Practice.* 2nd ed. Hoboken, NJ: John Wiley & Sons, Inc.; 2019:481–499. Steenkamp G. Oral biology and disorders of tusked mammals. *Vet Clin North Am Exot Anim Pract.* 2003;6(3):689–725.

TUSK OVERGROWTH

See also Chapter 7

Overview: The canine teeth, or tusks, grow continuously in the male and may require regular trim to prevent traumatic damage to the face, other animals or people, or to address malocclusion that interferes with opening and closing of the jaw. Long tusks may become caught on fencing or furniture, and sharp tusks may cause serious traumatic injury to other pets or humans; even blunted tusks can cause bruising. The roots of these teeth in the female close around 2 years of age, and growth ceases, so regular trim is unnecessary.

Signalment	Male, usually 2–3+ years	Tusk growth may slow or cease in older males (12–15+ years), possibly due to damage from infection.
History	Owner reports tusks catching on fencing, furniture, clothing; razor-sharp edges have caused traumatic injury to people or other animals; overgrown tusk is rubbing, or growing into, the face	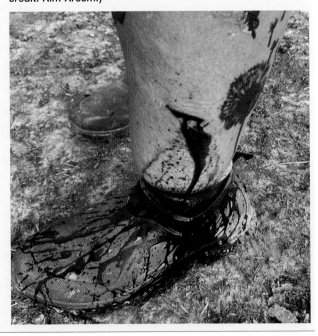 **Fig. 10.66:** Accidental injury caused by sharp tusks. (*Photo credit: Kim Kreem.*)

Physical Exam Findings	Long tusks curving back towards the face and abrading or penetrating the skin of the cheek (see Fig. 6.9); friction when the pig opens and closes the mouth (may not be evident in an awake animal but identified under sedation); razor-sharp edges

Fig. 10.67: Overgrown lower tusk penetrating the skin; note poor alignment between upper and lower tusks due to a shortened maxilla—a very common finding in these proportionate dwarves.

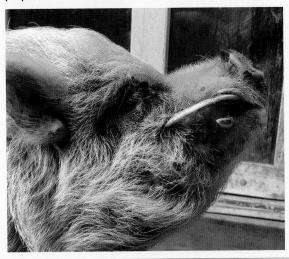

Diagnostics	NA
Treatment	Trim using dehorning/obstetric saw wire (aka gigli wire) or a dental drill ± smooth edges with the grinding attachment of a rotary tool; clip and clean wound(s)

Tusk growth is slow, allowing scar tissue to develop, so even deeply penetrating injuries are readily treated by a simple tusk trim and wound cleaning. Systemic antibiotics are not generally indicated.

Fig. 10.68: (A) An overgrown mandibular tusk has penetrated the skin. (B) The lower tusk has been trimmed about 1.5 inches (3.8 cm) above the gumline, and both upper and lower tusks have been rounded/smoothed with an abrasive rotary tool attachment. The well-granulated wound in the cheek was cleaned with an antiseptic wipe; no further treatment was necessary.

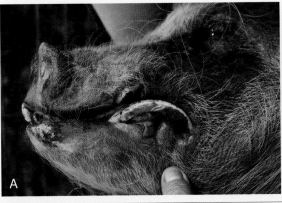
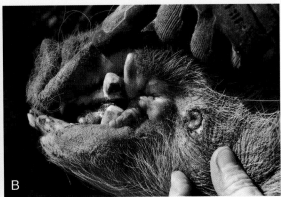

Differentials	None
Other	See Chapter 7 for details on tusk trimming technique.
References	Eubanks DL, Gilbo K. Trimming tusks in the Yucatan minipig. *Lab Anim*. 2005;34(9):35–38.

ULCERATION, GASTRIC (STOMACH ULCERS)

Overview: Gastroesophageal ulceration is extremely common in commercial breed swine (reportedly as high as 90% depending on feeding and husbandry practices); the problem is multifactorial, and risk factors include fine particle size of feed, fasting or interruption of feed intake, alteration of normal gastric microbiota, environmental stressors, and genetics for lean, fast growth. Miniature pet pig genetics, feeding practices, and husbandry reduce or eliminate many of these risk factors, and miniature pigs are less commonly affected than domestic pigs. However, it is ideal to treat— at least prophylactically—sick, hospitalized, or otherwise stressed minipig patients for gastric ulceration. While stomach ulcers can be a primary issue, there may be another underlying disease process, and further investigation may be warranted.

Signalment	Any	
History	Depression, anorexia, teeth grinding, occasional vomiting may be reported	
Physical Exam Findings	Depression; lip-smacking, teeth grinding, excessive salivation, and/ or pressing the snout to the floor may be indicative of nausea; melena	Pepto Bismol (bismuth subsalicylate) is a common over-the-counter medication that an owner may give prior to presentation—this can cause dark feces, which mimics melena.
	Tense abdomen, kicking at the abdomen	
	Heart and/or respiratory rate may be elevated in a painful pig.	

Diagnostics   CBC, serum chemistry; fecal occult blood; gastroscopy ± biopsy

Depending on other suspected underlying disease, additional testing may be warranted.

Fig. 10.69: (A) The pars esophagea in this pig is white and glistening though slightly corrugated/thickened. This is clinically insignificant, though hyperkeratosis can precede erosion and ulceration. (B) The pars esophagea bears a small, reddened area of erosion *(arrow)*.

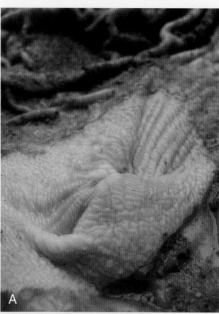

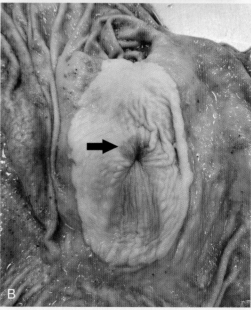

Continued

ULCERATION, GASTRIC (STOMACH ULCERS)—cont'd

Treatment	Proton pump inhibitor (i.e., omeprazole, pantoprazole, esomeprazole) Histamine type-2 receptor antagonist (i.e., famotidine, cimetidine) Sucralfate, preferably administered as a suspension ± Maropitant (Cerenia) Environmental modification to remove stressors Diet change (i.e., eliminate corn, add fiber) Treat underlying illness as indicated	Medications used to treat gastric ulceration are not intended for long-term use (Marks). Also, keep in mind that many of these drugs can interfere with the absorption of other medications. Grains such as oat or barley are protective; there is conflicting data concerning wheat. Corn is considered ulcerogenic. In general, factors that increase the fluidity of stomach contents or increase the speed of emptying increase ulcer risk.
Differentials	Eosinophilic or lymphoplasmacytic gastritis Polyps (rare) Neoplasia (rare)	
Other	In contrast to humans and dogs, ulceration in the pig is most common in the stratified squamous epithelium of the pars esophagea rather than in the glandular mucosa. Normal pars esophagea is white and glistening but becomes thickened and corrugated due to hyperplasia, which precedes erosion and ulceration. While I have occasionally seen minor hyperplasia in hundreds of minipig necropsies, I have identified gastric ulceration only a handful of times, even in the face of protracted illness or long-term NSAID or steroid use where adverse gastrointestinal effects might be expected.	
References	De Witte C, Demeyere K, De Bruyckere S, et al. Characterization of the non-glandular gastric region microbiota in Helicobacter suis-infected versus non-infected pigs identifies a potential role for Fusobacterium gastrosuis in gastric ulceration. *Vet Res*. 2019;50(1):39. doi:10.1186/s13567-019-0656-9. Gottardo F, Scollo A, Contiero B, et al. Prevalence and risk factors for gastric ulceration in pigs slaughtered at 170 kg. *Animal*. 2017;11(11):2010–2018. Marks SL, Kook PH, Papich MG, et al. ACVIM consensus statement: support for rational administration of gastrointestinal protectants to dogs and cats. *J Vet Intern Med*. 2018;32(6):1823–1840. Thomson JR, Friendship RM. Digestive system. In: Zimmeran JJ, Karriker LA, Ramirez A, et al., eds. *Diseases of Swine*. 11th ed. Hoboken, NJ: John Wiley & Sons, Inc.; 2019:234–263.	

URINARY TRACT OBSTRUCTION; UROLITHIASIS

Overview: Crystalluria is occasionally identified in miniature pigs, and crystalline debris or discrete uroliths can lead to obstruction in the male. Non-surgical treatment is difficult as urinary catheterization is extremely challenging due to penile anatomy—the penis remains permanently sheathed in castrated males and accessing the tip for catheterization can be problematic, urethral diameter is narrow, and the sigmoid flexure and urethral recess are major hurdles as well. Prognosis is fair to guarded as problems may recur even if initial treatment is effective.

Signalment	Male, especially middle-aged to older animals	
History	Frequent straining, often with pronounced abdominal effort; agitation; inability to get comfortable (i.e., frequently lying down then rising again, standing with the tail held straight out); inappetence; lethargy	Straining to urinate and tenesmus can be difficult to distinguish. As the former is more common and more likely to constitute an emergency, any straining pig should be evaluated as soon as possible.

Physical Exam Findings	White crystalline material may be noted on the long hairs at the preputial orifice; dysuria, stranguria, dribbling; pain on abdominal palpation; tachypnea; fever	The bladder may be difficult to palpate in an awake pig patient, and the abdomen is especially tense in these animals.
Diagnostics	Radiographs; ultrasound; positive-contrast study such as cystography or urethrography; urethral endoscopy; urinalysis ± culture, CBC, serum chemistry	The urinary bladder will be greatly enlarged on imaging; discrete stones may or may not be apparent as "sandy" crystalline material can also cause obstruction.

Fig. 10.70: (A) Small calculi can be seen within the enlarged bladder as well as lodged along the urethra *(arrows)*; (B) Contrast urethrogram confirms obstruction at site of urethral stones. (*Photo credit: Exotic Animal Medicine Service, North Carolina State University Veterinary Teaching Hospital.*)

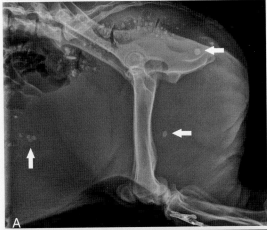

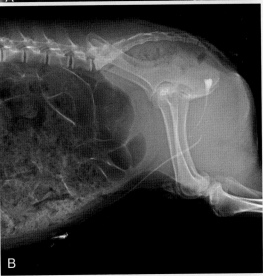

Continued

URINARY TRACT OBSTRUCTION; UROLITHIASIS—cont'd

Treatment	Difficult! Catheterization can be attempted to relieve the blockage, but symptomatic relief through decompressive cystocentesis is helpful while a diagnostic plan is made. A percutaneous transabdominal catheter is another option to allow medical management prior to more invasive treatment (Chigerwe). Surgical correction is necessary in many cases. NSAID, analgesic (opioid, gabapentin), antispasmodic (prazocin, diazepam), antibiotic IV fluids to correct electrolyte and acid-base imbalances Urinary acidification (i.e., oral methionine or ammonium chloride) if warranted Husbandry modifications to promote fluid intake (i.e., provide fresh water at all times, add water to pelleted feed at meals, offer water flavored with juice on occasion); increase outdoor access to promote frequent urination Tube cystotomy is most commonly recommended for treatment of obstructive urolithiasis (as in the goat); however, other treatment options such as percutaneous cystolithotomy or urethroscopy and laser lithotripsy have been described (Coutant; Halland). Other surgical options include perineal or prepubic urethrostomy (León), penile amputation, or urethrotomy. Urethral rerouting through extrapelvic urethral or urethropreputial anastomosis has also been successfully performed (Mann). Retropulsion is reportedly ineffective as stones tend to become trapped in the urethral recess rather than moving into the bladder, eventually returning to an obstructive position. Pigs readily scar and stricture, so less invasive methods are preferred when possible.
Differentials	Constipation; cystitis or urethritis; other causes of urethral obstruction (i.e., polyp, mucus plug, traumatic insult)
Other	The underlying etiology of urolithiasis in pet pigs is unknown though it is likely multifactorial with genetics, diet, restricted water intake, etc., playing a role. Crystal formation is common in non-clinical animals as well. Females may also be affected but are less likely to become clinical due to urethral anatomy. Tip: Tissue forceps can be inserted through the preputial orifice and used to blindly grasp a horn of the preputial diverticulum adjacent to the penis. Gentle traction will then move the tip of the penis into view, where it can be grasped with gauze.
References	Chigerwe M, Shiraki R, Olstad EC, et al. Mineral composition of urinary calculi from potbellied pigs with urolithiasis: 50 cases (1982–2012). *J Am Vet Med Assoc* 2013;243:389–393. Chigerwe M, Heller MC, Balcomb CC, Angelos JA. Use of a percutaneous transabdominal catheter for management of obstructive urolithiasis in goats, sheep, and potbellied pigs: 69 cases (2000–2014). *J Am Vet Med Assoc* 2016;248:1287–1290. Coutant T, Dunn M, Montasell X, Langlois I. Use of percutaneous cystolithotomy for removal of urethral uroliths in a pot-bellied pig. *Can Vet J.* 2018;59(2):159–164. Halland SK, House JK, George LW. Urethroscopy and laser lithotripsy for the diagnosis and treatment of obstructive urolithiasis in goats and pot-bellied pigs. *J Am Vet Med Assoc* 2002;220:1831–1834. Helman RG, Hooper RN, Lawhorn DB, Edwards JF. Urethral polyps in Vietnamese pot-bellied pigs. *J Vet Diagn Invest.* 1996;8(1):137–140.

León JC, Gill MS, Cornick-Seahorn JL, et al. Prepubic urethrostomy for permanent urinary diversion in two Vietnamese pot-bellied pigs. *J Am Vet Med Assoc.* 1997;210(3):366–368.

Mann FA, Cowart RP, McClure RC, Constantinescu GM. Permanent urinary diversion in two Vietnamese pot-bellied pigs by extrapelvic urethral or urethropreputial anastomosis. *J Am Vet Med Assoc.* 1994;205(8):1157–1160.

McClure SR, Welch RD, Johnson TL. Use of an implant for intraosseous infusion as supportive therapy for a Vietnamese pot-bellied pig with urethral obstruction caused by a polyp. *J Am Vet Med Assoc.* 1992;201(10):1587–1590.

Needleman A, Videla R. Urolithiasis in a female miniature potbellied pig. Needleman A, Videla R. *Vet Rec Case Rep.* 2019; doi:10.1136/vetreccr-2018-000809.

Parsons DA, Lawhorn B, Walker MA, et al. Incomplete urethral obstruction associated with dilatation of the urethra, cystitis, and pyelonephritis in a Vietnamese pot-bellied pig. *J Am Vet Med Assoc.* 1998;212(2):262–264.

VOMITING

See also Gastrointestinal Tract Obstruction; Neoplasia—Intestinal; Ulceration—Gastric

Overview: Vomiting in minipigs is diagnostically evaluated as for any companion animal species. Similar treatments are used, with drug dosages extrapolated from the dog if porcine doses are unavailable. Dietary indiscretion that leads to vomiting can result from natural rooting and nesting behaviors that lead to inadvertent ingestion of bedding or carpet pieces; owners may feed inappropriate items such as fruits with large pits or corn on the cob. Inflammatory bowel disease (eosinophilic or lymphoplasmacytic) has been identified in minipig patients, while underlying metabolic disease (i.e., renal or hepatic disease) is uncommon to rare.

Vomiting is often a transient condition of undetermined etiology that resolves with supportive care. However, repeated and continued vomiting warrants further investigation, and intractable vomiting should be considered an emergency that may require surgical correction (i.e., torsion, volvulus).

Signalment	Any
History	Episodes of regurgitation or vomiting; anorexia; reduced fecal output; lethargy
	Thorough history is needed to determine likely differentials and owners should be questioned on the bedding habits of the patient (i.e., Is the pig bedded with blankets and does the pig tend to rip or tear them?) as well as food items given (i.e., Could the pig have eaten fruits with large pits, corn on the cob?); is there any possibility of toxin ingestion (i.e., ant or rat bait, medications)?
Physical Exam Findings	PE may be unremarkable other than a reported history of vomiting
	Lethargy, depression
	Lip-smacking, teeth grinding, excessive salivation, head down with snout pressed to the ground (indicative of nausea)
	Vitals may be normal, or heart and/or respiration rates may be elevated due to pain and/or nausea
	Abdominal distension, abdominal discomfort on palpation, palpable abdominal mass

Continued

VOMITING—cont'd

Diagnostics	Imaging: abdominal radiographs, ultrasound	Marked gas distension of bowel loops likely warrants exploratory celiotomy immediately if clinical condition is severe. See Figs. 10.33 and 10.71.
	Endoscopy ± biopsy	
	CBC, serum chemistry	

Fig. 10.71: Right lateral (A), ventrodorsal (B), and left lateral (C) views of a pig presenting with chronic, intermittent vomiting of 3 weeks duration. At initial (in the field) presentation, the pig was depressed but physical exam was otherwise unremarkable (normal vitals, non-painful abdomen). Conservative treatment included subcutaneous fluids, flunixin (NSAID), maropitant (Cerenia) and acupuncture. Injectable formulations were used initially and replaced with oral medication once the pig began eating. Improvement was noted but clinical signs continued to wax and wane, so in-hospital radiographs were recommended. Radiographic findings warranted exploratory celiotomy, and a mid-jejunal stricture was identified, with an associated "knot" of adhesions between jejunal segments; bowel proximal to the stricture was markedly dilated and peristalsis was absent. After releasing adhesions, resection and anastomosis was performed with removal of approximately 8 cm of bowel. The pig was hospitalized for several days, and post-operative treatment included IV fluids, butorphanol, metoclopramide, maropitant, ceftiofur, and acupuncture. A full recovery was made. Etiology in this case was suspected to be scarring secondary to traumatic damage from ingested foreign material. Refer to Fig. 10.5 for normal abdominal radiographs.

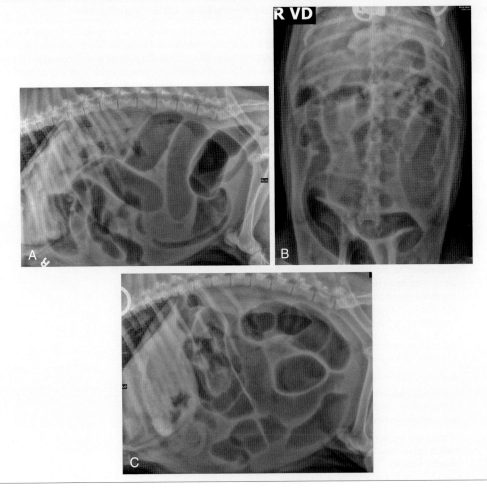

Treatment	Depends on suspected etiology and severity of clinical condition:	Pigs readily scar and form abdominal adhesions that may lead to a recurrence of clinical signs (and, possibly, additional surgery), so care should be taken to minimize risk—use atraumatic surgical technique, keep tissue moistened, lavage, use a protective lubricant such as intraperitoneal hyaluronic acid or carboxymethylcellulose, close the dense peritoneum separately from the body wall, and give anti-inflammatory drugs post-operatively.
	Nothing by mouth (NPO) for a limited period (~12–24 h) followed by slow introduction of oral fluids and bland solid foods such as rice or oatmeal	
	Rehydrate (IV fluids if possible but SQ, IP, or rectal are other options)	
	Antiemetic medication such as maropitant (Cerenia) or ondansetron	
	GI protectants such as a proton pump inhibitor (i.e., omeprazole), histamine type-2 receptor antagonist (i.e., famotidine), sucralfate	
	Prokinetic drugs such as metoclopramide (contraindicated with obstruction)	
	+/− Analgesia including opioids and gabapentin, avoid NSAIDs if ulceration is suspected	
	Exploratory celiotomy with appropriate treatment as needed (gastrotomy/enterotomy, resection and anastomosis); if negative explore, consider biopsy of GI tract!	
	Acupuncture	
	Toxin ingestion: contact Animal Poison Control Hotline if available; emetic or charcoal as indicated for ingestion of certain toxins	
Differentials	Foreign body	
	Neoplasia	
	Dietary indiscretion (i.e., moldy feed, overeating)	
	Intussusception, stricture, fecal impaction, torsion, mesenteric volvulus	
	Toxin ingestion (i.e., flavored insect or rodent bait, irritant plant, medications)	
	Gastritis, pancreatitis, inflammatory bowel disease, other? Etiology may be undetermined, and the condition resolves with supportive care	
Other	Although commercial breed swine are highly prone to gastric ulceration, this problem is much less common in minipigs as a primary issue. However, irritation from gastric contents with vomiting as well as the stress of being ill can damage mucosa, so gastric protectants are recommended.	

Continued

VOMITING—cont'd

References   Cain A, Kirkpatrick J, Breuer R, et al. A case of a linear foreign body removal in a miniature companion pig. *J Dairy Vet Anim Res*. 2020;9(1):6–9.

Chandel AKS, Shimizu A, Hasegawa K, Ito T. Advancement of biomaterial-based postoperative adhesion barriers. *Macromol Biosci*. 2021;21(3):e2000395. doi:10.1002/mabi.202000395.

Ehrle A, Gillespie A, Rubio-Martinez LM. Management of a linear foreign body gastrointestinal obstruction in a miniature pig. *Vet Rec Case Rep*. 2019; doi:10.1136/vetreccr-2018-000791.

Ludwig EK, Byron CR. Evaluation of the reasons for and outcomes of gastrointestinal tract surgery in pet pigs: 11 cases (2004–2015). *J Am Vet Med Assoc*. 2017;251(6):714–721.

McCoy AM, Hackett ES, Callan RJ, Powers BE. Alimentary-associated carcinomas in five Vietnamese potbellied pigs. *J Am Vet Med Assoc*. 2009;235(11):1336–1341.

Sipos W, Schmoll F, Stumpf I. Minipigs and potbellied pigs as pets in the veterinary practice–a retrospective study. *J Vet Med A Physiol Pathol Clin Med*. 2007;54(9):504–511.

Index

Page numbers followed by 'f' indicate figures, 't' indicate tables, 'b' indicate boxes.

213